# DANCE

## and American Art

*this book was published with a lift from*

FIGURE FOUNDATION

# DANCE
## and American Art

### A Long Embrace

Sharyn Rohlfsen Udall

THE UNIVERSITY OF WISCONSIN PRESS

The University of Wisconsin Press
1930 Monroe Street, 3rd Floor
Madison, Wisconsin 53711-2059
uwpress.wisc.edu

3 Henrietta Street
London WC2E 8LU, England
eurospanbookstore.com



Printed in Canada

Library of Congress Cataloging-in-Publication Data
Udall, Sharyn Rohlfsen.
Dance and American art : a long embrace / Sharyn R. Udall.
p. cm.
Includes bibliographical references and index.
ISBN 978-0-299-28800-6 (cloth : alk. paper) —
ISBN 978-0-299-28803-7 (e-book)
1. Dance in art. 2. Art, American—Themes, motives. I. Title.
N8217.D3U33 2012
704.9'4979280973—dc23
2011042650

Rita Dove's poem "American Smooth" first appeared in *The New Yorker*
(February 3, 2003) and was subsequently collected in her poetry book
*American Smooth*, W. W. Norton, New York, © 2004 by Rita Dove.
Reprinted by permission of the author.

Book design and composition: David Alcorn, Alcorn Publication Design

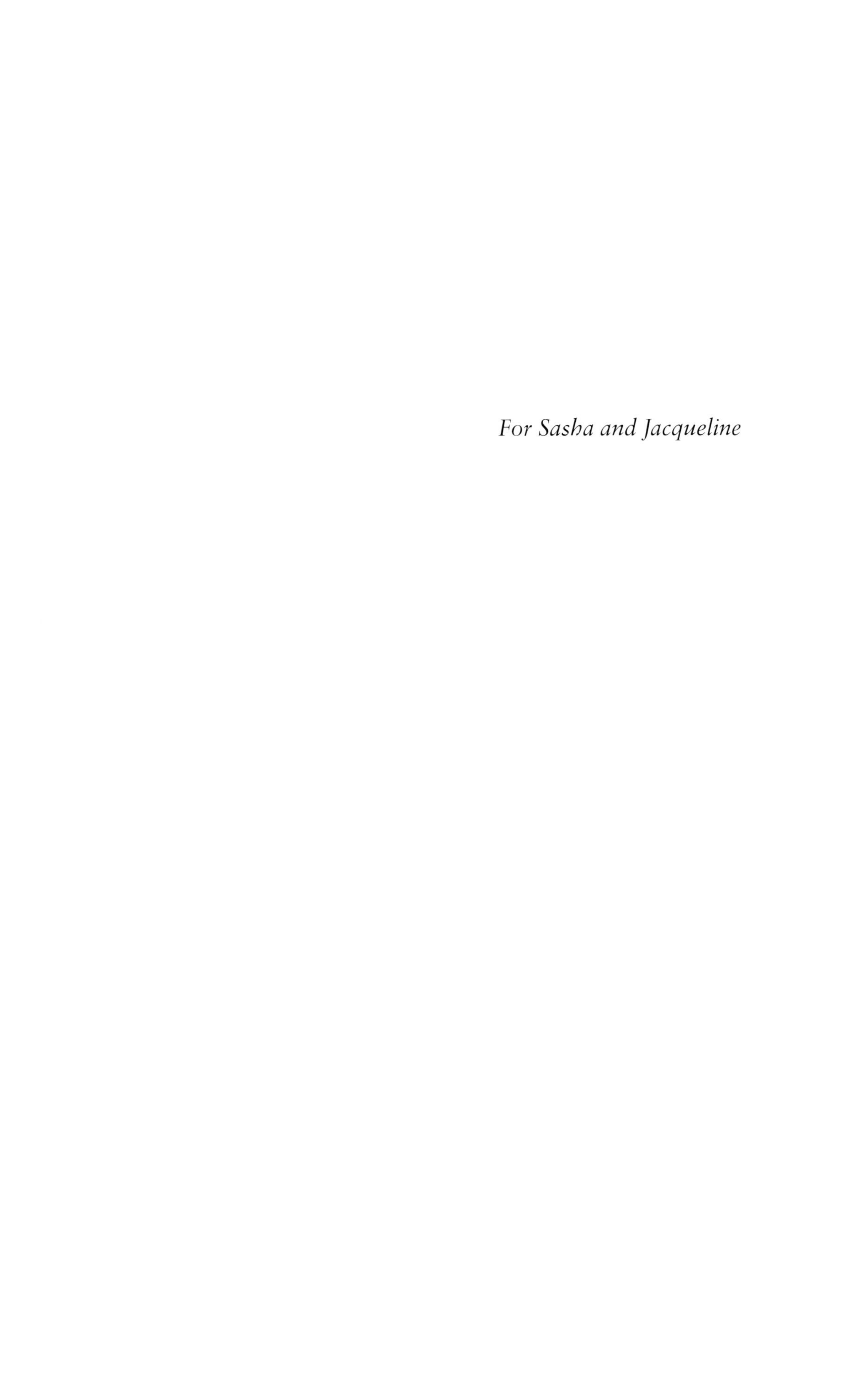

*For Sasha and Jacqueline*

We were dancing—it must have
been a foxtrot or a waltz,
something romantic but
requiring restraint,
rise and fall, precise
execution as we moved
into the next song without
stopping, two chests heaving
above a seven-league
stride—such perfect agony
one learns to smile through,
ecstatic mimicry
being the sine qua non
of American Smooth.
And because I was distracted
by the effort of
keeping my frame
(the leftward lean, head turned
just enough to gaze out
past your ear and always
smiling, smiling),
I didn't notice
how still you'd become until
we had done it
(for two measures?
four?)—achieved flight,
that swift and serene
magnificence,
before the earth
remembered who we were
and brought us down.

    —Rita Dove, "American Smooth"

# Contents

# Illustrations

# Preface

This book grew out of a curiosity about the affinity of visual art and dance. During two decades of teaching and looking at American art, I began to notice the surprising frequency and quality of visual representations of dance in painting, sculpture, prints, and photographs. Why, I asked myself, were so many artists drawn to the subject?

As my research began in earnest, I quickly decided that I was neither competent nor desirous of attempting a new study of dance history per se. Experts in that field have continued to produce useful and provocative interpretations of dance history, notably the comprehensive volume by Nancy Reynolds and Malcolm McCormick, *No Fixed Points: Dance in the Twentieth Century* (2003). And volumes of critical theory, academic in tone, appear regularly from scholars of the dance. There have even been a few exhibitions, especially of Degas's dancers, in recent years. Art and Dance (1982), at Boston's Institute of Contemporary Art, looked at the modern art–dance dialogue. Its emphasis was heavily European.

By contrast, my focus is primarily on American art and extends forward from the early nineteenth century, when visual representations of dance began to appear in significant numbers. The approach is new in that it keeps visual representations at the center and asks repeated questions, both general and specific, about why artists have been drawn to dance and dancers. Driven by the images themselves, the investigation led where the artists wandered—into many, but not all, corners of the dance world. The artists' curiosity became my own; their focus—or indeed, their neglect—of certain dancers or styles itself a spur to further questions. Over a period of years I looked at hundreds of dance representations, a visual record on one hand as idiosyncratic as the individual artists, on the other as broad as the visual culture of America. Indeed, while far from complete as a broad history of dance, the wide-ranging body of images grouped themselves around several insistent themes, pervasive in American consciousness, that eventually became the basis for the book's organization: American art and dance as expressions of the real or imagined heritage of a nation; dance and the legacies of Romanticism in American culture; dance, time, and the immediate cultural moment, or expressions of modernity; and dance, the liberated body, and America's cultural revolutions.

Within each of these sections I have tried to frame the cultural context in which certain dance forms developed, with special attention to how certain visual artists came to focus on those forms or their performers. Often the discussion proceeds in two ways, seeking both depth and breadth. Moving from in-depth analysis of a central work of art, discussed in either iconographic or stylistic terms, the argument gathers additional examples to reinforce, extend, or amplify aspects of the same idea.

Although the book is structured thematically rather than chronologically, I have, whenever possible, proceeded along chronological lines following the artists, not the dancers. Thus, in chapter 4, for example, late nineteenth-century visual artists such as Eakins, Cassatt, and Sargent, who portrayed Spanish dance and dancers of their own time logically precede Joseph Cornell, a mid-twentieth-century artist. Yet Cornell reached back, in a deliberately nostalgic mode, for dance subjects from the mid-nineteenth-century Romantic Ballet. For the same reason, certain dancers precede their teachers in the discussion according to the way each was taken up by visual artists. In short, while the separate histories of dance and visual art can be written chronologically, it has not been possible to retain neat chronological sequences when combining them. Instead, what I have written comprises *episodes* from a specialized history of American art focusing on dance. To help readers deal with that episodic structure and the art-centered discussions, I have provided a separate extensive chronology. There, and throughout the text, I've tried to maintain a flexible balance between art history and dance history, knowingly crossing interdisciplinary boundaries while remaining firmly grounded in the viewpoint I know best, the contextual history of art.

A few words about the scope of this book: dance in American art is a subject of prodigious breadth and depth. Like an exuberant young tree, it pops up with minimal encouragement and survives under adverse conditions. To deal with the subject in any meaningful or coherent way, one must impose limits—of time, genre, or place. Within the vast range of America's dance heritage, one necessary omission here is a comprehensive look at Native American dance, more accurately called ritual drama. For many Euro-American artists and dancers, Native American ceremonials modeled ideas about visual rhythm, patterning, and movement expressive of life's deeper verities—truths so compelling that whole artistic careers focused on Native American ceremonials. Still, despite its aesthetic and cultural importance, the sheer numbers of representations—by European, European American, and Native artists in all artistic mediums—preclude any adequate treatment in a study such as this. Instead, the book begins with only a brief look at two of the earliest images of Native American dancers by Europeans arriving on these shores, with brief mentions in later sections of the book. Fortunately, the profound influence of Native American ritual has already been explored in many previous books and catalogs.[1]

# Acknowledgments

Laura Addison, New Mexico Museum of Art; Jan Adlmann; Ana Archuleta and Molly Wagoner, Gerald Peters Gallery, Santa Fe; Susan Barger; Ellen Berkovitch; Mary Brannen; Merrill Brockway; Sarah Burt; Leslie Calmes, Center for Creative Photography, University of Arizona; Allison Colborne; Amy Conger; Lee Cox, San Francisco Performing Arts Library and Museum; Elizabeth Cunningham; Virginia Dehn; Tina Dickey; Teresa Ebie; Trevor Fairbrother; Richard and Dorothy Fitch, Old Maps & Prints & Books, Santa Fe; Shirley Frank; Elizabeth Hadas; Marilyn Hunt; Mary Jebsen, New Mexico Museum of Art; Paul Karlstrom; Helen Langa; Virginia Couse Leavitt; Samella Lewis; Wendy Lewis, Photo-Eye Gallery, Santa Fe, New Mexico; Andrew Lowe; Tom McGuire; Jackie M., The Georgia O'Keeffe Museum; Sandra Miller; Ron Moody, Dallas Museum of Art; Francis Naumann; Percy North; Kathleen Pyne; Ellen Bradbury Reid; Jerry Rightman; Arnold Rönnebeck; Lois Rudnick; Mary Anne Santos Newhall; Julie Schimmel; Marc Simmons; Signe and Joseph Stuart; Chip Ware, Jonson Gallery, University of New Mexico; Catherine Whitney, formerly, Gerald Peters Gallery; Zaplin-Lampert Gallery.

# Chronology

<table>
<tr><td>1774</td><td>First Continental Congress urges closing of all places of public entertainment.</td></tr>
<tr><td>1784</td><td>In Philadelphia, French dancer Mme. Gardie and American John Durang star in La Forêt noire, first recorded serious ballet production in the new nation.</td></tr>
<tr><td>1820</td><td>Famous Parisian dancing master Charles Blasis, writing in his Traité élémentaire, théorique et pratique de l'art de la danse (Milan, 1820), describes Spanish and American Negro dances.</td></tr>
<tr><td>1830s</td><td>Marius Petipa (1818–1907) visits United States. As master of the Russian Imperial Ballet, he refined romantic ballet with brilliant new technique and repertory, including 60 original works.</td></tr>
<tr><td>1832</td><td>Era of Romantic ballet inaugurated with Marie Taglioni's first performance in La Sylphide; lasts roughly until 1850.</td></tr>
<tr><td>1838</td><td>American dancer Augusta Maywood, age 15, achieves overnight success dancing in Paris; later choreographs a version of Uncle Tom's Cabin performed by her own company in Italy.</td></tr>
<tr><td>c. 1840</td><td>Polka introduced in United States, bringing on a "polka mania" among all classes of New York society.</td></tr>
<tr><td>1840–41</td><td>American tour of the celebrated Austrian ballerina Fanny Elssler, known as the "Pagan Viennese."</td></tr>
<tr><td>1842</td><td>First Dodworth Academy established in New York, becomes arbiter of fashionable social dancing for nearly a century.</td></tr>
<tr><td>1844–45</td><td>American dancer Mary Ann Lee studies ballet at the Paris Opera; returns to perform Giselle in Boston and Philadelphia; becomes America's first classical ballerina of international reputation.</td></tr>
<tr><td>1849</td><td>Electric lighting ("fairy lighting") installed at Luna Park, Coney Island, ushering in new era of possibilities for artificial theatrical illumination.</td></tr>
<tr><td>1851</td><td>Irish-born "Spanish" dancer Lola Montez performs on a Broadway stage in New York.</td></tr>
<tr><td>1866</td><td>The Black Crook first produced at Niblo's Garden in New York. A variety stage show, it features ballet and musical acts, becoming the prototype for American musical comedy, burlesque, and</td></tr>
</table>

vaudeville. In revivals and nationwide tours, Crook runs more than 40 years, employing nearly every American dancer of the period.

Winslow Homer sails to France, spends a year in Paris, shares a studio in Montmartre, produces wood engravings of Paris dance halls for *Harper's Weekly.*

1871 New York's Metropolitan Museum of Art opens in temporary quarters at 681 Fifth Avenue, in an elegant building formerly housing the Dodworth Academy of Dance.

1876 Philadelphia Centennial Exhibition gives Americans a first opportunity to see a large collection of Japanese art objects.

1880 John Singer Sargent paints his monumental *El Jaleo,* a dramatic composition of a gypsy dancer and her accompanists.

1882 American Mary Louise (later Loïe) Fuller tours with Buffalo Bill Cody's troupe of Wild West performers in the eastern United States.

Sargent's *El Jaleo* shown at the Paris Salon, praised as a tour de force by many artists, generally disliked as "ugly" by the public.

1885 Allen Dodworth publishes his book *Dancing and Its Relation to Education and Social Life,* a manual of manners, morals, and health for Americans.

1889 Twelve-year-old Isadora Duncan dances in touring variety show throughout California.

1890 Brazilian *maxixe* introduced in Europe.

During a visit to New York, expatriate American painter John Singer Sargent paints a full-length portrait of the famous Spanish dancer "La Carmencita"; William Merritt Chase paints her the same year.

1892 Loïe Fuller goes to Paris, creates sensation at Folies Bergères for her Fire Dance, Lily Dance, Butterfly Dance, and Serpentine Dance, all enhanced by her own lighting inventions, frosted glass, and yards of swirling silk in extravagant motion; seen by many visual artists, including James A. McNeill Whistler, who makes drawings of her in motion.

1893 World's Columbian Exposition in Chicago reintroduces Americans to Japanese Cherry Blossom dances, and extensive Japanese installations extend American familiarity with Japanese aesthetics, first seen at 1876 Philadelphia Centennial Exposition. Also at Chicago, dances are performed by Senegambian, Native American, South Sea Islander, Bedouin Arab, Spanish, Cingalese, and ragtime groups. Crowds are entertained by "Little Egypt," belly dancers (the "Hootchy Kootchy"), and other vaguely defined "Oriental" dances, setting off interest in Egyptian, Indian, Asian aesthetics.

1894     Parisian dealer Siegfried Bing (1818–1905) introduces Japanese art to New York.

1895     International introduction of recorded sound; first commercial moving-picture shows in Paris, December 28.

1896     Loïe Fuller brings her triumphant solo dance spectacles from Paris to New York, San Francisco.

First commercial moving-picture show in New York, April 23.

Isadora Duncan leaves California for the East Coast, performing in New York's commercial theaters.

Javanese dancers appear in Paris.

Craze for Cakewalk begins, making dance more visible among America's performing arts.

1897     Duncan abandons Broadway music halls for an artistic career as a salon soloist; begins "to compose her own dances in her little Greek tunic."

One of Loïe Fuller's imitators, the dancer Annabella, is filmed by Thomas Edison, who hand paints each frame of the film to simulate the varicolored light effects invented by Fuller.

1899     Scott Joplin's *Maple Leaf Rag* published; nearly a century later (1990) Martha Graham would use it as the inspiration for one of her last dances.

1900     Loïe Fuller performs in her own Art Nouveau theater at the Paris Exposition Universelle, a cavelike structure adorned by swirling drapes and a monumental statue of herself; seen by Isadora Duncan and Ruth St. Denis.

Famed Japanese actress Mme. Sadi Yacco performs at Paris Exposition Universelle, inspiring Ruth Dennis (later Ruth St. Denis) to create a solo dance sketch, "Madame Butterfly," produced in New York by vaudeville impresario David Belasco, and setting off a wave of U.S. interest in Japanese dance-drama.

Also at the Paris Exposition Universelle, American ragtime music and dance introduced by John Philip Sousa, followed shortly by such dances as the One-Step or Turkey Trot.

Pablo Picasso, drawn to Paris from Barcelona by the exposition, immerses himself in art galleries and the dance halls of Montmartre; paints *Le Moulin de la Galette* (Guggenheim Museum, New York), his first Parisian painting.

Isadora Duncan seeks new sources for her art in Europe; begins to dance to Chopin, other serious music.

Freud publishes *The Interpretation of Dreams*.

1902      Robert Henri and Arthur B. Davies share as model the dancer Jesseca Penn, and both produce portraits of her.

Isadora Duncan, adored among Germans as "Die Erste Barfuss Tänzerin" (the first barefoot dancer), makes her debut in Munich. At the close of her wildly successful visit there, learned professors at the Künstlerhaus (home of German Art Nouveau or Jugendstil) crown Duncan with a laurel wreath, and painter Fritz von Kaulbach publishes his full-length pastel portrait of her on the cover of *Jugend*. In Budapest she dons red tunic and dances in support of Hungarian revolutionaries.

1903      Nouveau Cirque in Paris presents Cakewalk *(danse du gâteau)* and ragtime.

American dancer Maud Allan makes solo debut in Vienna wearing Greek tunic like Duncan's and "visualizing" Bach, Beethoven, Schubert, et al.

In June, Isadora Duncan debuts at Théâtre Sarah-Bernhardt in Paris. A few days later she dances in the open air at a *banquet champêtre* in the woods at Vélizy, viewed by Rodin.

Loïe Fuller organizes exhibit of Rodin's work at the National Arts Club, New York, followed by his exhibition later that year at the Metropolitan Museum of Art.

Wright Brothers make first successful flight.

1904      Duncan premiers Beethoven's *Seventh Symphony* at Trocadéro, Paris.

Duncan, already famous throughout Europe, invited to perform dances to Wagner's operas at Bayreuth Festival.

Duncan travels to Saint Petersburg, beginning her influence on the Russian Ballet, to which she delivers (according to Diaghilev) "a shock from which it could never recover." She returns there in 1905, 1907, and 1909.

1905      Ruth St. Denis conceives her dance *Radha,* based on Indian legend of god Krishna's love for the mortal maid Radha; combines skirt dancing with mime and tableau, performs for both vaudeville and society audiences in New York.

Isadora Duncan's performances in Saint Petersburg make a deep impression on choreographer Michel Fokine and present a challenge to the supremacy of classical ballet.

Fokine creates solo dance *The Dying Swan* for Anna Pavlova; it becomes her most famous role, performed in Europe and on coast-to-coast tours in U.S.

Einstein publishes *Special Theory of Relativity.*

New York Hippodrome, with capacity of 5,000 spectators, opens in New York; its huge stage controlled by hydraulic elevators becomes site of grandiose performances of all kinds, including ballet and stage shows featuring as many as 280 chorus dancers.

1906–9    Ruth St. Denis dances to triumphal acclaim in Berlin, London.

1906    Inspired by Isadora Duncan's dance, Paris couturier Paul Poiret introduces experimental dress-reform gowns based on visions of women's bodies in motion, employing modern neoclassical forms based on Greek sculptures in the Louvre. He names some of these newly shaped costumes, which fall straight from underarm to ankle, after dancers: the "Lola Montez," the "Isadora," etc. Eventual result of Poiret's flowing designs is widespread change in women's walk, posture, gestures. Especially among American women, it emphasizes new concerns with health and physical ease.

Cambodian dancers perform in Paris, inspiring drawings by Rodin.

Composer Claude Debussy incorporates elements of African American music in his "Golliwog's Cakewalk," part of his piece *Children's Corner.*

1907    Florenz Ziegfeld introduces the American chorus girl in his Ziegfeld Follies.

Franz Lehár's operetta *The Merry Widow* debuts in New York; features dance segment that forecasts integration of dance into American musical theater.

Metropolitan Opera mounts Richard Strauss's *Salomé* for one performance only; seen as too shocking by backers J. P. Morgan, W. K. Vanderbilt, and August Belmont, who withdraw support. Banished from opera, Salomé idea picked up by Florenz Ziegfeld for vaudeville; he casts Mlle. Dazie (Daisy Peterkin of Detroit) as Salomé, who in turn trains and sends a whole spate of Salomés touring the country's vaudeville circuits.

1908    Rodin makes several portraits of the young Japanese dancer Hanako, introduced to the sculptor by Loïe Fuller.

Duncan performs at Metropolitan Opera, New York, dancing to the music of Beethoven, including his *Seventh Symphony,* which the composer himself had called "the Apotheosis of Dance."

Henry Ford manufactures assembly-line cars.

Marinetti publishes Futurist Manifesto.

1909    Ballets Russes first appears in Paris.

Charles H. Caffin publishes article "Henri Matisse and Isadora Duncan" in *Camera Work,* vol. 25.

Loïe Fuller and her troupe make first of three appearances at Metropolitan Opera House, New York, November 30.

Max Weber sees Duncan perform at Carnegie Hall.

**1910**    In February, Russian dancers Anna Pavlova and Mikhail Mordkin debut at Metropolitan Opera House, then move to New Theatre to perform programs, including scenes from *Coppélia* and a frenzied Bacchanale, to music from Glazunov's *The Seasons*. New Theatre sells out an opera/dance performance for the first time in its existence.

In November, Pavlova and Mordkin return for more performances at the Metropolitan Opera House, then launch tour of U.S. and Cuba.

Spanish dancer La Guerrero introduces the Argentine tango to audiences of mostly English and American tourists at the Marigny Theatre, Champs Elyseés, Paris. Born in Buenos Aires and partly inspired by the Cuban *habanera,* the tango features crossing and flexing steps along with dramatic pauses in midglide. Tango becomes a dance sensation lasting more than 20 years, with subsequent revivals in Europe and U.S.

Henri Rousseau's work shown at Stieglitz's Gallery 291, arranged by Edward Steichen.

**1911**    Pirated versions of Fokine's Ballets Russes productions presented in U.S. by dancer Gertrude Hoffman with a troupe of about 100 Russian and French dancers; new Russian dance techniques, according to dancer Theodore Kosloff, were intended "to do what modern Russian painters and poets have done—invest our art with realism and life."

During Ballets Russes performances in London, John Singer Sargent makes charcoal drawings of two star dancers, Vaslav Nijinsky and Tamara Karsavina.

Isadora Duncan's *Orpheus* personifies classic Greek revival in dance.

Michio Ito (1892?–1961) leaves Tokyo to study voice; sees Nijinsky dance in Paris, Isadora Duncan in Berlin, and decides to become a dancer.

First major appearances of elegant ballroom dance couple Irene and Vernon Castle.

The year's "dance craze" introduces a flood of new social dances: Texas Tommy, Bunny Hug, Turkey Trot, One-Step, Camel Walk.

**1912**    May 29: Debussy's *L'Après-midi d'un Faune* premieres in Paris, choreographed and danced by Nijinsky; Rodin attends.

Nijinsky's ballet *Jeux* premieres in Paris, the first "sports ballet."

Foxtrot introduced.

Michio Ito enrolls at Dalcroze Institute near Dresden, stays until 1914 studying dance, music, drama.

1913  Stravinsky's *Sacre du Printemps,* choreographed by Nijinsky with sets by Nicholas Roerich, makes its scandalous debut in Paris; audience riots.

Rodin writes "La Danse de Civa" (Shiva), published in 1921 as the preface to the catalog *Ars Asiatica.* Rodin's text concerns the sacred dance of India, and his own collection contains several wood sculptures of dancers from the East Indies.

Ruth St. Denis premieres *O-Mika,* her ethereal, stylized Japanese-inspired dance-drama in New York.

Ted Shawn and Norma Gould appear in Edison film *Dance through the Ages,* with Shawn as director.

The Foxtrot is the latest dance sweeping the United States.

Armory Show (International Exhibition of Modern Art) opens in New York, travels to Chicago and Boston; introduces American audiences to some of Europe's most avant-garde art; includes many dance subjects in painting and sculpture.

Apollo Theatre opens in Harlem.

1914  Photographer Baron Adolf de Meyer to U.S., having already photographed many dancers, including the Ballets Russes, Nijinsky, and the Denishawn troupe.

W. C. Handy publishes the classic *St. Louis Blues.*

American collector Isabella Stewart Gardner acquires Sargent's *El Jaleo;* has a special room, the Spanish Cloister, built for it in her Boston home, later the Isabella Stewart Gardner Museum.

Radical periodical *The Masses* sponsors a fund-raising ball in Greenwich Village; other exotic-themed balls follow, including the Liberal Club's "Pagan Routs," attracting both bohemian and uptown New York crowds.

Panama Canal opens.

1915  In February, Spanish dancer La Argentina makes first American appearance at Maxine Elliott Theatre, New York; reviewed by Carl Van Vechten.

In the spring, Macbeth Gallery in New York features an exhibition of dance subjects by a number of sculptors and dance drawings by Arthur B. Davies.

May 7: German U-boat torpedoes British liner *Lusitania* off Ireland, stimulating anti-German sentiment in United States.

May 9: Isadora Duncan, deep in debt from her staged performances of Greek tragedies and solo concerts at the Metropolitan Opera and the Century Theater, sails for Europe with her students, "the Isadorables," away from the "philistine darkness" of New York.

June 1: Loïe Fuller and her troupe begin multiple dance performances to packed audiences and critical praise at the Panama-Pacific International Exposition, San Francisco, where the Italian Futurists also exhibit many dance-themed paintings.

In September, Dada publication *Rogue* stages a benefit costume ball in New York, awarding first prize for costume to illustrator Clara Tice.

New York School of Dalcroze Eurhythmics opens with European faculty; teaches a rhythmic movement system that eventually is taught by hundreds of physical education teachers in American colleges.

Ruth St. Denis and Ted Shawn establish Denishawn School, incorporating many ideas of Delsarte and Dalcroze into their musical "visualizations."

1915–18   Arnold Genthe photographs Duncan many times in New York; later (1929) publishes a portfolio of his Duncan photos.

1916   Americans embrace the new music of jazz; Bill "Bojangles" Robinson stars in vaudeville.

From January to May, Post-Panama Pacific Exposition Exhibit at San Francisco's Palace of Fine Arts provides forward-looking exhibition of European and American art, including Arthur B. Davies's Cubo-Futurist dance murals.

Duncan dances in Paris at the Trocadéro, performing the *Marseillaise* in solidarity with the French effort in World War I; repeats performance the following year in New York.

Nijinsky rejoins his Ballets Russes company in U.S., performing two seasons at the Metropolitan Opera House in New York. Nijinsky premieres *Till Eulenspiegel,* a ballet set to symphonic poem by Richard Strauss; set designed by Robert Edmond Jones. Ballets Russes sets out on cross-country American tour (1916–17) of four months' duration, to 56 cities with more than 100 dancers and musicians.

Man Ray moves from Ridgefield, New Jersey, to Manhattan, begins to incorporate more urbanized themes into his painting.

Dancer Ted Shawn photographed wearing animal skins, perhaps in emulation of Nijinsky in *L'Après-midi d'un Faune.*

Michio Ito arrives in New York, begins performing there.

*Prima ballerina assoluta* Anna Pavlova appears at New York's Hippodrome in *The Sleeping Beauty,* sharing billing with a flying piano act.

Marcel Duchamp judges costumes at the Rogue Ball in New York, held to celebrate the second series publication of the Dadaist periodical *The Rogue.*

1917    Cubist ballet *Parade* premieres in Paris, written by Jean Cocteau, choreographed by Léonide Massine, and designed by Picasso, with score by Erik Satie.

In March, Duncan dances a "war program" at Metropolitan Opera, New York, featuring the *Marseillaise*; program ends with Duncan draped in an American flag during the "Star-Spangled Banner"; performances encourage recruitment for American war effort.

In April, rumblings of revolution in Russia inspire Duncan's danced response, her *Marche Slave,* danced to the music of Tchaikovsky at Metropolitan Opera House in New York. Later in the year, Russian revolution disrupts traditional patronage machinery of Imperial Russian ballet, effectively making Ballets Russes dancers permanent exiles.

April 12: Katharine Dreier organizes a Latin Quarter Ball in New York to benefit the Red Cross.

April 20: The Independents Ball, with guests costumed as schools of art, held concurrently with New York's Independents Exhibition, in which Man Ray's *The Rope Dancer Accompanies Herself with Her Shadows* is first seen.

May 25: Blindman's Ball, a riotous Dada dance, held in Greenwich Village; Beatrice Wood (later famous as a ceramic artist) performs Russian dances.

Spanish dancer La Argentina returns to New York, sharing a bill with Doloretes at the Park Theatre; reviewed in superlatives by Carl Van Vechten, who compares the dancers to those in the paintings of Goya, Manet, and Zuloaga and reinforces American interest in elaborate rhythms of Spanish music.

C. J. Jung publishes *Psychology of the Unconscious.*

Original Dixieland Jass Band makes its first recordings, paving the way for mass cultural reception of jazz.

D. W. Griffith's film *Intolerance* features hundreds of Denishawn dancers in its Babylon sequences.

c. 1918    The Shimmy (descended from the Fox Trot) is introduced; the Charleston (according to some sources brought to New York from South Carolina) follows within a few years.

1920    Marcel Duchamp, Katherine Dreier, and Man Ray found the Société Anonyme to display and promote modern art.

Coco Chanel introduces low-waisted chemise dress, worn without a corset; short skirts become fashionable.

Ted Shawn creates vaudeville spectacle *Xochitl,* which he dances with Martha Graham on tour throughout the American West and Canada. Based on an Aztec legend, *Xochitl* is hailed as the "first native American ballet" due to its decor and strong "virile" dynamic in dancing; influences Graham's later choreographic subjects from American earth and legend.

Ruth St. Denis and her student-collaborator Doris Humphrey create *Soaring,* a danced "musical visualization" set to classical music.

1921    Duncan invited to open a school in the Soviet Union; begins extended stay there.

Russian dancer/choreographer Adolph Bolm performs Slavic war dance at Santa Fe Fiesta, reciprocated by Zuni Pueblo dancers.

First regular radio broadcasts by KDKA, Pittsburgh; by 1922 three million American homes have radios.

Man Ray, discouraged by the reception of his work in New York, sets sail for Paris, where he remains for most of the next nineteen years.

New York State passes law allowing a state commissioner to censor dances.

Rudolph Valentino (1895–1926), Italian immigrant who became the renowned exhibition dancer "Signor Rodolfo," achieves movie stardom performing an erotic tango in *The Four Horsemen of the Apocalypse.*

1922    Harlem nightclub the Cotton Club opens at 142nd Street and Lenox Avenue; most performers are African American.

Discovery of Tutankhamen's tomb in Egypt popularizes geometric design, which in turn influences new shapes in decor, fashion, and popular dancing, perhaps including Egyptian-type angular arm movements in the Charleston.

Degas's sculptures, including many dancers, shown in New York at the Grolier Club and at Durand-Ruel Galleries.

Adolph Bolm stages New York production of *Krazy Kat,* jazz pantomime based on George Herriman comic strip.

Adolph Bolm offered post of ballet master of Chicago Civic Opera, moves on to direct Chicago Allied Arts, creating new ballets for small orchestra.

Duncan makes last appearances in America, including her dance in red tunic to *La Marche Slav* in celebration of Russian revolution.

1923  Les Ballets Suédois (Swedish Ballet) performs modernist ballet *The Skating Rink* in the United States, with Cubist-inspired costumes and sets by Fernand Léger.

Across America dance marathons become the rage, encouraging couples to "dance until you drop."

New York's Prohibition Enforcement Act repealed.

1924  Religious mystic Georges I. Gurdjieff (c. 1874–1948) brings a troupe of his dancers to New York, where they perform dances, purportedly of ancient and sacred origins, before audiences of American intellectuals in modernist salons. Writers and artists such as Aaron Douglas attend.

Louvre gives Loïe Fuller a *Retrospective Exposition, 1892–1920* of her dyed and painted fabrics, presented as *Studies in Form, Line and Colour for Light Effects*.

Chicago Allied Arts presents ballet-pantomime *Foyer de la Danse*, based on a Degas painting of a ballet rehearsal at the Paris Opéra in 1870.

Women's bobbed haircuts sweep the U.S.

Fernand Léger's abstract film *Ballet Mécanique* completed.

Picabia's Dada ballet *Relâche* performed in Paris.

Pavlova makes last American tour 1924–25.

1925  The Charleston sweeps across America.

African American dancer Josephine Baker makes sensational debut in La Revue Nègre in Paris.

In Washington, D.C., 40,000 Ku Klux Klansmen march, watched by 200,000 spectators.

International Decorative Arts Exposition in Paris draws attention to Art Deco or *moderne,* the new style of geometric modes in art and design. At the opening, Loïe Fuller stages a new abstract visual arts/dance performance, *The Mighty Sea,* repeated in San Francisco in September.

1926  Black Bottom introduced.

1927  Duncan dies near Nice, France, strangled by a long scarf caught in her car wheel.

April 10: New York premiere of George Antheil's *Ballet Mécanique, Jazz Symphony,* and other pieces at Carnegie Hall, with Joseph Mullen's backdrop of African American couple doing the Charleston for the *Symphony. Ballet Mécanique* plagued with technical problems; many in the audience walk out.

1928    Stuart Davis travels to Paris, paints there for over a year.

African American Dance Marathon, staged at Manhattan Casino in Harlem, introduces the new Lindy Hop.

1929    Martha Graham achieves first important dance recognition, performing the part of the Chosen One in the American premiere of Stravinsky's *Le Sacre du Printemps,* conducted by Leopold Stokowski and choreographed by Massine.

Isamu Noguchi makes two portrait heads of Graham.

1941    Michio Ito resides in Los Angeles, choreographing and performing; returns to Japan following America's entry into World War II.

Mexican-born José Limon, studying painting in New York, sees dance performance by Harald Kreutzberg and determines to become a dancer.

1930    Martha Graham begins her own company; travels to the American Southwest, visiting the Pueblos of Isleta and Santo Domingo, as well as Taos and Santa Fe, absorbing Native American rituals and Hispanic dance elements. In Santa Fe, stays with writer Mary Austin, whose ideas about an American rhythm and dance drama Graham absorbs.

1931    Graham premieres two new works, *Primitive Canticles* and *Primitive Mysteries,* the latter based on her perception of Native American connections to the earth. Again visits Mary Austin in Santa Fe.

Adolph Bolm's *Mechanical Ballet* performed to great acclaim in Hollywood Bowl; features gears, dynamos, fly wheels, and switches as characters.

1932    Graham premieres *Ceremonials,* also inspired by the Southwest, receives the first Guggenheim Fellowship awarded to a dancer, again visits New Mexico this year and in July 1933 as guest of Taos hostess Mabel Dodge Luhan.

Frederick Ashton choreographs *Foyer de Danse* in London, based on Degas's painting of the Paris Opéra.

African American modern dancer Katherine Dunham performs *Fantaisie Nègre* at an Artists Ball in Chicago.

1933    George Balanchine arrives in U.S. from Russia.

In New York, Julien Levy Gallery exhibits *Twenty-Five Years of Russian Ballet,* a collection of original material (sets, costumes, miscellany by prominent artists who worked with Diaghilev) acquired from the Ballets Russes by dancer-choreographer Serge Lifar.

Fan dancer Sally Rand (formerly with the Denishawn company) appears at Chicago World's Fair, causing an obscenity scandal.

1934    Ninette de Valois choreographs *Bar aux Folies-Bergère,* based on Manet's eponymous painting.

George Balanchine and Lincoln Kirstein found School of American Ballet in New York.

American dance-mime and visual artist Angna Enters (1897–1989) receives Guggenheim Fellowship to study Greek art, mime, and music forms, resulting in exhibitions of her paintings and drawings in New York, Minneapolis, and Rochester, N.Y., with a simultaneous exhibition and performance at the Worcester, Mass., museum. Following year she receives second Guggenheim to continue art and mime studies in Egypt, again resulting in many new performance and visual art compositions presented throughout the U.S. and Europe.

1935    Martha Graham asks Alexander Calder to design mobiles for her productions *Panorama* and *Horizon* (1936).

1936    Martha Graham performs *Lamentation-Dance of Sorrow,* a work showing her awareness of contemporary art. Choreographed to music of Zoltan Kodaly, it is performed at opening events of Colorado Springs Fine Arts Center.

At Bennington College, Vt., Erick Hawkins comes to study and perform with the Martha Graham company, initiating a long professional and personal relationship with her.

Lincoln Kirstein founds Ballet Caravan to perform new ballets on American themes.

1937    Martha Graham's company first performs her *El Penitente,* with themes of sin, suffering, and atonement arising from the flagellant practices of the Penitente (rural, lay Catholic) brotherhood of the Southwest.

Tenth Memorial Exhibition for Isadora Duncan features Walkowitz drawings at Park Art Galleries, New York (Sept. 27–Oct. 29).

1939    Lincoln Kirstein founds the dance archive at the Museum of Modern Art, America's first resource of the kind.

1940    Julien Levy Gallery, New York, opens a solo show of Joseph Cornell's work, introducing his work on the Romantic ballet.

| | |
|---|---|
| 1942 | Periodical *Dance Index* appears, published by Lincoln Kirstein and Donald Windham; continues until 1948. |
| 1944 | With his set for *Appalachian Spring,* Isamu Noguchi begins a collaboration with Martha Graham that would encompass 22 productions, lasting intermittently until 1967. |
| 1945 | Graham's *Herodiade* (set by Noguchi, music by Hindemith) debuts at Coolidge Festival, Washington, D.C. |
| 1950 | Herbert Ross choreographs *Los Caprichos,* based on Goya's etchings, for Choreographer's Workshop and American Ballet Theater. |
| early 1950s | College Art Association mounts *The Dance in Modern Art,* an exhibition of paintings, prints, and sculpture by contemporary artists, shown at Washington County Museum of Fine Arts, Hagerstown, Md. |
| 1977–78 | California Palace of the Legion of Honor mounts *In Celebration of Loie Fuller,* a festival of performing arts and exhibition of visual representations inspired by Fuller and executed by Rodin, Rivière, Larche, and Cheret. |
| 1979 | Virginia Museum of Fine Arts, Richmond, mounts *Loïe Fuller: Magician of Light* exhibition with more than 140 works of art reflecting Fuller and Art Nouveau. |
| 1982 | Institute of Contemporary Art, Boston, mounts *Art and Dance,* a series of exhibitions, performances, and screenings exploring relationships between twentieth-century art and dance, with emphasis on European art. |

# DANCE
## and American Art

# Introduction

Why have visual artists looked so often and so insistently at dance? In its largest sense, dance has interested visual artists as part of the moving surface of the world, and it is clear that the dancer's will to move has been, in many cases, no less urgent than the visual artist's will to record that movement. The visual artist has often been faced with the paradox of trying to fix—to make permanent—an image of the dance, while at the same time sustaining the fiction of motion. All of this resonates across American culture to find a literary echo in William Faulkner's famous assertion that "the aim of every artist is to arrest motion, which is life, by artificial means and hold it fixed so that a hundred years later, when a stranger looks at it, it moves again since it is life."[1] Thus, in their paintings, sculptures, prints, and photographs, American artists have grappled with the essence of movement, asking probing visual questions about how dance movements differ from other forms of movement.

In this book I have challenged myself to trace, from the nineteenth into the twentieth century, what visual artists have revealed about and through dance. In that process, I have come to believe that dance, like visual art, is capable of bestowing, guarding, and conveying deep cultural meaning. Within their own disciplines, dance historians already know that capability, as do art historians. Still, in writing the present volume I have concluded that the intertwined history of American art and dance is even more revealing, more visually complex, more culturally nuanced, and more interesting than has yet been acknowledged by historians of either dance or art. Artists and dancers have delighted in taking up old and new themes, playing them off against each other, teasing but at the same time taking each other seriously as they move in and out of an evolving cultural embrace. In every conceivable style and medium, artists' innovative formal responses to rhythmically moving bodies have enriched American art. And, as the extended discussions in the text relate, many dance subjects in art have lain just below the surface, emerging only now to alter, in ways large and small, the shape of American art history. The discussions focus on American art, on its fluid conversations between "high" art and vernacular expression, on its historical encounters among diverse cultures, and on the way dance subjects have contributed to a visual construction of American nationhood. Along the way, it has been important to acknowledge the significant exchanges, borrowings, and appropriations from European sources that have vitalized our cultural heritage. We begin in the early nineteenth century, when visual representations of dance began to appear in significant numbers in the work of American painters, sculptors, printmakers, and, later, photographers. Sometimes their focus was sustained, as in the work of James A. McNeill Whistler, John Singer Sargent, Robert Henri, or Malvina Hoffman. Other visual artists gave fleeting attention to the dance, inspired by famous performers who visited the United States from abroad or whom the artists encountered on their own travels. In such instances their exposure to dance might be as fleeting as a tourist's glimpse. But sometimes that cursory experience planted the seed for the artist's prolonged study of a particular dancer, the performance of a captivating step, or the sheer challenge of expressing something of the energy of the dance. In rare instances, such as that of Isamu Noguchi's long collaboration with Martha Graham, choreography and artistic design were tightly interwoven. More often, visual artists have responded to the act of performance itself or to the physical presence of a dancer offstage.

Still, the dialogue between visual artists and dancers extends well beyond the study of movement, beyond the look of the dancing body, even beyond the aesthetic realm itself. When, where and how dance happens is also of interest as embodied social practice. It is clear that visual artists have—sometimes unknowingly—uncovered deep connections between dance and the social, historical, and even ideological contexts it inhabits. Through their paintings, sculptures, photographs, and prints they have explored many questions: Who dances with whom, and what gets danced? How have stylistic developments in American visual art paralleled cultural change and articulation? To what extent have individual artists been able to foreground dance as a central cultural experience? How do social, commercial, and theatrical dance styles lend themselves to visual representation? How have dance movements been expressive of class, race, or nationality?

Dance's attraction for visual artists has been, at least for some, an exploration of an old question that has resonated through all the arts in this country: what, if anything, is quintessentially American here? There can be no doubt that the United States has given the world a broad range of dance forms. In the nineteenth century, fresh variants of older European theatrical and social dance preceded the evolution of American musical theater, ballroom innovations, jazz dance, and hip hop, to name just a few. But the question of national styles lingers. In broad general terms, celebrated choreographer Paul Taylor draws a distinction within theatrical dance, seeing modern dance as an essentially American form, ballet as European. Comments Taylor: "There is something about dance that represents life. There is a dichotomy in this country's attitude to dance. It will never be popular like sports, but it will never die out either."[2] Taylor has used American themes, such as in his 1965 dance *From Sea to Shining Sea*, in which Pilgrims trod on Indians, and a tiny American flag became a distress signal. "I'm patriotic enough to kid my own country," adds Taylor. His is only one voice in an extended conversation about dance's place in American visual culture. A recurrent question has concerned changing perceptual experiences of each generation: how, for example, have perceptual shifts affected choices in medium, style, and technique? Throughout American history dance has demonstrated a visible relationship between art and mass society, moving ideas and innovations back and forth from cultural undergrounds to the most visible centers of artistic production. Like the other arts, dance does not simply reflect history but also participates in it, capturing and texturing cultural change. Beginning in the nineteenth century, certain dancers were numbered among the celebrities of their day, faced—like visual artists—with answering the expectations of their audiences while stretching the limits of their modes of expression. Not a few visual artists discovered that dance subjects helped to keep their art fresh and vital while still addressing certain intellectual challenges.

The processes by which American dance and visual art engaged with each other are sometimes hidden, but occasionally emerge with a welcome clarity. Here, let me cite a single incident to demonstrate the potential richness of such exchanges, one of many described at length in my text. Robert Henri (1865–1929), one of the most influential painters and teachers of his day, was, like many of his colleagues, a fan of all kinds of dance. Henri's fascination with live performance led him to seek out and to portray many dancers. On one occasion in the 1920s, Henri, in company with his artist friends John Sloan (1871–1951) and George Bellows (1882–1925), went backstage following a performance by the talented mime dancer Angna Enters (1897–1989), now mostly forgotten but then the toast of Broadway. She had performed one of her new pieces, a tribute to the sensational American Cakewalk dance. Recalled Enters: "Up until this time the Cakewalk was performed in minstrel and variety shows. My point of departure was that the Cakewalk had been taken into the ballroom, and was danced by whites as well as by Negroes. I tried to show the effects on the Negro form in being danced by whites." Much taken with her performance, Henri asked how she had arrived at her lively interpretation. How, specifically, did she know that it had been done "just so" back in 1897? Enters's reply was deduced from the music and the clothes worn; Cakewalkers, she told Henri, "*must* have moved that way, just as today a rhumba dictates its own style."[3] In preparing her performance Enters had studied the surviving visual evidence, such as it was—old posters, sheet music, photographs. From those sources she had been able to reconstruct the costume, setting, and music of the earlier era. She may also have known, as Henri and his artist friends certainly did, an ebullient monoprint of the Cakewalk by another of their circle, George Luks (*Cakewalk*, 1907, Delaware Art Museum, Wilmington). What is also important to know here is that Enters, besides being a dancer and mime, was a painter of considerable talent, who created her dance "compositions" with careful attention to visual aesthetics. Certainly not all dancers knew, or cared about, the connections between painting and their own art. But for those who did—beginning long before and extending well after the Henri–Enters encounter—such associations have lent depth and richness to their work across artistic disciplines.

Henri's question to Enters points to an irony and a difficulty at the heart of dance history. While it is a highly visual aesthetic form, dance is generally the most ephemeral of the arts, existing mainly in the moment of its performance and resisting, always, becoming a fixed object. In that sense it differs significantly from painting, architecture, and most sculpture, which exist in space, and from music and poetry, which exist in time. The most fragile of the arts, dance lives at once in time and space, its rhythmic patterns of movement and active use of space created in and by the dancer's own body. Compared with the human clay molded by the choreographer, a painter's pigments or a sculptor's marble are profoundly stable. By contrast with those mediums, whose traditional products are objects, and unlike carefully notated (and therefore repeatable) forms of music, dance has been preserved by a kind of "oral" transmission, passed from "body to body" as in ancient cultures. As dance critic Joan Acocella has observed, "Dance is a chain, with each link attached only to the last."[4] In recent years improved methods of dance notation, in symbols, on film and videotape, have helped to preserve dance. But each time an important choreographer or dancer passes from the scene, as with the death in July 2009 of Merce Cunningham, the thorny question of posthumous dance preservation arises again.

In past centuries the issue was addressed to some extent by visual artists who sought to preserve the look and feel of dance performance. Legendary Russian ballerina Anna Pavlova (a favorite subject of American visual artists) knew that without a visual record her legacy could not survive: "My art will die with me," she told a photographer. "Yours will live on when you are gone."[5] She understood, like Martha Graham, that one art can unlock the secrets of another. Said Graham, "The only record of a dancer's art lies in the other arts. . . . A painting or a work of sculpture can give the world another artist's concept of a dancer. Photographs present more tangible evidence of a dancer's career. Photographs, when true to the laws that govern inspired photography, reveal facts of feature, bodily contour, and some secret of his power."[6] Graham's statement—that photography can reveal essential aspects of dance—is itself revelatory, for she believed that dance is, perhaps above all else, *communication*. Like many twentieth-century visual artists, she tested a simultaneously dawning principle of communicating thoughts and feelings by means of abstraction and symbol, whether that visual spectacle existed on canvas or in the stylized body movements of mute characters on a stage.

The visual artists who worked with Pavlova and Graham witnessed and interpreted the dance of their own day. Others, looking back into American history, tried to imagine an even earlier era in which transplanted Europeans adapted old dances to reflect the places and character of a new nation. Asher B. Durand, for example, in his dance scenes taken from the *Knickerbocker Tales*, portrayed an early instance of the American immigrant experience glimpsed through dance. Many more followed, extending well into the twentieth century, and representing an important segment of this book. Dance, as part of the immigrant experience, revealed much about powerful sociocultural implications: to cite just one, American social hierarchies, of much shorter duration than Europe's, often ignored the strict segregation of "high" and "low" dance forms. While class has registered its influence in many other aspects of American culture, both social and theatrical dance, as seen repeatedly in the images considered here, often blurred such distinctions. Indeed, as more American artists trained their gaze on dance, they revealed much about the nation's regional differences, the mobility of large numbers of its people, and the fluidity of American culture in general, within which popular and more esoteric artistic forms of dance, like those in American art, continually and profoundly influenced each other. Recognizing that such nebulous concepts as "American culture"—with its implications of stereotyped national characteristics—are in many ways outdated in the early twenty-first century, they contain ideas germane to their day and to evolving ideas about national identity, authenticity, nativism, cultural change, and community, as well as to the importation and export of culture.

In this book then, the spotlight has been trained on a manageable, if still broad, range of American dance and visual art from the early nineteenth century to 1950, after which the explosion of new forms, especially performance art, video, and other electronic media, transformed dance into movement experience of a new order. Both dance and visual art, entering this postmodern period, gathered inspiration from every corner of American experience and embraced such a myriad of styles that they have defied any kind of unified aesthetic. That profusion I have merely suggested in an epilogue, included primarily to assert the continuing importance visual art and dance retain for each other. There too, several later American reprises of such iconic pieces as Matisse's *The Dance* testify to the recurrent power of images produced many decades earlier.

The geographic focus throughout the text is mainly on American art and dance, but even that guideline has required occasional trespass. The visual appeal of certain American dancers abroad, notably Isadora Duncan, Loïe Fuller, and Josephine Baker, can be understood best by assembling and comparing images from a range of American and European artists. Beyond that, protean figures such as Duncan must be considered in multiple thematic as well as geographic contexts: as neoprimitivist innovator, as counterculture rebel, as transatlantic link between French and American dance culture. Thus, while Duncan is discussed primarily in part 4, she also appears more briefly in several other chapters. Another consideration is travel: many American artists spent considerable time abroad, finding compelling dance subjects in foreign cities. Thus, this study, while primarily of American dance and art, has necessarily wandered across national boundaries for fuller understandings of the uniquely American blending so typical of our culture.

Renewing itself with each decade, the enduring cultural embrace between dance and visual art in America has given us an intensely visual form of theater. As choreographer Mark Morris reminds us, "Dance is a visual art."[7]

# Part One

# Art, Dance, and American Consciousness

Americans, blending heritages from Europe, Africa, and Asia, have invented and reinvented their culture repeatedly. Nowhere is this more visible than in the words printed on every American dollar bill: *Novus ordo seclorum*, a new order of the ages. Because of our relatively recent formation as a nation, Americans have often seemed less constrained by history, or guided by it for that matter, than other peoples. Change, newness, and selective resistance to old social models were built into American identity from its earliest days. Regardless of skin color or ancestral origins, Americans have embraced the possibility—indeed the necessity—of change in many aspects of their culture. Often they have equated change with renewal and have woven it, together with sustaining values such as a strong work ethic and the centrality of spirituality, into the fabric of a new society. In American places of all kinds, from the early seaboard settlements to newly minted cities, through the waves of westward migration, that notion of cultural renewal can be traced both in the written saga of the nation and in all its artistic developments. In painting, music, literature, and dance, Americans have pictured themselves, their places, their changing aspirations and entertainments. From early portraits to the advent of American landscape painting, culture and nature have contended and simultaneously reinforced each other, documenting new ways of relating to the natural world and to each other. If America's landscape, as has often been observed, embodied the early promise of what the country might become, the cultural activities of its people imprinted the landscape with human traces. Matthew Arnold argued in his 1869 *Culture and Anarchy* that Britons and Americans needed to find a new cultural birthright in the arts. "Do not tell me only of the magnitude of your industry and commerce," he admonished Americans, "tell me also if your civilization—which is the grand name you give to all this development—tell me if your civilization is *interesting*."[1]

In America's arts and entertainments, I will argue, we find captured some of its most *interesting* aspects of identity: its aspirations and dreams, its sense of uniqueness and destiny, its discoveries of cultural realities both compelling and unforeseen. This chapter traces ways in which dance, in a sustained if discontinuous dialogue with the visual arts, first extended, then challenged, America's status as cultural appendage to Europe. Throughout the ensuing discussion, one thing is abundantly clear: the development of an American cultural consciousness occurred in fits and starts, eluding the historian's desire for seamless and readable continuity. Instead, that cultural movement lurches from one significant moment to another, dictating an episodic approach to the structure of this book. More, if America's cultural history is episodic in its chronology, it is also disjointed geographically: it was written and painted and sculpted—but also danced—in every corner of the country. Tracing dance through visual images helps to illuminate both the broad paths and the niches and byways of the nation's cultural history.

One of the early points of confluence for dance and the visual arts begins on the East Coast, where Southerners, New Englanders, and groups such as the Shakers incorporated dance into their secular and religious lives. In urban centers, as populations grew, Americans strove to reconcile their desire for a new, classless society with the realities of social stratifications imposed by wealth, race, and occupation. Dance, at times a leveling influence, at other times a mark of social status, was learned and performed in many contexts, and visual artists were there to record and comment on many of them. America's immigrants, from the New Amsterdam Dutch to the street performers of later ghetto neighborhoods, flavored evolving American identities (for they are multiple), dancing into the paintings, sculptures, and photographs of many visual artists.

As the ensuing pages relate, American art's love affair with dance has taken a meandering course, reaching repeatedly across boundaries between "high" and "low" art, between theatrical and social dance, between elite and popular audiences. And it has flourished in all kinds of communities. Outside the cities, nineteenth-century Americans adapted imported dances and invented new ones to suit their rural circumstances. Where musicians were in short supply, a single fiddler might suffice, and visual artists exercised their own creativity to record simple scenes of solo or couple dances.

The saga of America's westward exploration has been told in countless ways, never more inventively than by visual artists who tracked dancers to the barns of rural farmers, to the riverboats of the Missouri, and eventually to the burgeoning communities of the California gold rush era. In their subjects are exposed the founding and sustaining myths of the American frontier, brought vividly to life through the energy of dance.

From there the dancers and the artists leap forward in time, sometimes by decades, as we follow Arnold's advice to seek the *interesting* in America's cultural heritage. American places, including the legacy of the frontier, engaged dancers and visual artists into the twentieth century. In that later period the account will focus for the first time on a dancer-choreographer, Martha Graham, whose deep connections to American

places spanned several decades and inspired innovative visual responses. In her dances, and in the many responses to them by visual artists, we see that American national identity has been related in part to arrangements and control over space, demonstrated both in broad geographic terms and in manipulating smaller spaces in performance. Moreover, in dances ranging from *Primitive Mysteries* to *Frontier*, Graham took on some of the thorniest issues of American identity: the social role of ritual and religion, and the struggle between individual and community. Those issues provided Graham with an important point of entry into the feel of American reality. In the decade of the 1930s, that era when American themes obsessed many artists, writers, and dancers, she would devote three-quarters of her attention to probing further into those subjects. "The dance reveals the spirit of the country in which it takes root," said Graham. "No sooner does it fail to do this than the dance begins to lose its indispensable integrity and significance."[2]

Finally, in our efforts to explore America's multiple identities as expressed in dance and the visual arts, we will turn to African American dance. Its rich history, from Africa to colonial America, from minstrelsy to the Harlem Renaissance, attracted visual artists both within and outside the African American community. Paintings, sculpture, prints, and photographs interpret the vitality of African American dance culture, while opening up new questions of black identity, ritual legacies from black Africa, and the creation of cultural stereotypes through visual imagery and dance. Among the artists discussed are Aaron Douglas, Meta Vaux Warrick Fuller, William H. Johnson, Richmond Barthé, and James VanDerZee. The many visual representations of Josephine Baker, by both black and white artists, expose the complex cultural politics surrounding the body of the black dancer. By placing African American dance in the foreground of experience, not as secondary to white efforts, it becomes clear that in the broader process of dance making, the African American presence is primary, from all kinds of modern social dance to Balanchine ballets. Black vernacular dance, in fact, dominated Broadway during much of the 1920s and 1930s, when musicals and revues featuring the Charleston, Lindy, and Black Bottom drew huge audiences. As critic Carl Van Vechten correctly pointed out in 1930, "Nearly all the dancing now to be seen in our musical shows is of Negro origin, but both critics and public are so ignorant of this fact that the production of a new Negro revue is an excuse for the revival of the hoary old lament that it is a pity the Negro can't create anything for himself. . . . This, in brief, has been the history of the CakeWalk, the Bunny Hug, the Turkey Trot, the Charleston and the Black Bottom."[3] Even though the popularity of such shows declined with the Depression, later choreographers have kept alive the influence of black show dance. And sensitive visual artists of all races have helped to recognize that primacy, while simultaneously acknowledging the socially constructed categories of race and gender that can be read through dancing bodies. What follows, then, is a wide-ranging array of significant moments within a long American dialogue in which art and dance engaged, generating conversations as expansive and as varied as American culture itself.

# 1

# Expressing the Real or Imagined Heritage of a Nation

## Prelude to the Dance: American Beginnings

From the earliest arrivals of Europeans on the shores of what would become the United States, a scattering of visual artists stepped off ships to gaze for the first time on new landscapes and their indigenous inhabitants. Artists' images of Native American ceremonials were among the first records of what they saw. Often referred to as dances, they were more properly ritual enactments of ancient connections to nature and the spiritual realm. Such ritual dramas were fascinating in their diversity and their broad communal participation, and as pure visual spectacle. Despite the frequent prohibition against on-site recordings, artists often could not resist drawing or painting what they saw, working out of mere curiosity on one hand or, more subtly, as a means of experiencing more fully the unfamiliar pairings of rhythmic sacred movement and its profound connections to newly encountered places.

Our intent here is not to survey that vast range of imagery, but rather to look selectively at just a few early and visually compelling responses to Native American ritual dance subjects. English artist-cartographer John White (fl. 1585–93), arriving in the coastal territory of Virginia in 1585, made detailed watercolor drawings of the inhabitants and natural environment, with an intent to attract future settlers to the area. White's elevated view of a circle of ceremonial dancers, *The Dances at Their Great Feasts* (c. 1590; fig. 1), was made into an engraving by Theodor de Bry (1528–98). White himself captioned the scene as "a ceremony in their prayers with strange gestures and songs dancing about posts carved on the tops like men's faces." Male and female dancers form a circle defined by the posts, in the center of which three Native women stand together. Clearly the indigenous carvers, artists themselves, created important links between their sculpted images and their ritual dance. White and his expedition colleagues, including Walter Raleigh and Thomas Hariot, were not sure what to make of the dancing they saw, but they readily associated it with nature worship. And they were right, to an extent. The proximity of ritual object and dance evokes associations facilitated by a shaman. Shamans are people with special powers, perhaps artists and dancers, who mediate between the human and the spirit world. Typically they enter trance states during which they fly, receiving communications from spirit guides in the form of animals or birds.

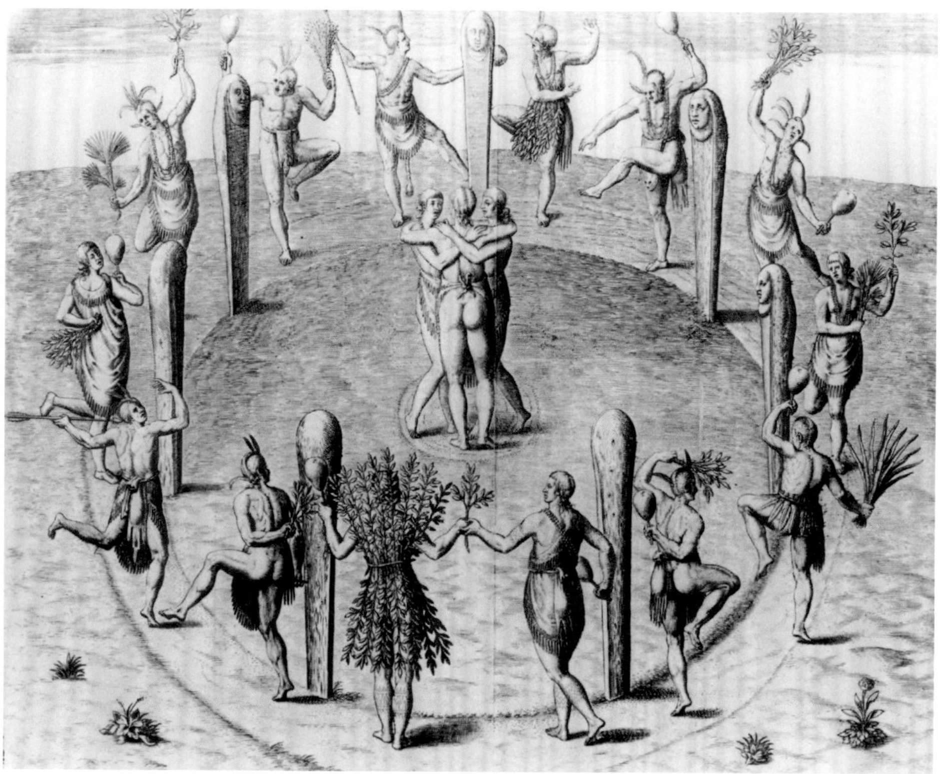

**Figure 1** Theodor de Bry, *The Dances at Their Great Feasts*, 1590, engraving after water-color by John White. (photo courtesy Library of Congress, LC-USZX62-40055)

Another indigenous figure John White painted during his years in Virginia seems to be demonstrating just that form of ancient and widespread power. In fact, White captioned his shamanic dancing figure *The Flyer* (c. 1587–88; fig. 2). In this reproduction of a watercolor in the British Museum, White's *Flyer*, with his upraised arms and active stride, enacts more of the "strange gestures" the artist had noted in the ritual circle. Of special note in the watercolor is that White's *Flyer* wears a small bird attached to the side of his head, likely a spirit guide and emblem of his shamanic power. The key word here is *power*, a palpable presence inhabiting the *Flyer* and invoking a certain awe, even fear, in sixteenth-century white observers. As White's companion Hariot noted, "They have sorcerers or jugglers who use strange gestures and whose enchantments often go against the laws of nature. For they are very familiar with devils."[1] White's careful visual record, part of a body of work with promotional as well as reportorial motives, may have helped to unleash another kind of promotional zeal: the Christian missionary impulse, which would propel many a future expedition among Native Americans. Whatever else they signify, the *Flyer*'s movements are unmistakably a kind of ritual *dance* in its broadest sense, that is, a form of powerful, rhythmic movement. In its performance and in White's urgent visual translation, we see further evidence of the combined power of dance and visual art to extend the boundaries of human thought, feeling, and perception.

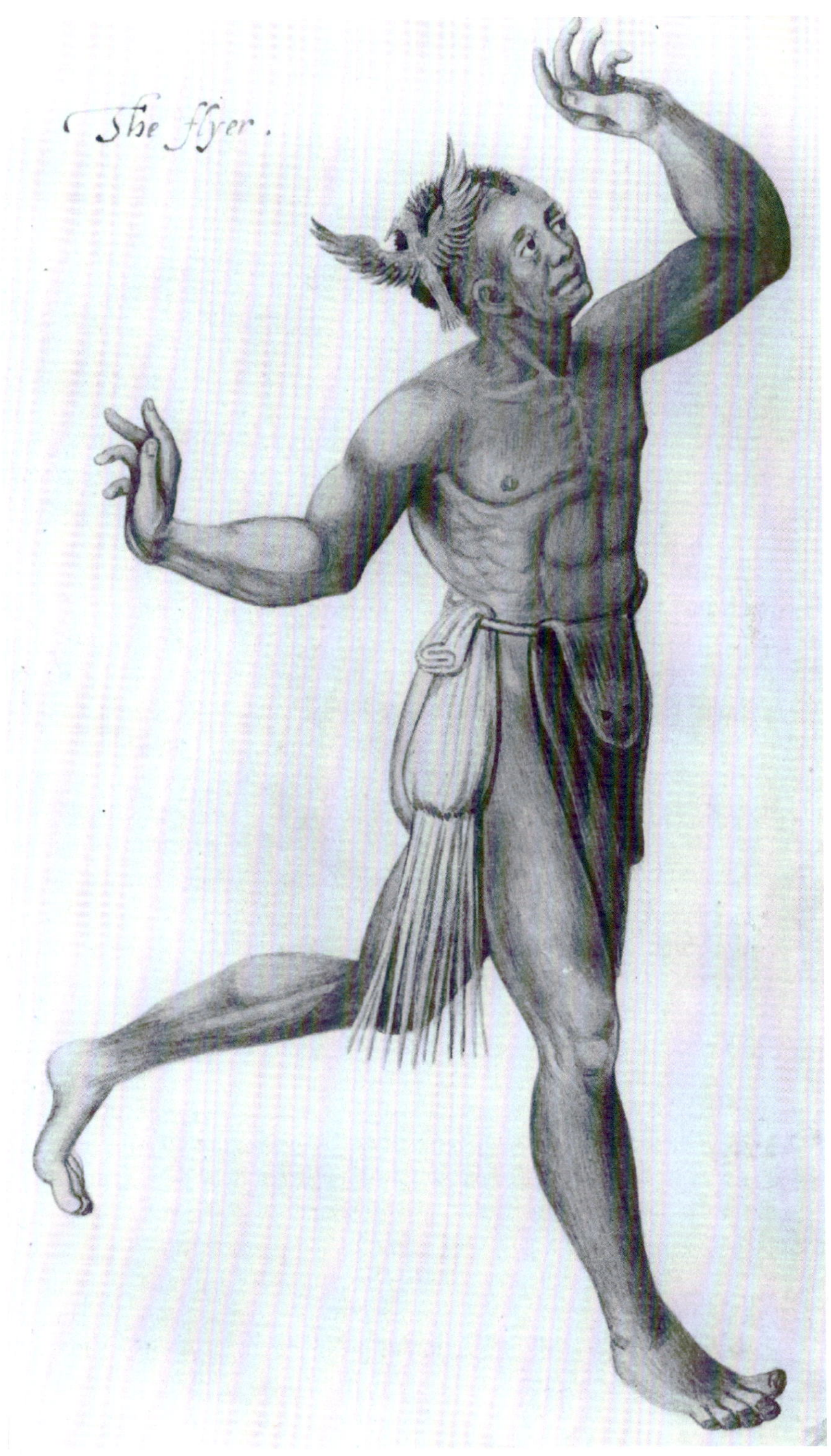

**Figure 2** Reproduction of *The Flyer* [*The Sorcerer*] by John White, c. 1587–88, watercolor, 9¼ × 6 inches. (original in the British Museum, photo courtesy Library of Congress, LC-USZ62-584)

White's images are likely not the first representations of Native American dance by Europeans, but when circulated widely in the form of engravings, they established long-lasting European views of indigenous ceremonies.[2] And, especially in their exquisitely detailed anthropological accuracy, they anticipate elements for which later visual artists would strive.

## European Dance Arrives on American Shores

By 1735, when an Englishman named Henry Holt staged the first ballet ever presented in Charleston, South Carolina, the form already had a considerable history in European courts.[3] Paving the way nearly a century earlier at Versailles, some celebrated French amateurs had donned disguises and taken on dancing roles in court productions. One of them, Louis XIV, was cleverly cast as the Sun King in *La Nuit (Ballet of the Night)* by the court composer Jean-Baptiste Lully.[4] It was as serendipitous a choice as the ambitious Lully ever made: perhaps recognizing his own limitations as a dancer, the stage-struck monarch in time renounced his own terpsichorean aspirations and endowed a Royal Academy of Music and Dancing, which undertook to train France's first corps of professional dancers. They, their successors, and their counterparts in other European capitals would spread the gospel of theatrical dance to audiences everywhere. And where they went, their visual representations followed. Artists, who had long attempted to preserve the fleeting memory of live performance, now found growing audiences for their dance images. Whether in Paris or Charleston, dancers exerted broad appeal, at least among the elites. Holt's 1735 Charleston performance was merely the first of that city's many subsequent pantomimes and staged spectacles throughout the century. Following the French Revolution, many dispossessed aristocrats crossed the Atlantic. Lacking practical skills, but well trained in the social niceties, they soon discovered they could earn a livelihood in America's larger cities as dancing masters. One later historian of the dance credited this post-revolutionary "French invasion" with bringing to Americans pianos, French pastries, and an army of French dancing teachers.[5]

Southerners, especially those of aristocratic descent, engaged in frequent dancing, while their northern counterparts, progeny of religious dissenters, were less inclined to tolerate dancing. Colonial America inherited varying attitudes about dance, despite its inclusion for centuries—in England as well as France—as one of society's necessary cultural refinements. Ease in dancing had been a marker of social class as far back as medieval times, when Chaucer's squire could "juste and eke dance and well pourtraie and write."

If the English colonials in early America had mixed views of dance, those diverse views reflected their class, religious affiliation, and geographical placement. Among early political leaders, for example, civic virtue was linked to a work ethic that accommodated little diversion. Frivolity in general and dancing in particular were widely suspect. Benjamin Franklin, through his fictional character Silence Dogood, disparaged the education conveyed at Harvard College (a school he had been unable to afford) by linking it to the folly of dancing: "[Harvard students] learn little more than how to carry themselves handsomely, and enter a room genteely (which might as well be acquired at a dancing school)." Apparently there was a grain of truth in Franklin's aspersions, for John Quincy Adams, while a student at Harvard a few decades later, indulged in bouts of late-night dancing, after which he once conceded: "When the feet are so much engaged, the head in general is vacant." In purely pragmatic terms, many Americans mistrusted dancing as an enticement away from more productive pursuits.

If Franklin and Adams both regarded dance as a youthful distraction, there were more serious objections in other quarters: dance's imagined association with lascivious behavior raised many an American eyebrow, as dance historians have long recounted. The country's early religious leaders expressed profound unease with the seductive power of dance, imagined agent and exemplar of all manner of sensual temptations. In early Pennsylvania, for example, the Quakers rigorously opposed dancing as a potentially corrupting agent of children. Attitudes varied from one colony to another: in Connecticut dancing was commonly accepted, while definitely frowned upon in nearby Massachusetts. Yet even there its condemnation was not universal among Puritan divines. Reverend John Cotton, a leading Boston minister, said,

> Dancing (yea though mixt) I would not simply condem. For I see two sorts of mixt dancings in use with God's people in the Old Testament, the one religious . . . the other civil, tending to the praise of conquerors. . . . Only lascivious dancing, and amorous gestures and wanton dalliances, especially after feasts, I would bear witness against, as a great *flabella libidinis*.[6]

Other clergy were less forgiving of anything resembling "wanton dalliances." In seventeenth-century New England, court records often mention severe punishments for mixed dancing or dancing in taverns. Such objections were no doubt related to deeper Puritan ambivalence about sexuality, dress, and display of the body, and the lingering notion that dance belongs to a dissolute way of life. That Puritan heritage, augmented by the Victorian denial of the body's sensuality, poisoned many modern Americans against their Puritan forbears, whose excesses, they charged, stunted American dance for generations. Visual artists, dancers, and writers led the twentieth-century assault on old puritanical attitudes, a struggle explored in chapter 9.

In the era of the American Revolution a new kind of dancing appeared in small communities known as Shakers, who sang, shouted, stepped, and whirled as part of their ritualistic worship. Organized under the mystic "Mother" Ann Lee, they developed into eleven communities by 1792, each centered around a meetinghouse where emotion-laden "exercises," were performed by those granted divine "gifts." But they were also presented publicly for prospective converts in that era of salvation seeking. The curious, including visual artists, flocked to the Shaker settlements at Niskeyuna, New Lebanon, New York, and beyond. Shaker dancers and singers appeared onstage at the American Museum in New York for seven weeks in the 1840s. Varieties of Shaker dancing evolved

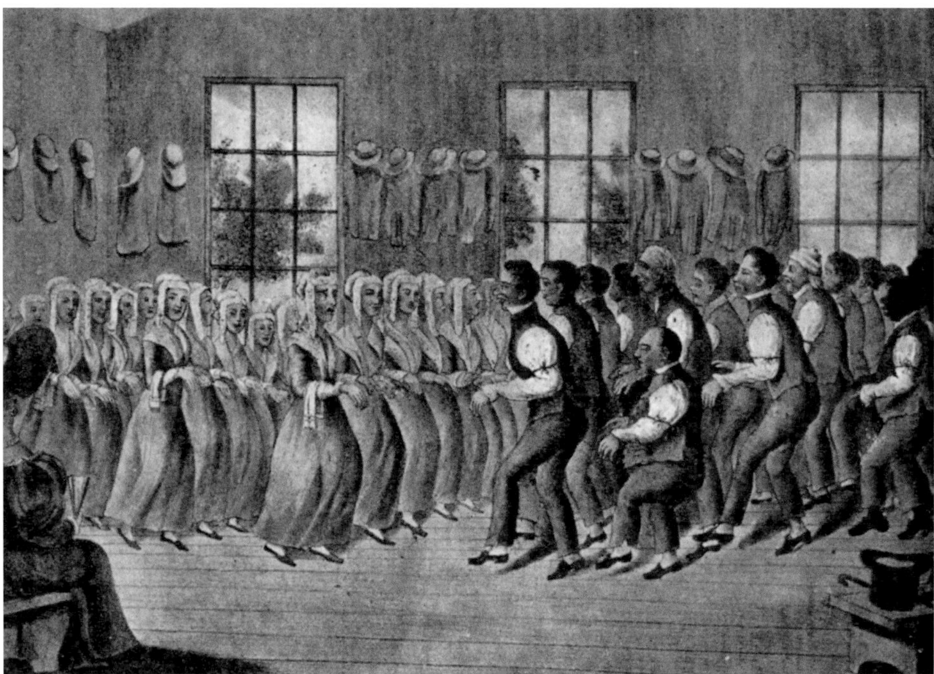

**Figure 3** Currier & Ives, *Shakers near Lebanon: A Square-Order Dance*, after 1825, hand-colored lithograph.

as leadership changed: the sedate "square-order shuffle" was patterned according to a vision of angels dancing around God's throne. Drawn by an observer, the scene was turned into a hand-colored lithograph as early as 1825, then distributed widely by Currier & Ives, who freely pirated such prints (fig. 3). A more joyous, ecstatic level of dance swept Shaker practice in later decades, accelerating the square-order tempo into a "skipping manner." In rooms lit by flickering candles or oil lamps, floor markings guided increasingly precise maneuvers that replaced the advancing and receding lines of male and female dancers in earlier configurations. Marches and ring dances appeared, relaxing stiff earlier gestures into more graceful waving or clapping, and adding complexity to earlier floor patterns (1855; fig. 4).

For nineteenth-century Americans, it was the efforts of visual artists that revealed (and preserved) the order, plainness, recreation, and spiritual release that dancing afforded the Shaker communities. Visually, the pure shapes of evolving Shaker ritual—embodiments of rational, orderly forms—have been likened to the simple lines and graceful proportions of Shaker design in furniture and architecture. "The wheeling of ranks," writes one dance historian, "had the same polished but simplified perfection as the turning on the posts of a table or chair."[7] Appreciation for Shaker design would emerge later in American history, eventually bringing their artistic production to a broad and appreciative audience.[8] That legacy, perpetuated in objects, parallels the long lineage of early dance representations swept into the evolving braid of American cultural identity. Shakers, as millennialist communities in post-revolutionary America, steadfastly rooted

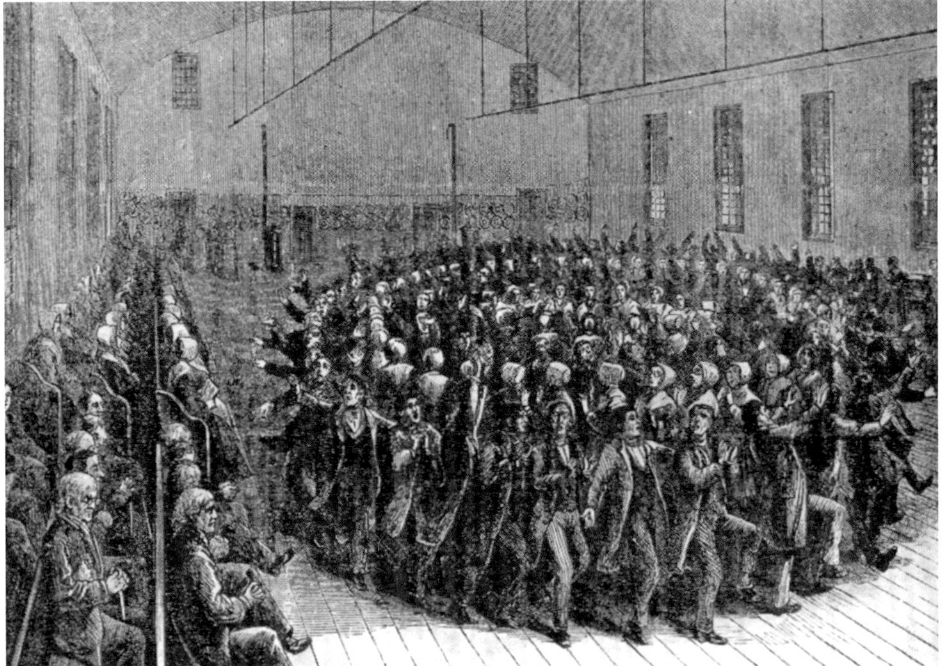

**Figure 4** Attributed to Joseph Becker, *Shaker Religious Exercises in Niskeyuna, Wheel within a Wheel Dance*, from *Leslie's Popular Monthly*, 1885.

themselves in the soil of rural America, yet their ecstatic dance signaled a twin attachment to the spiritual. Both loyalties—to soil and to spirit—have formed important, and sometimes seemingly contradictory, aspects of Americans' cherished cultural identity. Harmless enough to encourage a self-congratulatory tolerance among most Americans, the Shakers, equally fascinating in situ or on the concert stage, intrigued all manner of observers, including Charlotte Cushman, the early American stage star, who puzzled over the Shakers in an ode: "Mysterious worshippers! Are you indeed the things you seem to be, / Of earth—yet of its iron influence free . . . ?"[9]

## Stepping Ashore: Artists Glimpse the Urban Immigrant Experience through Dance

The Shakers were a small, distinctive group of American immigrants whose dancing, a part of their participatory rituals of worship, never passed into general use. To visual artists, Shaker dance was something of a curiosity, a kind of metaphysics made visible, which they were eager to record. On the other hand, there were immigrant groups whose secular dance traditions spread, developed, and survived as rich documents in the cultural history of the United States. If early visual images of dance remained scarce, that paucity reflects both the small number of trained artists and the arduous lives of early immigrants, whose days and nights were seldom given over to leisure pursuits.

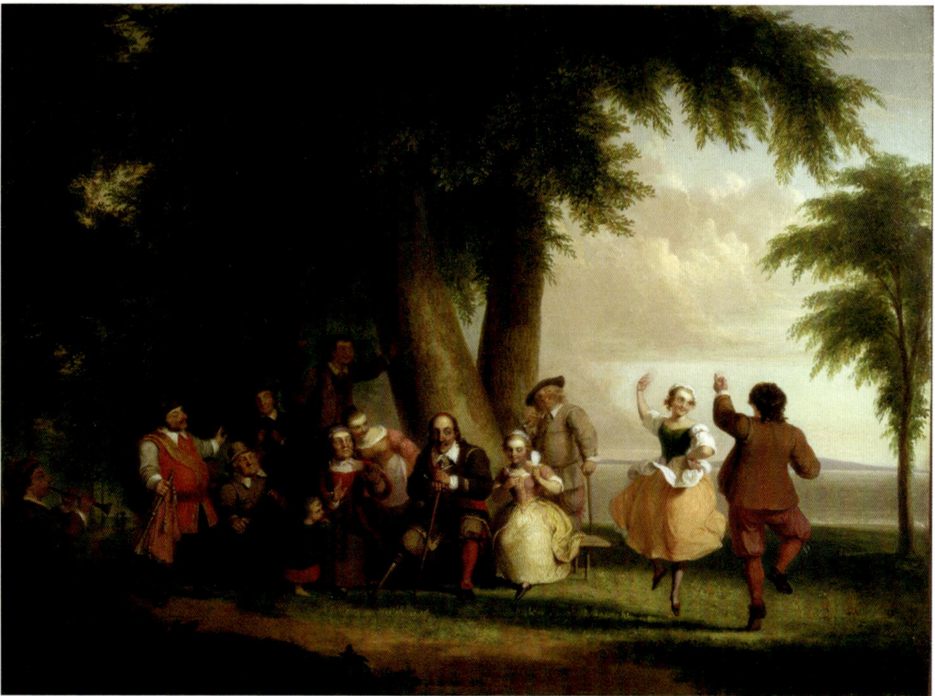

**Figure 5** Asher B. Durand, *Dance on the Battery in the Presence of Peter Stuyvesant*, 1838 (depicting c. 1650), oil on canvas, 32 × 46 inches. (Museum of the City of New York, Gift of Jane Rutherford Faile through Kenneth C. Faile, 55.248)

When put down on canvas—often long after the fact—artists such as Asher B. Durand (1796–1886) had to work largely from written descriptions augmented by their inventive imaginations. He and his colleagues, then, are among the first to draw on American history, real or imagined, as a "usable past" with which to underpin a developing cultural nationalism.[10] Still, despite (or perhaps because of) their reconstruction from literary sources, the best of these visual images of early dance in America possess a spontaneous feel, as if high spirits and the desire to celebrate swept people into lively stepping. Qualities cherished subsequently as "American" are often embedded in these early dance images: a certain freshness, inventiveness, and rhythmic vigor, and an eclectic viewpoint.

Durand, best remembered as an engraver and a leading light of the Hudson River School of landscape painting, was also skilled in painting genre scenes based on real and invented historical moments. His *Dance on the Battery in the Presence of Peter Stuyvesant* (1838; fig. 5), depicts a scene from about 1650 taken from the droll *Knickerbocker's History of New York*, Washington Irving's 1809 imaginary history of New Amsterdam. In the painting, Durand places the crusty, peg-legged Stuyvesant under a vast tree around which a circle of burghers erupts into dance. Along with his dancers, Durand also gives seventeenth-century American history a positive spin, for the controversial Dutch director-general was almost constantly at odds with his constituents, who ultimately refused to support him against a British takeover that transformed New Amsterdam into New

York. Here, however, jollity and good feelings prevail in this "season for the lifting of the heel as well as the heart," as described by Diedrich Knickerbocker, Irving's fictional narrator. Knickerbocker describes a gathering at Manhattan's southern tip, where a fetching young woman, newly returned from the Netherlands, performs a lively jig, attired in "not more than half a dozen petticoats, and these of alarming shortness." Reportedly, as the dour Stuyvesant looked on, an errant breeze lifted those skirts into a shocking "display of her graces." With tongues firmly in cheek, Irving and Durand poke a bit of fun at the hyper-respectability of the proper Dutch Calvinists, while at the same time appreciating the nostalgic charm of a Dutch country scene translated into a new American idiom.[11]

Durand's contemporary John Quidor (1801–81) used dance to convey a different view of the Dutch in New Amsterdam, training a withering parodic gaze on Stuyvesant and escalating the high spirits of Durand's battery dance into burlesque social comedy. Quidor's *Antony van Corlear Brought into the Presence of Peter Stuyvesant* (1839; fig. 6) exposes the incipient American rift between social privilege (represented by the irascible Stuyvesant) and an emerging Jacksonian-era individualism in the person of Antony van Corlear, one of Irving's more flamboyant characters from the *Knickerbocker History*.[12] Stuyvesant, seeking to consolidate his power in New Amsterdam, has clamped down on his constituents' "unreasonable habit of thinking and speaking for themselves," and has summoned before him a perceived troublemaker, the city's "matchless champion," Antony the Trumpeter. Calling Antony to account for himself, Stuyvesant demands, "How didst thou acquire this paramount honor and dignity?" Antony's reply, dripping with parodic metaphor, is that "like many a great man before me, simply by sounding my own trumpet," whereupon he "put his instrument to his lips, and sounded a charge with such a tremendous outset, such a delectable quaver, and such a triumphant cadence, that it was enough to make one's heart leap out of one's mouth only to be within a mile of it."[13] Among those electrified by Antony's trumpet are Stuyvesant himself, a howling dog, and two men—an old gent behind Stuyvesant and an African American at the far left—who erupt into dance. The flavor of the response is unmistakably (and farcically) sexual, from Stuyvesant's phallic accoutrements of saber, erect peg leg, and cane, to the nervous, undisciplined energies of the two men, white and black, who enact a dance of chaotic and libidinous release triggered by the trumpet. Stuyvesant, it appears, is undone, his desire to protect his power from the masses undercut by the energies (here caricatured by Quidor) of early American individualism. Quidor's African American dancer, not a part of Irving's original account, functions as a trope of potent new forces, political and social, stirring in America. He is also the prototype of a subject to which we will return, the African American dancer of minstrelsy, whose talents would stir a later generation of visual artists.[14]

Dancing in New York, long after Stuyvesant's era and well after Durand's own time, mirrored important social, historical, and economic change. Even as the worship of commercialism spread across the continent, American civic leaders, concerned about their children's readiness to take their place in a civilized society, initiated the cultural awakening called for by Matthew Arnold. To offset the

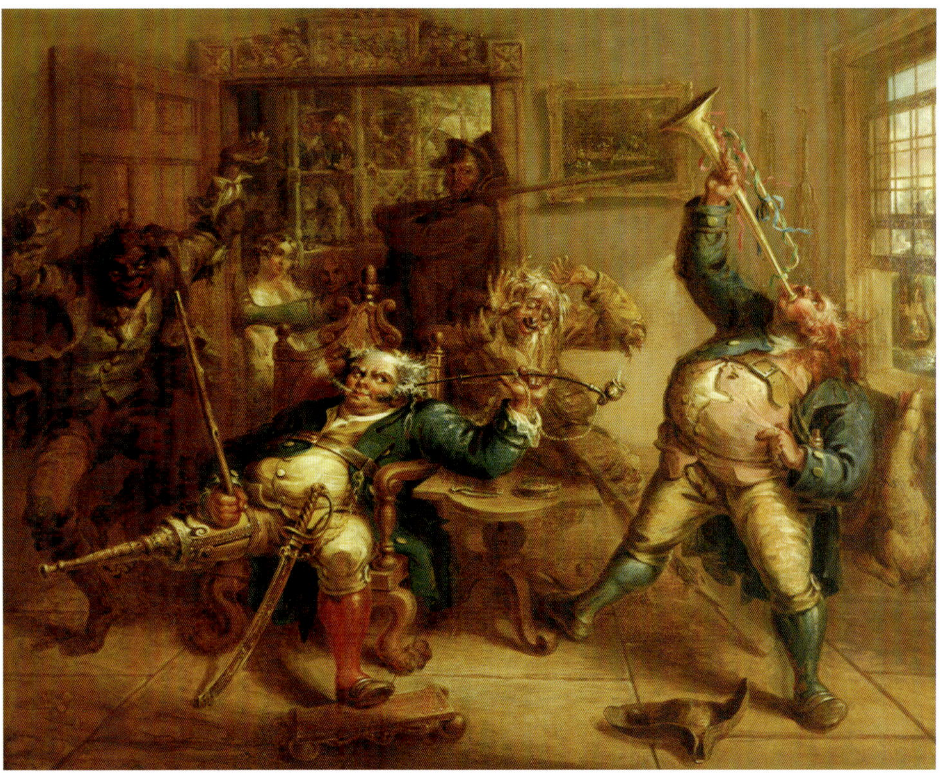

**Figure 6** John Quidor, *Antony van Corlear Brought into the Presence of Peter Stuyvesant*, 1839, oil on canvas, 27⅜ × 34¹⁄₁₆ inches. (Munson-Williams-Proctor Arts Institute, Museum of Art, Utica, New York, 63.110)

moneyed impulse of hard-driving business, they looked to the arts as a necessary medium of education and cultivated behavior. And dance, as an aspect of culture, good manners, and gentle living, was seen as an important aspect of that social evolution.

Almost from the beginning of the nineteenth century, books on proper social dancing had appeared, and magazines such as *Godey's Lady's Book* printed regular articles on dancing, etiquette, and music as requisites of cultivated behavior. In American cities society balls began to be staged, and dancing entered the drawing rooms of the well to do. New dances appeared regularly, including contradances and quadrilles, the gallopade and the notoriously wicked waltz, regarded by many as "the devil's greatest invention." About 1840 the polka bounced onto American shores, a rollicking hop-skip-slide unburdened by social restraints. A polka mania ensued, sweeping Americans of all social levels into a generalized free-for-all of popular dance. Dance halls sprang up in New York and elsewhere, places where impoverished young women were hired to teach the polka and its variants. As one critic sniffed, "The young women willing to be employed were naturally those to whom the small amount paid was of importance; they, therefore, exercised little, if any, improving influence upon those who practiced with them . . . Small rooms were generally used, so that the crowding and squeezing . . . [were] not conducive to delicacy, to say the least."[15]

Into that landscape of eroded propriety, like an acolyte of the tasteful Terpsichore, stepped Allen Dodworth (1817–96), a dancing teacher destined to become America's arbiter of decorous social dancing for over half a century. Dodworth would attempt to restore fashionable dancing to its rightful place among the arts, taking its place alongside music and painting in the galaxy of American cultural refinements. He began not far from Stuyvesant's old neighborhood in lower Manhattan, setting up the first Dodworth Academy on Broome Street about 1842. There, in groups of up to 150, carefully selected young people were taught not merely the steps of social dance, but a social philosophy that related dance to the other arts and to the gentle life. Indicative of Dodworth's success in raising the status of social dance, his academy moved uptown with the migration of fashionable New Yorkers. Perhaps its apex of cultural status was reached in the grandly proportioned rooms of an elegant Fifth Avenue mansion later occupied by the Metropolitan Museum as its first, temporary home in 1871 (fig. 7). As the museum's official history recorded it, "A sky light let into the ceiling of the large hall where the poetry of motion had been taught to so many of the young men and maidens of New York converted it into a picture gallery."[16] Crossing paths, symbolically, in those rooms, American social dance—long the stepchild of American cultural practice—swept into the rarefied sphere inhabited by visual art. For ambitious social dancers like Allen Dodworth, it was a triumphant, if tentative, pas de deux.

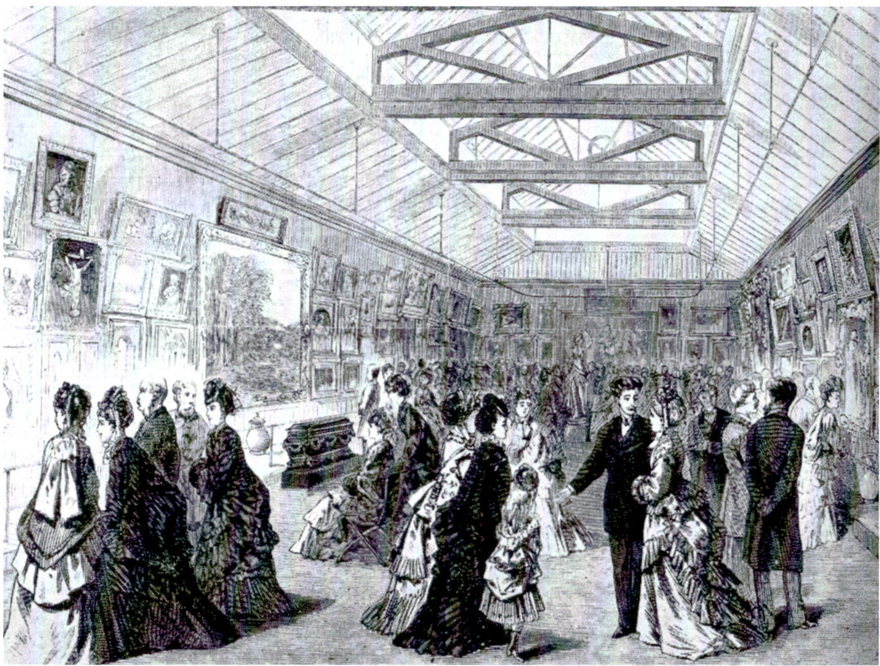

**Figure 7** Anonymous, *First Opening of New York's Metropolitan Museum of Art in the Former Dodworth Dancing Academy on Fifth Avenue*, wood engraving, 1871.

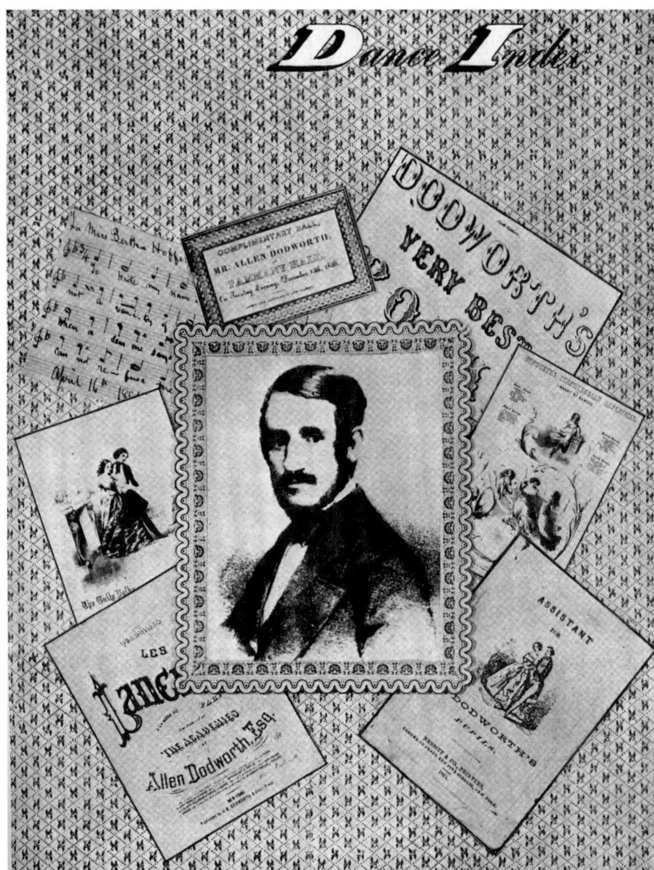

Figure 8 Joseph Cornell, photomontage of Allen Dodworth, 1940s.

Besides his farsighted approach to dance as a social force, Allen Dodworth also helped to found the New York Philharmonic Society, in which he played as a violinist. Son of a musical family of immigrants, Dodworth had been brought from his native Sheffield, England, to America in 1825 at the age of eight. Using their musical skills, the Dodworths began to contribute significantly to New York's fledgling cultural life, and were the unmistakable leaders in promoting dance in American life of their day. Much later, American artist Joseph Cornell (1903–72), aficionado of all forms of dance, created a photomontage of Allen Dodworth framed by the stylish lace and Victorian wallpaper of his era. Around the dancing master's head Cornell tucked programs, sheet music, tickets, and title pages of Dodworth's writings, which together constitute a veritable "how-to" guide for the upwardly mobile in nineteenth-century American society (1940s; fig. 8).

The acceptance and success enjoyed by the English-speaking Dodworths was hardly typical for American immigrants, however. Most endured not only grinding poverty, but suffered a wrenching rupture from the language, customs, and entertainments they left behind. Yet dance links the Dodworths with a survival strategy common to most immigrants, as seen in a series by photographer Lewis Hine (1874–1940), who captured some of the tens of thousands who arrived

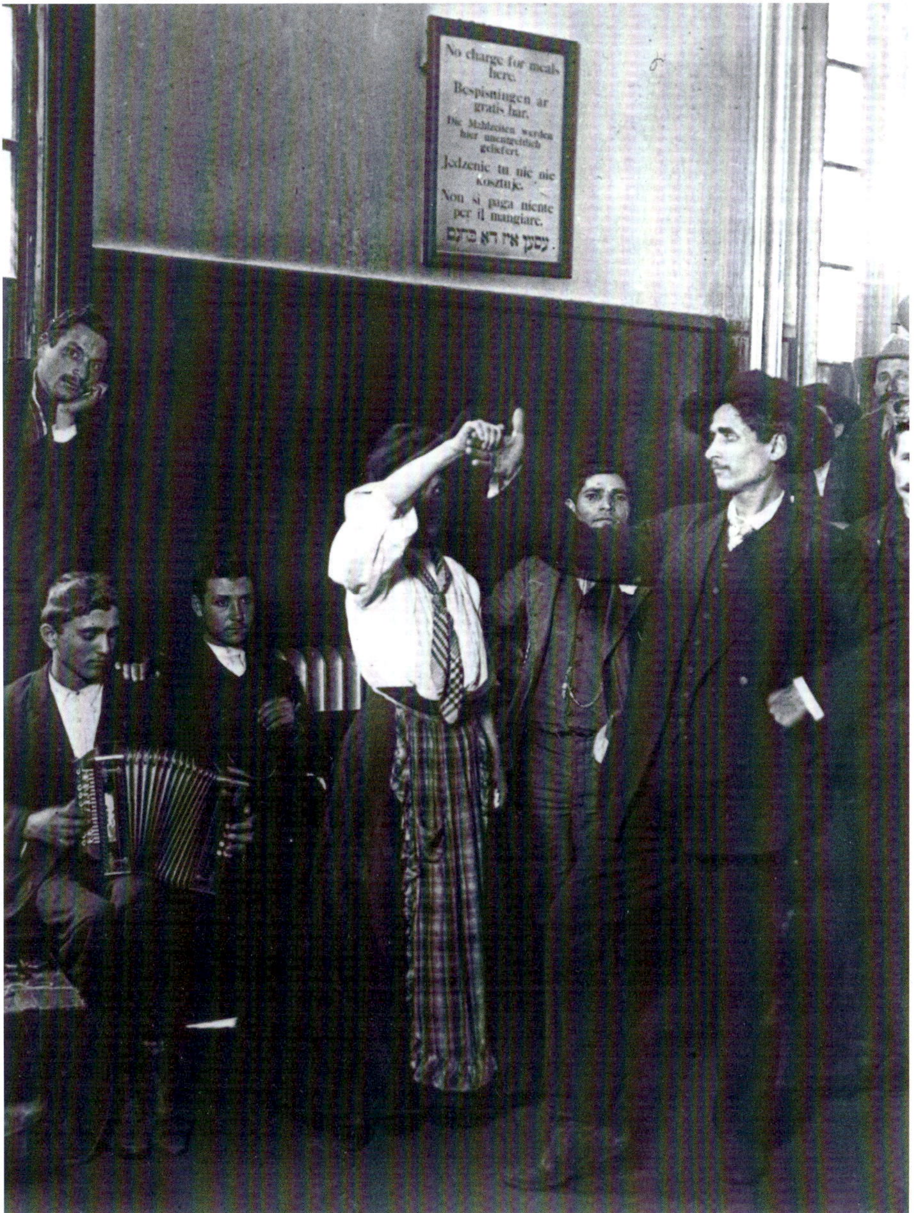


**Figure 9** Lewis Hine, *Music and a Little Dance while Waiting at Ellis Island*, n.d. (photo courtesy George Eastman House)

in the years before the First World War. A sociologist by training, Hine was ever alert to the negative social ills of his era, but he looked as well at positive human qualities wherever he found them. He took his 5-by-7-inch camera to Ellis Island, where one day his lens framed a group of immigrants who generate their own music and dance while awaiting processing after their long voyage (fig. 9). Hope, relief, anxiety, and a bit of familiar entertainment—Hine shows us that these ingredients too were part of the American immigrant experience.

Working in the same years as Lewis Hine, painter George Luks (1866–1933) also explored the ways American popular culture absorbed, through dance, the flavors of its varied ethnic groups. Luks favored themes drawn from vaudeville or from American ghetto life, especially the lively street scenes of New York's bustling neighborhoods. A good example of Luks's warm appreciation for immigrant life is his painting *The Spielers* (1905; fig. 10). In this work, originally titled *East Side Children Dancing to Hand Organ Music,* the Ashcan painter captured the exuberance of two young girls dancing together on the sidewalks of New York. Luks's subject has been interpreted in several ways. Robert Snyder and Rebecca Zurier point out that spielers were sometimes "tough girl" types who danced alone or with a partner, hoping for a tossed coin, or perhaps for a first break into vaudeville.[17] Most often German- or Irish American, the girls blended street-savvy with a certain fresh-faced innocence. Art historian David Bjelajac, with slightly different emphasis, explains that spieling (also called "pivoting") began as a working-class, German-style social dance: "In contrast to the upper-class waltz, which involved elegant, graceful movements, spieling brought couples into close physical contact as they swirled wildly across the dance floor."[18] That closeness and the fact that the girls' or women's skirts

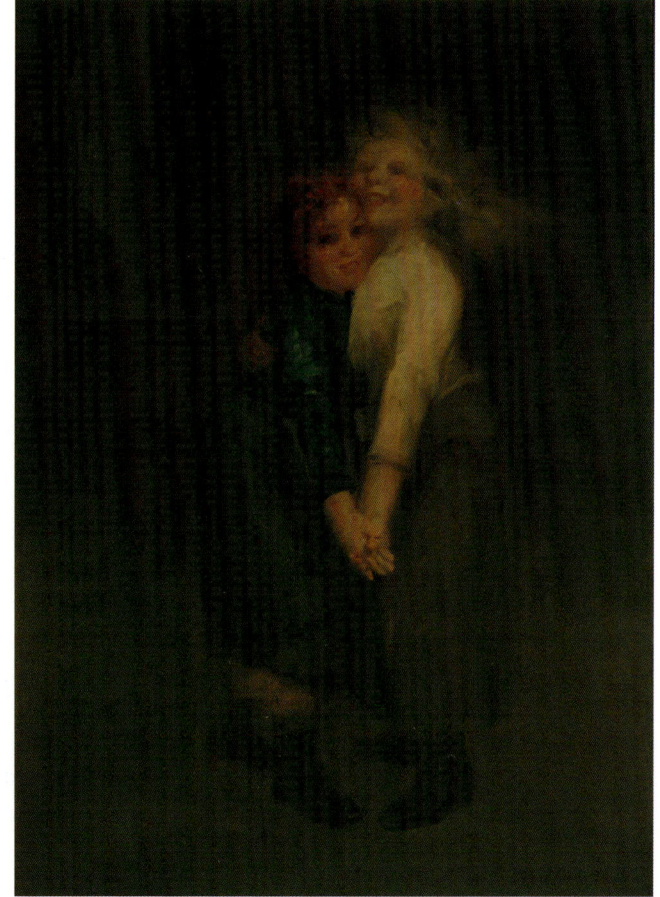

**Figure 10** George B. Luks, *The Spielers,* 1905, oil on canvas, 36 1/16 × 26 1/4 inches. (Addison Gallery of American Art, Phillips Academy, Andover, Massachusetts, Gift of anonymous donor, 1931.9)

were "blown immodestly high" while spieling undoubtedly contributed to its censure by social moralists of the day, who found it a lascivious dance.[19] In Luks's painting, however, adult spieling turns into a kind of innocent play—perspiration supplanting passion—when danced by his sturdy child-spielers. All here is charged by pure adrenalin and high spirits, not by sexuality. Whichever interpretation one favors, it is clear that Luks and his Ashcan colleagues pursued, in dance subjects, some of the exotic flavor of immigrant life, a bottom-up view of New York's turn-of-the-century energy and diversity. Unlike many other narratives of immigrant life, their paintings reveal as much about what the newcomers held onto as what they gave up in their process of assimilation into the American mainstream.

Just two years later Abastenia St. Leger Eberle (1878–1942), a sculptor who moved from Ohio to New York in 1899, created an equally lively three-dimensional counterpart to Luks's *Spielers*. Like him, she also worked in the circle of the Ashcan school, translating into sculpture its broad, reportorial, almost caricatured style. From every angle, Eberle's *Girls Dancing* (1907; fig. 11) bounces with playful energy, skirts and hair lifted in laughing pleasure. A close observer of Lower East Side social life described the kind of scene Eberle saw:

> The sound of the hurdy-gurdy on a warm spring evening is the signal for all the children in the neighborhood to assemble and to turn the side-walk into an impromptu dance-hall. Children from eight to fourteen, with a natural feeling for rhythm, keep perfect step to the changing time of the music, from polka to waltz or schottische, as the grinder goes through his repertoire.[20]

Eberle's interest in portraying ghetto children arose in part from her observations of street life in Puerto Rico as a child and in Naples as a young adult. Trained at the populist Art Students League, Eberle came under the influence of Robert Henri's progressive views—especially the belief that artists should use their talents to effect positive social change. As Eberle said in 1913, "The artist has no right to work as an individualist. . . . He is the specialized eye of society. . . . Artists must see for people—reveal them to themselves."[21] Eberle's commitment to those values led her to set up a studio in a settlement house on New York's Lower East Side, where she had ready access to neighborhood children. They and their poor immigrant mothers, together with old ragpickers and unemployed workers, became frequent subjects in her sculpture, now recognized as pioneering work in the social realist effort to reveal Americans to themselves.

Not far from the site of Eberle's studio on Manhattan's Lower East Side, William Gropper (1897–1977) was born into a large family of Eastern European Jewish immigrants. Poverty forced him to leave high school for work as a delivery boy and dishwasher, but he found time, beginning in 1912, for evening art classes with Robert Henri and George Bellows, who sharpened Gropper's observations of social and political injustice. For decades Gropper worked as a satiric cartoonist and illustrator, creating pungent visual critiques of society's ills and the hypocrisy of its leaders. Still, while bitingly cynical about certain aspects of

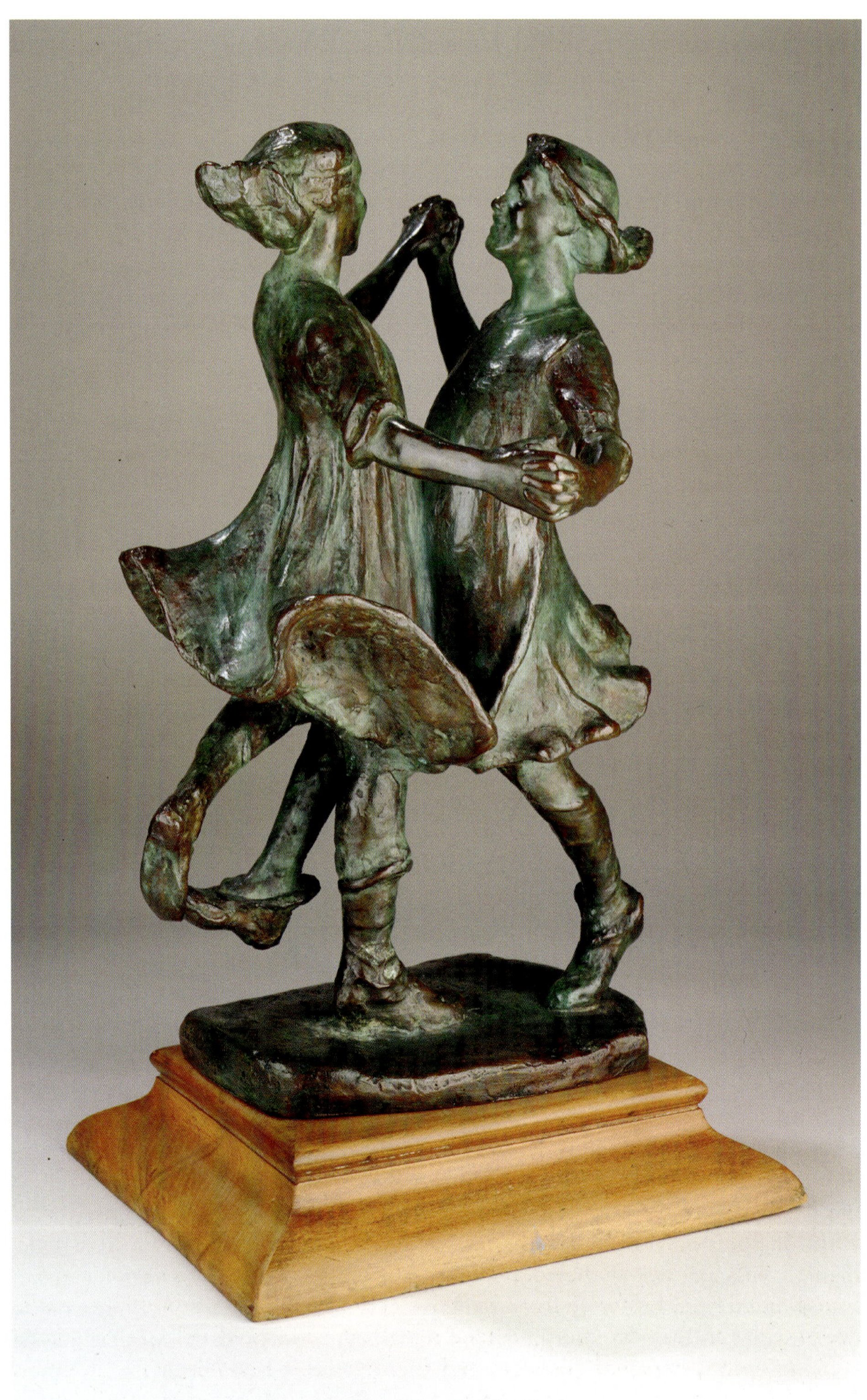

**Figure 11** Abastenia St. Leger Eberle, *Girls Dancing*, 1907, bronze, 13 × 7¼ × 7⁵⁄₁₆ inches. (Corcoran Gallery of Art, Washington, D.C., Bequest of the artist, 68.28.4)

society, Gropper always retained a humanitarian warmth in his cartoons, prints, and paintings, in which one readily discerns his sympathies for the underdog and the worker in America.

After touring Eastern Europe in 1948 and witnessing the aftermath of the Nazi Holocaust, Gropper began to dedicate one painting a year to the memory of ghetto victims, particularly in Warsaw. In those postwar years he also took a closer look at his family's own immigrant origins. In keeping with his intent to respond always to life, not to art styles, Gropper began to portray Jewish subjects from his own upbringing in his paintings and prints. His small etching *Hassid Dancing* (1968; fig. 12) resurrects his childhood memory of an exuberant dance by a member of the Hassidim, an Eastern European Jewish sect who expressed their piety in joyful acts. Their long, rich tradition of dance, song, and storytelling arrived with the boatloads of immigrants who passed through Ellis Island. Among the Hasidim, dance was seen as integral part of life, a joyous act permitting every part of the body to serve God. Sometimes the dances were repeated for hours, encouraging a feeling of ecstatic oneness with God that lasted until dancers and singers exhausted themselves. Such worshipful celebration defined Hasidism for its adherents, who liked to say of their sect that "the whole Jewishness comes with a happiness, with dancing and with singing." In their communities dance itself becomes a devotional act, transplanted from Eastern Europe to thrive in lower Manhattan. Gropper's memory of such occasions from his boyhood remained, undimmed, half a century later, evoking both a personal nostalgia and a group solidarity. Formally, Gropper's *Hassid Dancing* employs lessons learned early in his cartooning career: the artist caricatures the human form by de-emphasizing mass, using bold, supple lines to exaggerate postures and gestures. Arms upraised, legs bent in a lively cross-step,

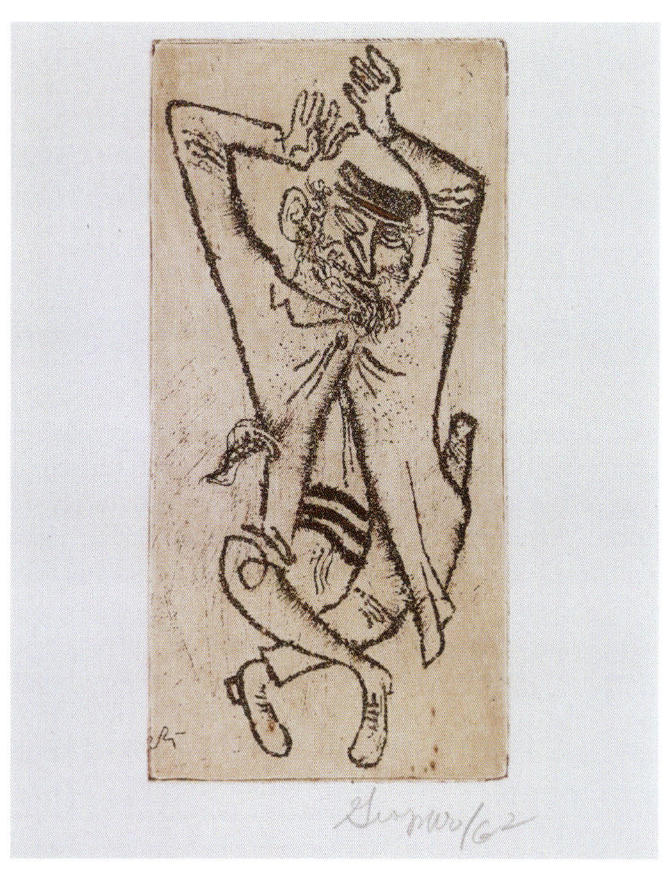

Figure 12 William Gropper, *Hassid Dancing*, 1968, etching on wove Rives paper, 5 ½ × 3 inches. (Terra Foundation for American Art, Chicago, Illinois, 2004.14; photo: Terra Foundation for American Art, Chicago/Art Resource, New York)

Gropper's smiling, bearded dancer vividly conveys his complete immersion in the dance, a fusion of Old World and American energies, at once social and religious.

Dances seen in New York's working-class immigrant neighborhoods—places deeply imprinted on the identity of generations of Americans—furnished artists with unforgettable subjects, rich with the diversity of their melting-pot streets. In the small sampling just discussed, it is evident that whatever the chosen medium—photography, painting, sculpture, or prints—capturing the motion of the dance, and its particular character, demanded the artist's best efforts. As difficult as it is to elicit the character of a face or figure in repose, the task of isolating the essential, telling moment within fluid human motion requires a supple, energetic hand at the service of an artist's keenest powers of observation. Whether interpreted by visitors to the Lower East Side, such as Hine, Luks, and Eberle, or by a resident such as Gropper, urban dances, as expressions of Americans' appetites for play, romance, nostalgia, or piety, help to frame our modern understanding of the ways cities and their diverse inhabitants shaped the evolving American character.


## Country Dance and the Visual Mythology of the American Frontier

As far back as the early nineteenth century, much of America's colonial-era ambivalence surrounding dance began to dissipate, allowing the activity to enter and take root in all levels of society. Outside the cities, dancing was not merely tolerated; often it was seen as a socializing virtue. Bringing scattered, isolated Americans together, occasions for dancing provided the social glue in many rural places. According to an anonymous social observer of the day,

> I really know among us of no custom which is so useful and tends so much to establish the union and the little society which subsists among us. Poor as we are, if we have not the gorgeous balls, the harmonious concerts, the shrill horn of Europe, yet we delight our hearts as well with the simple Negro fiddle.[22]

Context was crucial: the just-quoted anonymous observer would have been perfectly at home among the crowd in a dance scene painted by William Sidney Mount (1807–68), a Long Island–based painter of provincial genre. Mount's *Rustic Dance after a Sleigh Ride* (1830; fig. 13) packs several dozen revelers into a plain, candlelit interior festooned with simple garlands. In the room's center two couples step to the tune of an African American fiddler, while delighted onlookers surround them and still others peer in from a partially opened door. Such rustic narratives were typical of American genre painting of the 1830s and '40s, and Mount found a ready audience for his efforts to "paint for the many, not the few."[23] Yet his paintings, as Elizabeth Johns suggests, "made much of their mark by flattering the self-styled sophistication of his city audience," Manhattanites who could gently denigrate the countrified amusements of their Long Island neighbors. Sniffed one urban critic, Mount's subjects were not

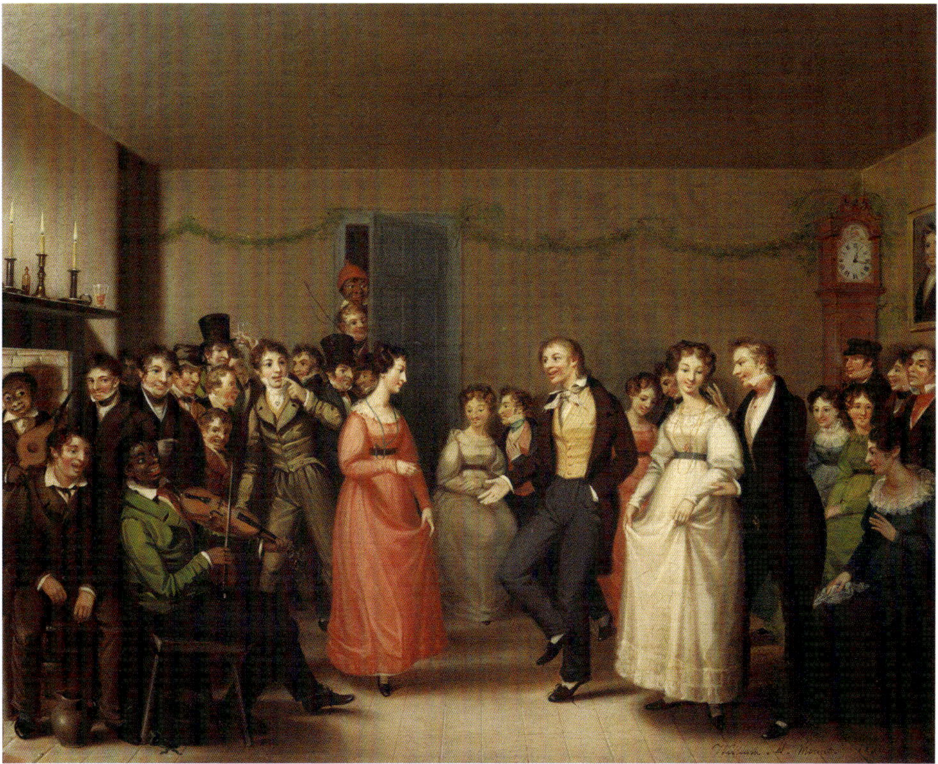

**Figure 13** William Sidney Mount, *Rustic Dance after a Sleigh Ride*, 1830, oil on canvas, 22 ⅛ × 27 ⅛ inches. (Museum of Fine Arts, Boston, Bequest of Martha C. Karolik for the M. and M. Karolik Collection of American Paintings, 1815–1865, 48.458)

*"gentlemen* and *ladies."*[24] Left unsaid, perhaps even unobserved, by critics of the day were Mount's revelations of other social realities: whites, particularly males, take center stage, while blacks are sidelined in service positions, as musician, coachman, and fireplace tender. For its range of American "types," Mount's canvas exudes authenticity, yet *Rustic Dance* reveals the painter's study of European art through engravings, plaster casts, and instruction books. The canvas was, in fact, based on John Lewis Krimmel's watercolor *Dance in a Country Tavern* (before 1822, Library of Congress, Washington, D.C.), a work known to Mount in lithographic form.[25]

Only a year after his *Rustic Dance*, Mount reinvented his portrayal of dance. *Dancing on the Barn Floor* (1831; fig. 14) is so bucolic by comparison that it makes the previous year's work look almost effete. But the new simplicity is deceptive. What Mount has done in the later work is to scale back the crowded, salon-style composition of *Rustic Dance* in order to take on new formal problems dealing with space and figure placement. To clear the way for that work, Mount reduced the figures to four: two dancers, a fiddler, and a woman at the partially opened back door. The dance steps themselves appear similar to those in the crowded *Rustic Dance*, but here the dancers have plenty of space within the nearly empty hay barn. Perhaps they practice their steps to prepare for a

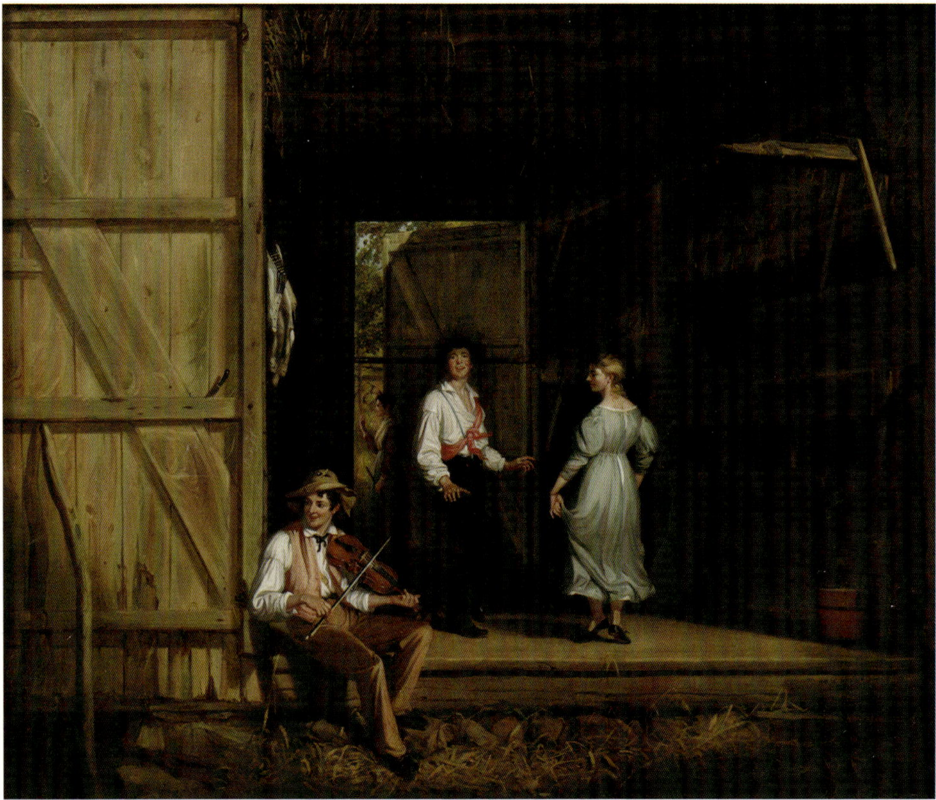

**Figure 14** William Sidney Mount, *Dancing on the Barn Floor*, 1831, oil on canvas, 25 × 30 inches. (Long Island Museum, Stony Brook, New York, Gift of Mr. and Mrs. Ward Melville, 1955)

more formal function; at least that is the kind of literary imagination applied to Mount's narrative subjects by contemporary critics. At least as likely is that Mount himself was rehearsing the serious artistic problems that would preoccupy him during much of the next decade. In the 1830s Mount made careful perspectival studies in his notebooks, studies in which he blocked out solid geometric projections of forms in deep space. Barbara Novak has discussed Mount's architectonic sense of space by comparing his works from the 1840s with those of the fifteenth-century Florentine painter Piero della Francesca. However, in *Dancing on the Barn Floor*, he has already initiated those geometric spatial organizations, perhaps empirically, with the front edge of the open barn precisely parallel to the picture plane. He would make a number of these compositions with an open barn door, near which figures sit or stand. The large open door enabled Mount to paint outdoor and indoor space within the same composition, feeding his essential tendencies toward plein-airism. "My best pictures," he wrote, "are those which I painted out of doors—I must follow my gift to paint figures out of doors as well as in doors, without regard to paint room. The longer an artist leaves nature the more feeble he gets."[26]

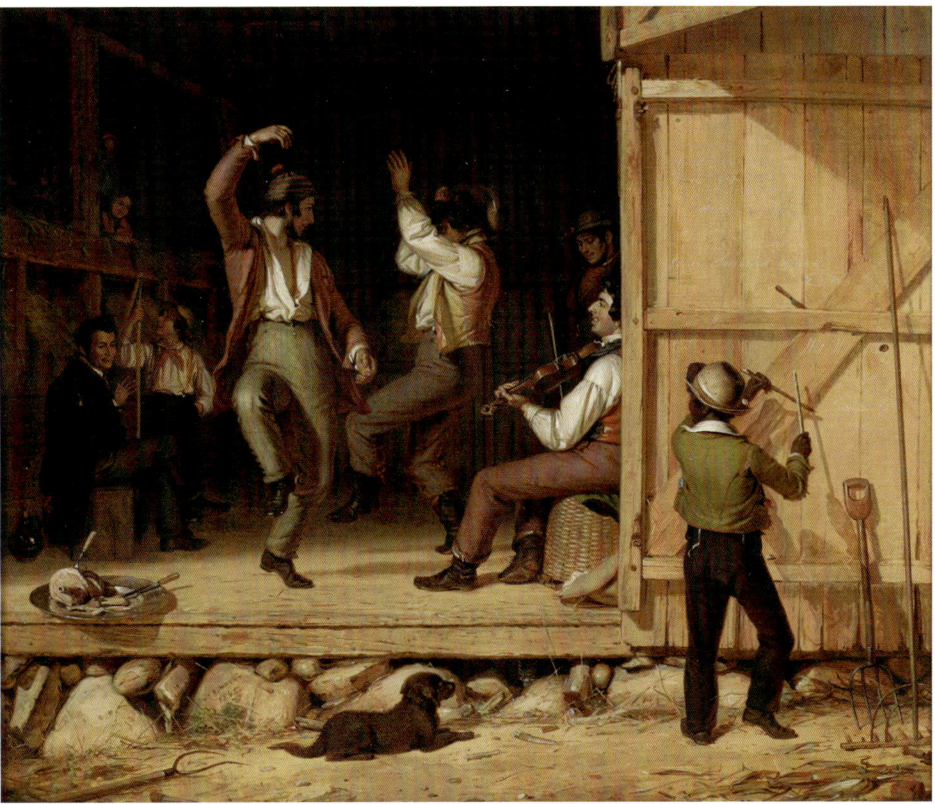

Figure 15 William Sidney Mount, *Dance of the Haymakers* or *Music Is Contagious* 1845, oil on canvas mounted on wood, 24 × 29 ¾ inches. (Long Island Museum, Stony Brook, New York, Gift of Mr. and Mrs. Ward Melville, 1950)

Mount's genre subjects of music and dance came in part from his own personal experience: after a day of painting, perhaps in company with his good friend Thomas Cole, the two—Mount on violin, Cole on flute—amused themselves with lively impromptu concerts. After two successive evenings of music at Cole's, Mount wrote, "My violin has been the source of a great deal of amusement."[27] Just that kind of informal music-making often gave rise to impromptu dancing, whether in the evening or during the midday break between long hours of farm work. In Mount's *Dance of the Haymakers* or *Music Is Contagious* (1845; fig. 15) the artist pays tribute to the power of music to enliven a leisure hour. Their pitchforks and noon repast set aside, two farmhands step out a lively rhythm just inside one of Mount's open barn doors. Released by the tune of a fiddler, music's contagion spreads to gleeful onlookers inside the barn and to a young black man who taps out the rhythm directly on the barn door. Mount's easily accessible narrative detail—the half-eaten ham on a platter, the brown jug, the companionable dog—testify to his fidelity to the concrete object. Those certainties, combined with the essentially planar structure Mount inherited from American folk tradition and his own Pieroesque mathematically based design, create compositions of firm, fixed stability. At the same time, as if to

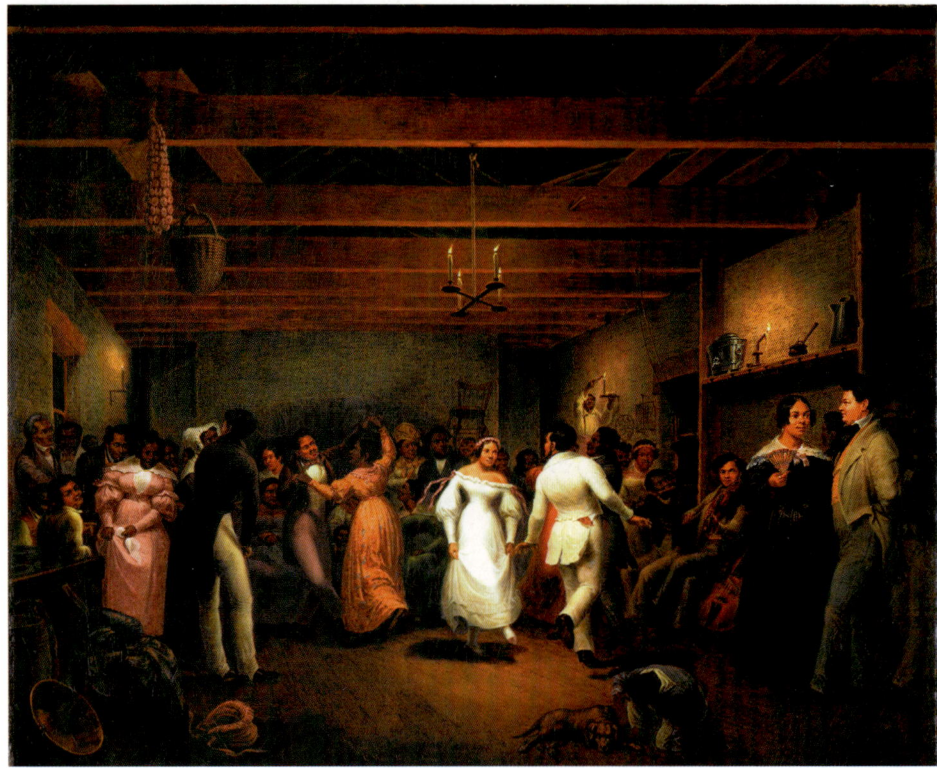

**Figure 16** Christian Friedrich Mayr, *Kitchen Ball at White Sulphur Springs, Virginia*, 1838, oil on canvas, 24 × 29 ½ inches. (North Carolina Museum of Art, Raleigh, 52.9.23)

leaven all that classical architectonic weight, Mount injects dance into his carefully structured setting—not the measured formal restraint of a parlor quadrille, but a raucous, foot-stomping jig. With each of these successive dance paintings, Mount has learned to loosen his figures. In *Dance of the Haymakers* he freed them fully—to respond physically to the music and with an energy that nearly defies gravity.[28]

Similarly rural, but with a distinctly different geographic flavor, is Christian Mayr's (c. 1805–51) *Kitchen Ball at White Sulphur Springs, Virginia* (1838; fig. 16). Beneath its portrayal of a country celebration, *Kitchen Ball* bridges, in fact, the conventions of rural and urban, black and white dance entertainments. Here, under the open beams of an expansive kitchen (not a barn) gather the servants—likely slaves—who have accompanied their masters to this Virginia resort, perhaps to celebrate a wedding. Young and old, lighter and darker skinned, they make merry, occupying center stage in the informal setting available to them behind the scenes. In their dance steps and dress Mayr's subjects emulate the social conventions of the whites they serve. Yet Mayr—perhaps because of his own status as German immigrant-outsider—endows these African American dancers with a grace and dignity far exceeding that of Mount's rustic Long Islanders. Mayr's dancers recreate, in a folksy American setting, the feel of sixteenth-century Flemish painter Pieter Bruegel's robust

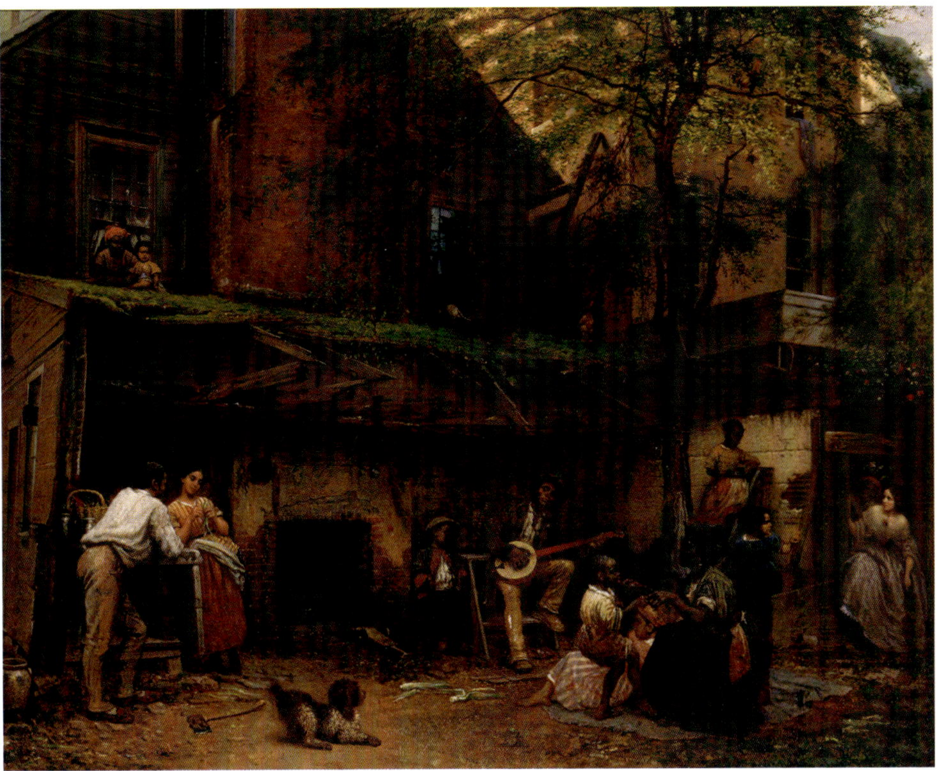

**Figure 17** Eastman Johnson, *Negro Life at the South*, 1859, oil on linen, 37 × 46 inches. (collection of the New York Historical Society, R. L. Stuart Collection)

country weddings. In both, dance lubricates the occasion, encouraging loosened collars, laughter, and plenty of perspiration.

More sentimental a genre subject is Eastman Johnson's (1824–1906) *Negro Life at the South* (1859; fig. 17), which, with its banjo player and young dancer, harks back to William Sidney Mount, while at the same time anticipating Thomas Eakins's 1878 *The Dancing Boy*, discussed below. In 1859, even as Johnson painted *Negro Life at the South*, the Civil War was already on the horizon. Curiously, however, Americans in both the North and South still seemed unready—at least in the visual arts—to confront the slavery question. Johnson provided what they still seemed to prefer: a benign gloss on the subject, in which dance and music lift his scene out of the obvious squalor in which it takes place. The painting was received uncritically when exhibited at the National Academy of Design, acclaimed by slaveholders and abolitionists alike for its evocation of a scene in which onlookers, both black and white, are momentarily brought together by an entertainment that reaches across the all-important racial divide in the South.

Beyond the varied sociopolitical implications of Mount's, Mayr's, and Johnson's rustic dancers, one sees in them glimpses of life in rural and frontier areas, where life had a rougher edge than in American cities. In contrast to the salons of New York, Boston, and San Francisco, where dancing masters, formal cotillions and rules of etiquette were de rigeur, such niceties were as scarce on the frontier as women dance partners. Outside the cities, raw energy usually trumped citified sophistication, and free-wheeling entertainment, usually in the form of dance, brought a climax to country fairs, quilting parties, and barn raisings. Hard work seemed to demand rousing Virginia reels, country jigs, and shakedowns—all undertaken with abandon and held wherever indoor space allowed.

Americans had danced to British jigs and hornpipes since the late eighteenth century, while other English country dances were gradually transformed into lively square dances. Such homespun dance entertainments were encouraged by the likes of Davy Crockett, the famous frontiersman who declared himself opposed to citified dance: "None of your straddling, mincing, sadying, but a regular sifter, cut-the-buckle, chicken flutter set-to. It is a good wholesome exercise; and when one of our boys puts his arm around his partner, it's a good hug, and no harm in it."[29] Crockett, Mount, and Mayr all seem to be tapping their toes to the same fiddle music.

As Americans moved west, they crossed boundaries between the familiar and the remote, imagining new futures while discovering that wherever they traveled much of their culture accompanied them. The frontiersman was no less a carrier of culture than the schoolteacher, the itinerant dance master, or the visual artist. Painters and printmakers, whether consciously or unconsciously, found unprecedented ways to reconcile freshly encountered contexts with the mythic traditions of American culture. One of those painters was George Caleb Bingham (1811–79). At a time when steamboats were already displacing the barge as cargo transportation to downstream markets, Bingham's *The Jolly Flatboatmen* (1846; fig. 18) celebrates the tranquil balance of humanity and nature on the unruffled surface of a broad American river. Suffused with golden sunlight, the luminist moment suggests time suspended just before the onslaught of "progress" in the westward expansion across the continent. In this brief idyll the artist paints a fragile harmony between the real and ideal. It is a self-contained moment, self-congratulatory and emblematic of America's optimism and exuberance, yet reminiscent too of Emerson's belief that "unlike all the world before us, our own age and land shall be classic to ourselves."[30]

Bingham's is indeed a classical frontier genre piece, in which compositional structure—wide horizontals supporting a stable pyramidal structure—supports that metaphor of classicism. Not unlike Mount's nearly contemporaneous barn dancers, Bingham's rivermen, in their positions and various levels of activity, represent the immediacy of a particular moment cast against the backdrop of a transcendent ideal. These tough-mannered types, with reputations for rambunctious behavior ashore, are here becalmed in an innocent fluvial arcadia, their energies channeled skyward through the upraised arms of a dancer. The figures at the base of the human pyramid sit or lie motionless; just above them, two members of the crew have pulled out banjo and fiddle to accompany a third—muscular, open-shirted—who rises to dance a lively jig atop the low-slung vessel. Bingham's dancer is among his most animated figures, like Mount's an antidote to the otherwise lugubrious weight and fixity of the composition. With his Michelangelesque physique and pose (at the apex of the pyramid

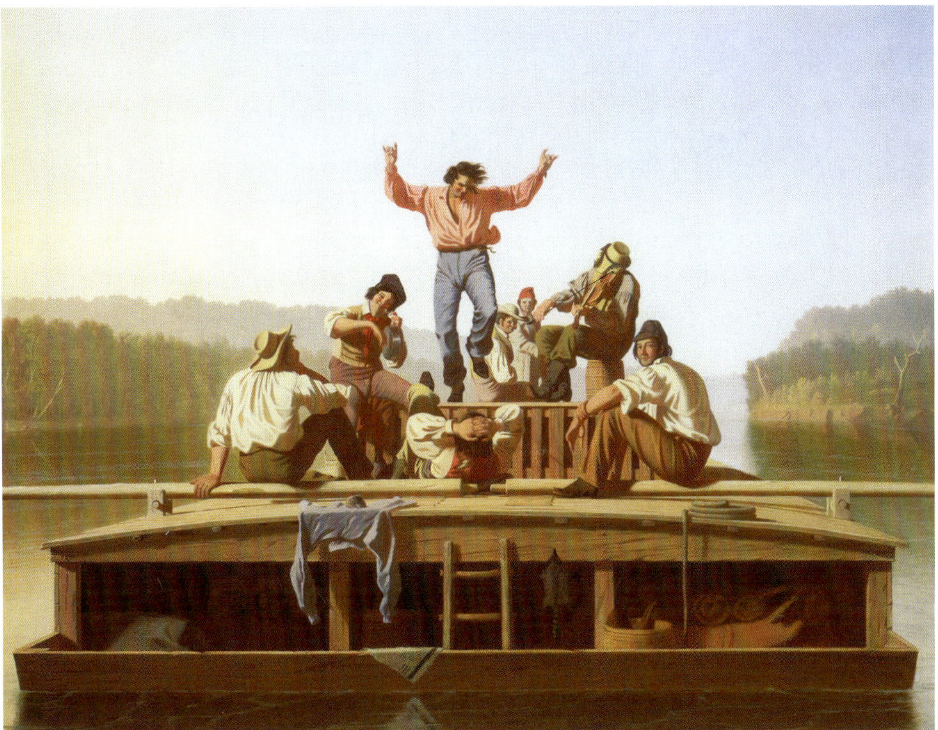

Figure 18 George Caleb Bingham, *The Jolly Flatboatmen*, 1846, oil on canvas,
38 ⅛ × 48 ½ inches. (Manoogian Foundation, New York; on loan to National Gallery
of Art, Washington, D.C.)

and at the pulse point of the action) Bingham's dancer bears a marked resemblance to the Italian master's *Last Judgment* Christ (1534–41, Sistine Chapel, Vatican).[31] In Michelangelo's Counter-Reformation fresco, Christ's upraised arm unleashes damnation on a dark, constricting world. Bingham, who surely knew the grimly moralizing Sistine Chapel fresco from reproductions, has here painted its obverse: a joyous hymn, borne aloft by music and dance, to the redemptive power of American nature. Painted for the American Art-Union, Bingham's *The Jolly Flatboatmen* brought him national fame when nearly ten thousand engravings of the painting were distributed to union subscribers. The work's populist message, untethered to a specific time and place, contains the cultural promise of the whole westering era and its myths of unfettered freedom, success, and social equality. Bingham's frontier boatmen are agents of that westward value transfer: in them we see respite earned after hard physical labor, and cultural pursuits (such as they were), mostly self-generated. In their largest sense, these dancers express the grand expanse of the whole American frontier idea, balancing nature and human endeavor in a kind of vital amplitude.

So popular were Bingham's riverboat dancers, and so revelatory of something vital in the American experience, that he would reprise their performances in the ensuing decades. In 1857, during a two-year stay in Dusseldorf, Bingham painted *The Jolly Flatboatmen in Port* (1857; Saint Louis Art Museum), and as late as

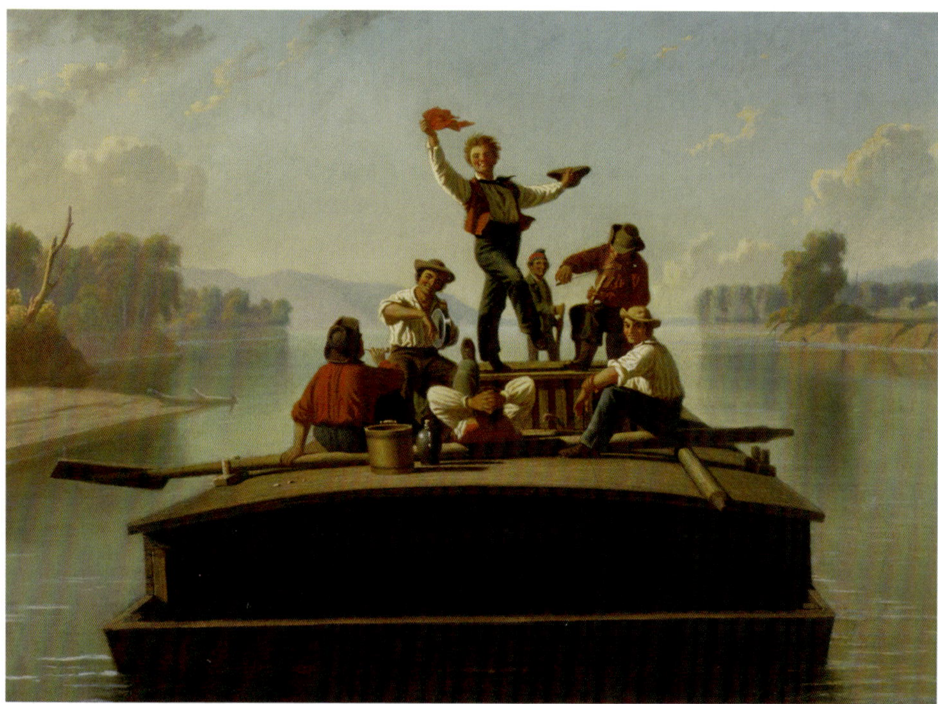

**Figure 19** George Caleb Bingham, *The Jolly Flatboatmen*, 1877–78, oil on canvas, 26 1/16 × 36 3/8 inches. (Terra Foundation for American Art, Chicago, Illinois, Daniel J. Terra Acquisition Endowment Fund, 1992.15; photo: Terra Foundation for American Art/Art Resource, New York)

the 1870s they reappeared (fig. 19). In the 1857 piece, as in his political subjects of that decade, Bingham masses many figures into a lively, theatrical scene. Lacking the frontality and essential calm of his boatmen from the previous decade, Bingham's complex perspectival scheme in the port scene, augmented by the low-slanting sun and the steamboat docked nearby, signal the passage of time to a new, bustling era on the river. One imagines that many noises accompany the dancer in port, in contrast to the thin melodies floated out from the isolated barge in the earlier version. In port, although the dancer still revels on the boat deck itself, figures and activity spill over everywhere onto the dock. All this makes for a dance of connection, joining riverlife to the faster-paced events of shorelife, and elevating Bingham's flatboatmen from narrative to what Barbara Novak has called a kind of "monumental contemporary history painting."[32] In Bingham's, as in Mount's compositions, architectonic pictorial structure is reworked in a distinctly American vein, leavening classical precepts with a good measure of optimism and exuberant national pride.

In Bingham's contemporary history paintings dance conveys much about the American character, at least as perceived on the frontier: his flatboatmen enact masculine exploits, with performances virile, vigorous, and direct. A Saint Louis newspaper critic, who had ample opportunities to observe the ubiquitous riverboatmen, described their diversity: "The western boatmen [are] a peculiar class in most of their habits, dress and manners. Among them, often in the same crew, may be found all the varieties of human character, from the amiable and intelligent to the stern and reckless man."[33] But that diversity did not extend to gender in the mid-nineteenth century; women are conspicuously absent among Bingham's river dancers. Males, in the prevailing gender stereotype of the day, could break into spontaneous dance with a kind of thumping sturdiness off limits to women, who were still defined largely by their domestic and maternal qualities. Ladies might dance in sedate indoor settings (as in Mount's post–sleigh ride scene) or watch males dancing outdoors, but in the mid-nineteenth century, respectable women were excluded from anything remotely akin to public dance performance. (Women who danced in theaters, as will be seen, only served to reinforce the prevailing distinctions between respectable and questionable female virtue.) Those mores and manners persisted late into the century, especially among those who equated the outdoors with masculinity.

While Bingham's dancers floated down America's great inland rivers, other frontier Edens beckoned American artists to the far West. In California, where the 1849 gold rush lured hordes of prospectors and turned hamlets into bustling towns, building was the order of the day. To feed the nation's appetite for lumber, California loggers took aim at the gargantuan trees inhabiting its forests. In 1853, for example, five men spent twenty-two days cutting down a two-hundred-foot tall sequoia in the Sierra Nevada.[34] Some twenty-four feet in diameter, the stump, when smoothed off, presented a platform for several possible uses. In actual fact, the stump became, at least temporarily, a dance floor on which dozens of people disported themselves in the midst of the forest. An obscure Massachusetts artist, F. R. Bennett, recorded the event in his painting *Dance on a Sequoia Stump* (c. 1875; fig. 20). In a style seemingly self-taught, or "naive," the artist spells out the features of a scene with narrative precision. He takes care to demonstrate the vast scale of the place, showing a surviving sequoia at the center, tunneled to allow horse-drawn wagons to pass through its vast trunk. Nearby, younger, smaller trees suggest the forest's future growth. From the brush of an artist schooled in more sophisticated perspectival unities, the looming trees might create an ominous, uneasy relationship with a group of tiny figures. But not here: precisely because they *dance* within nature, Bennett's people participate in an American allegory of progress, of humanity's subjugation of nature. Dancing on the remains of a tree more than a thousand years old, they seem to celebrate a victory over time and the primeval forest. Here is American enterprise writ large—nature tamed, not just by the saw, but by the civilizing power of dance. In a sense, Bennett's felled tree extends an American artistic legacy: earlier, better-known paintings by artists such as Thomas Cole and George Inness had included tree stumps as a well-recognized symbol of America's westward expansion.[35] *Dance on a Sequoia Stump* makes an even more explicit and assertive statement of cultural hegemony, its continuing history extending well beyond Bennett's canvas: from its beginnings as a dance floor, the stump's capacious expanse later became a lecture pavilion, then the foundation for a building used sequentially as a theater, hotel, bowling alley, and

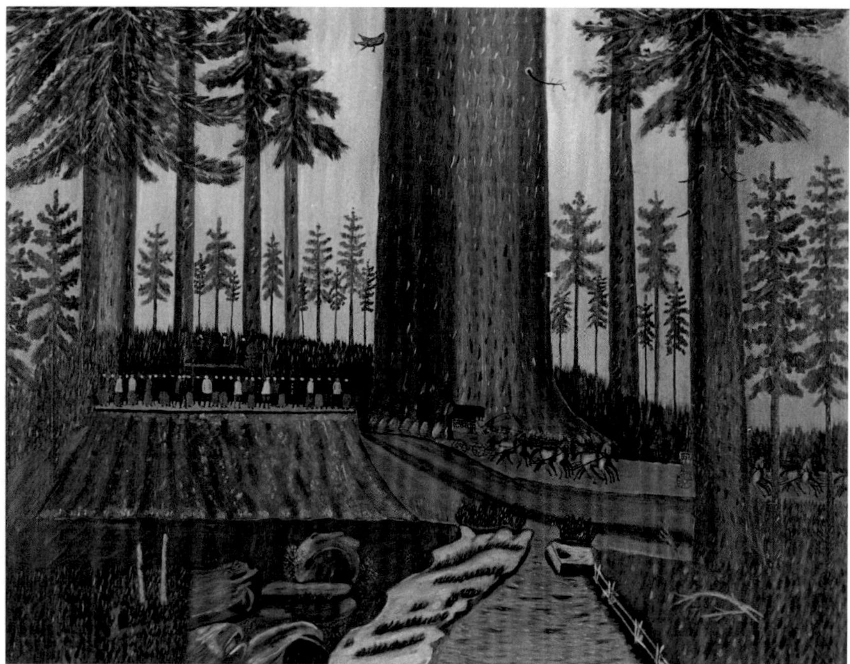

Figure 20 F. R. Bennett, *Dance on a Sequoia Stump*, c. 1875, oil on canvas, 20 ½ × 28 ⅛ inches. (Fenimore Art Museum, Cooperstown, New York, © New York State Historical Association, Cooperstown, New York)

newspaper office. Embedded within that broad range of human activities are some of America's prominent virtues and values: optimism, adaptability, and the dawn of an American consumer economy, which devours natural resources in the name of progress. All this is suggested by the contextual history of Bennett's painting, a canvas executed with an American primitivist's obsession for the linear, the whole, and the conceptual—that is, with more attention to the mind's knowing response than to the eye's. That this painting also has an appealing decorative rhythm in its lines and masses owes something, as does its iconography, to the minuscule, yet highly suggestible, spectacle of dance.

The American frontier lingered long in the nation's cultural imagination, reinvented at will to suit changing times. Missouri, which had provided frontier subjects to Bingham in the nineteenth century, had become the nation's settled heartland in the decades when Thomas Hart Benton (1889–1975) painted the American Scene. Well into the twentieth century Benton would mine a vein of nativism visible in both his subjects and his style. The Missouri-born artist studied in Chicago, then in Paris, where he was deeply affected by European modernism. Only after a stint in the U.S. Navy in 1918–19 did Benton arrive at the notion that art should grow from its environment rather than from ideas or styles imposed from outside. Thus American artists, Benton believed, ought to live in active connection with their heritage and environment. And his populist view—that ordinary individuals were at the root of America's development—led him to subject matter focused on American working life. During the 1920s and

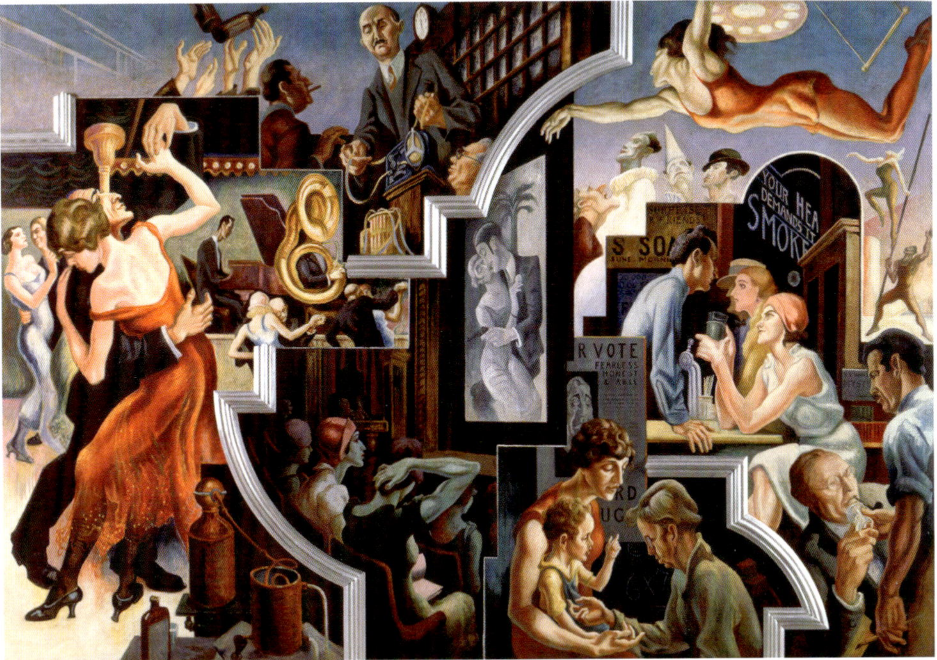


**Figure 21** Thomas Hart Benton, *City Activities with Dance Hall*, from *America Today*, 1930, distemper and egg tempera with oil glaze on gessoed linen, 92 × 134 ½ inches. (collection of AXA Equitable, New York)

1930s his American scene murals came to adorn many public buildings, expressing a broad range of labor and leisure activities, contrasting urban and rural themes. Benton's painting remained rooted in the figurative tradition, and he called himself a "painter of histories[;] . . . American histories rather than Greek or Roman or biblical ones."[36] A series he called *America Today* (1930), painted for New York's New School for Social Research, includes two murals devoted to recreational life. One of them, *City Activities with Dance Hall* (fig. 21), seems to take up old questions about who gets to dance in America; long after Bingham's flatboatmen have drifted into history, Benton turns his focus to dancing women. They are actresses, acrobats, and burlesque and social dancers, shown in a highly sexualized manner, as Frances Pohl has pointed out.[37] These women are urban sophisticates in an environment of questionable morals, and Benton seems to suggest that they dance for social or financial advancement. The most prominent female dancer in the mural is a woman in an off-the-shoulder, bright red gown. She sets up a telling contrast to another red-garbed Benton dancer, painted only two years earlier, but worlds apart in feeling. His oil *Country Dance* (1928, formerly, Danenberg Gallery, New York) seems to embody quite a different set of vestigial American mores—bucolic, innocent, far away from the corrupting influence of the big city. A blonde dancer in red dress (no low necklines here!) gazes up adoringly at her jeans-wearing partner. *Country Dance* is all rollicking pleasure—rural Americans kicking up their heels to the tune of a country fiddler. They are winsome remnants of a frontier nostalgia that became Benton's stock-in-trade, and they validate his retention of the figure, animated by dance, to explore American energies old and new.

Benton's nostalgic take on American history was not confined to his work, or even to painting. Rural America survived in the vital work of photographers employed by the Farm Security Administration (FSA), a federal agency established in 1935. Its historic photography project, which documented America during the Great Depression, would exert a strong influence on much subsequent documentary work later in the century.

Russell Lee was hired in 1936 by Roy Stryker, legendary head of the FSA photography project, and set out to record the successes and failures of the American dream through the lens of his camera. Working in New Mexico in 1939 and 1940, Lee photographed hardworking settlers relocated from Texas and Oklahoma. Often public events in obscure American places like Pie Town, New Mexico, offered Lee his best chance to explore their sense of community, their interactions, and their shared entertainments. To Lee, the community seemed a metaphor for pioneer aspirations throughout the nation's history. "In Pie Town," he wrote, "we could apply a twentieth century camera to a situation more nearly typical of the eighteenth century. We could picture the frontier which has unalterably molded the American character and make frontier life vivid and understandable."[38]

Lee's photograph *Jigger at a Square Dance, Pie Town, June, 1940* (fig. 22) captures just such frontier character, the kind portrayed by both Bingham and Benton. Caught up in the music generated by an unseen guitarist and fiddler, Lee's jigger kicks up his heels in a step very similar to that danced by Bingham's jolly flatboatman on the Missouri. Watchers, mostly women, look on from the sidelines, but in a companion photograph they rise to join the square dance, while an awkward adolescent looks on. Bingham's carefully constructed pyramidal composition gives way in Lee's photographs to the impression of sheer spontaneity. And that, in fact, is a strength of Lee's documentary work: his capacity to document an event without disrupting it. In that, he became a kind of performer himself. As J. B. Colson writes,

> Lee's proficiency was like that of a great dancer: his intuition had been developed through rigorous training, and he had a keen awareness of unfolding events. He moved with grace in response to action, synchronizing his photography with the movements of others.[39]

Lee's charge—and his great gift—was to capture the gritty realities of American places during the Great Depression, finding essential humanity in adversity, capturing communal virtues in the poetry of song, and preserving the joyous release of a timeless abandonment to dance. In their dance subjects from quintessential American places, visual artists such as Bingham, Benton and Lee searched out national character, real and imagined. With them, dancer-choreographer Martha Graham shared the frequent capacity to innovate from tradition, a perennial byword of American creativity. As seen in the following discussion, Graham would reveal still other components of an emerging

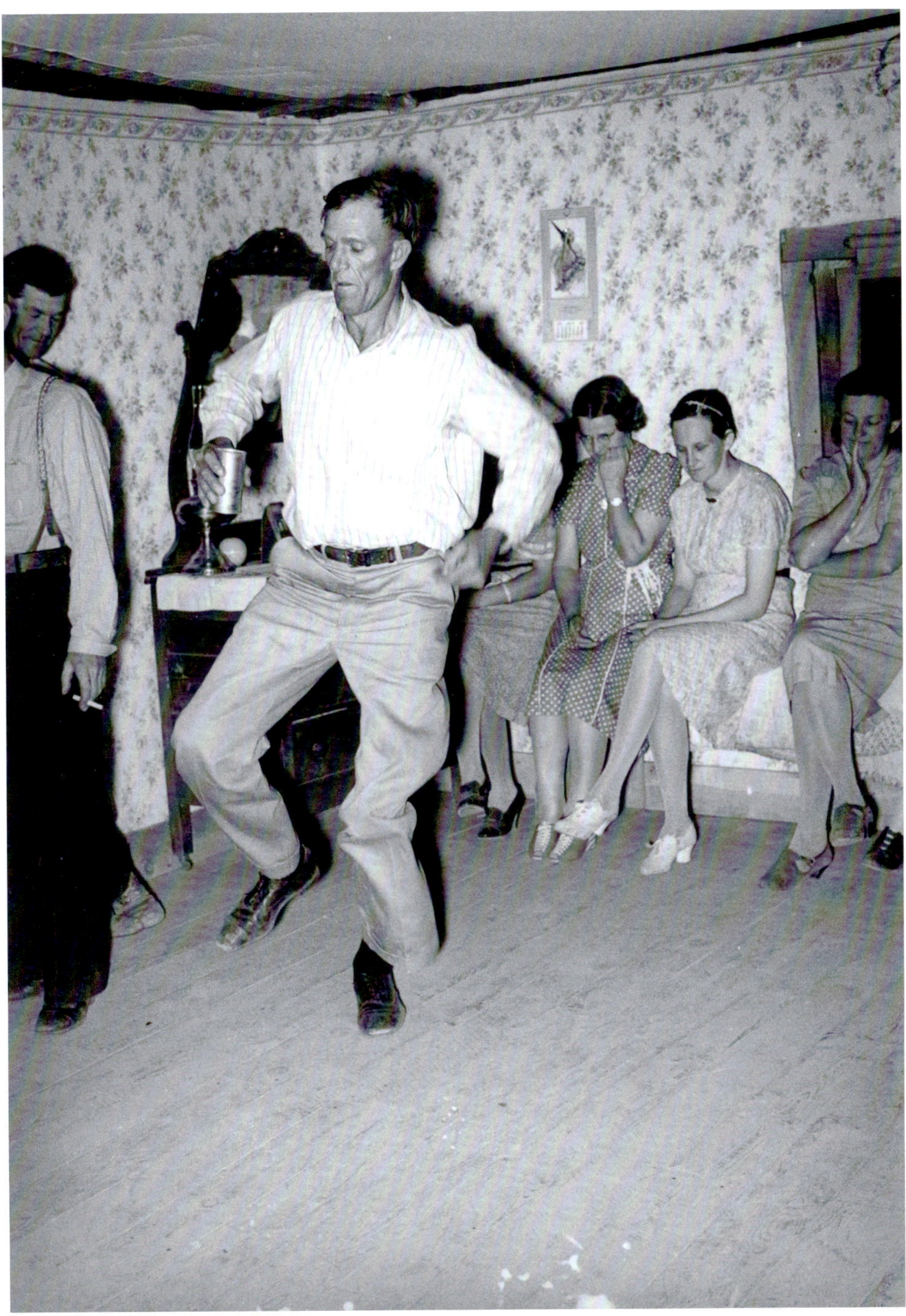

**Figure 22** Russell Lee, *Jigger at a Square Dance, Pie Town, June, 1940.* (Pinewood Collection of New Mexico FSA Photographs; photo courtesy Library of Congress, LCUSF34036912-0)

national identity, using movement, social history, and highly aesthetic visual settings to enlarge the expressive possibilities of concert dance performance.

## Reinventing American Places: Martha Graham and the Visual Artists She Inspired

Few dancers (or the visual artists who represented them) have paid closer attention to place and indigenous themes than Martha Graham (1893–1991). In 1920, while still a young dancer with the Denishawn company of Ruth St. Denis and Ted Shawn, Graham starred in the century's first ballet created on a North American theme, the exotic *Xochitl*, based on the Toltec legend of an emperor's lust for a dancing maiden. Francisco Cornejo, an authority on Aztec-Toltec art, designed the scenery and costumes for *Xochitl*, while Homer Grunn, a southwestern Indian music expert, wrote its score. Ted Shawn's "virile" choreography was stylized in the manner of Aztec reliefs, and critics acclaimed the whole production for its aesthetic excellence. Graham went on to dance in the 1929 American premier of Stravinsky's *Le Sacre du Printemps*, performing the part of another sacrificial maiden, The Chosen One. Due, at least in part, to her involvement with these folkloric productions, Graham became exquisitely attuned to the power of indigenous dance drama.

Graham's exposure to native themes deepened in 1930, when she traveled for the first time to the American Southwest. There, in Santa Fe, she paid a visit to writer Mary Austin (1868–1934). Graham was already an admirer of Austin's work on aboriginal dance drama and of her book *The American Rhythm* (1923), in which the writer attempted to capture patterns of color and community in the rituals of Spanish and Indian culture.[40] Both Austin and Graham discerned that Americans were ready to glimpse a premodern spiritual world as spectators of Indian dances, of shrines, and of the Hispanic penitente ritual. As far back as 1893, when throngs of Americans had visited the World's Columbian Exposition in Chicago, the most popular painting on view was of fifteenth-century Spanish flagellants, prototypes of the new-world penitentes. Part of its lure was undoubtedly antimodern escapism. One literary critic explained, "As the visible world is measured, mapped, tested, weighed, we seem to hope more and more that a world of invisible romance may not be far from us."[41] Jackson Lears sees a darker, more sensual side in America's rising fascination with folk tale, myth, archaic fantasy, and unsettling experiences with the darkly supernatural. "In its capacity to inspire dread," writes Lears, "the folk tale contained an erotic appeal similar to that of saintly 'excess.' . . . [Both] betrayed a taste for titillation but also constituted implicit critiques of the spiritual blandness diffused by liberal Protestant culture."[42] As an embodiment of "saintly excess," ritualized suffering such as that of the penitentes made the fantastic imaginings of secret rites and dances come alive.

Austin's and Graham's shared interests in rhythm and emotion-laden ritual, especially embodied in the rites of the penitentes, informed Graham's next dance work. *Primitive Mysteries* (1931) is a uniquely American blend of ritualistic elements, carved Hispanic *santos*, and the legacy of early Christian mystery plays. Graham's choreographed ritual proceeds from adoration of the Virgin to the Virgin's grief and final exaltation. She and her dancers moved in patterns, pausing in stiff vertical postures that framed the virgin (Graham) like a carved *bulto* (sculpture) of the Virgin of Guadalupe surrounded by her radiating mandorla (fig. 23). Diving deeply into the wellsprings of religious imagery, Graham found there a bold new answer to one of dance's abiding conundrums: how to capture the true character of raw movement. *Primitive Mysteries* is a dance triptych built around stark economy of gestures, the juxtaposition of Christian and pagan themes, and powerful connections to the earth. Its stylized simplicity and cold, yet ecstatic ritual seemed a newly minted miracle play, recognized instantly, in the words of one historian, "as a masterpiece of modern art and an indisputably American creation."[43]

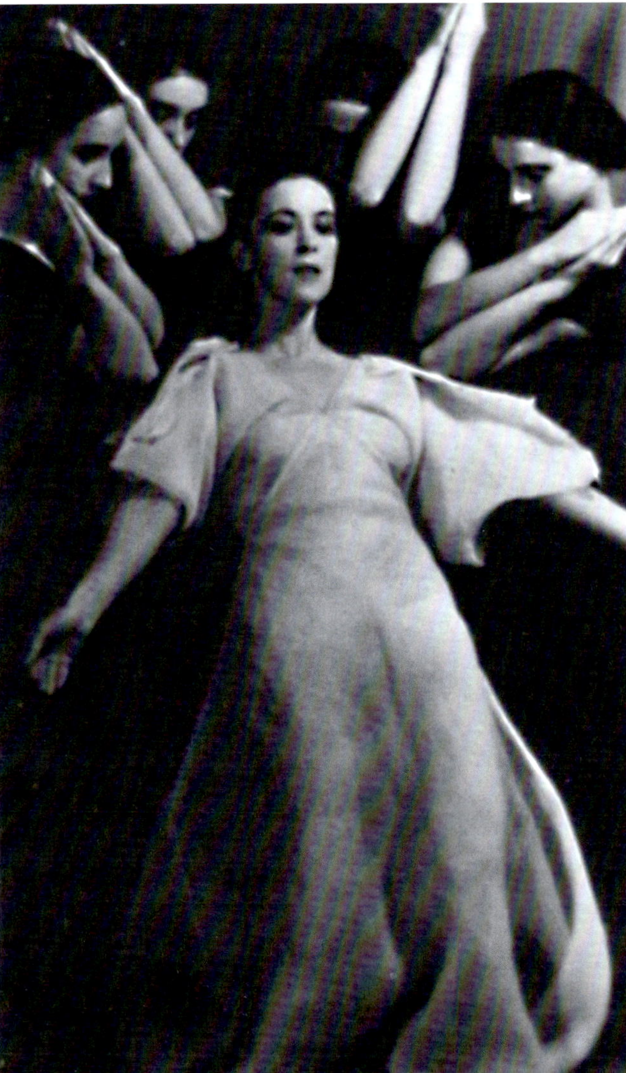

Figure 23 Martha Graham performing in *Primitive Mysteries*, 1931, photo by Edward Moeller. (courtesy Jerome Robbins Dance Division, The New York Public Library for the Performing Arts, Astor, Lenox, and Tilden Foundations)

By the 1930s, Graham was becoming a living embodiment of the avant-garde, bringing a fresh breeze of modernism everywhere she traveled. She presented new challenges to audiences, even to visual artists, in the ways she allied her dance with modern visual art. *Lamentation* (1930) alludes poignantly to the grieving women of Käthe Kollwitz and to the palpable tragedy of Ernst Barlach's sculptures. For those who missed such connections, Graham shared the critical fate of many a modern artist: her work was dismissed by some as inaccessible, even fraudulent.[44] Still, there were those who followed Graham's winding linkages between dance, place, and visual art: From those years also come dozens of "Dance Improvisations"—drawings of Graham by modernist painter Abraham Walkowitz (1878–1965) (1930s; fig. 24). These spare linear studies, some of which seem drawn in one continuous line without lifting the pencil, range from the curvilinear to the highly angular. All capture Graham's sharply defined movements, emphasizing the abstract visual qualities of her dance while preserving her powerful emotional gestures. As she wrote in 1933, "Since the dance form is governed by social conditions, so the American rhythm is sharp and angular, stripped of unessentials. It is something related only to itself, not laid on, but of a piece with that spirit which was willing to face a pioneer country."[45]

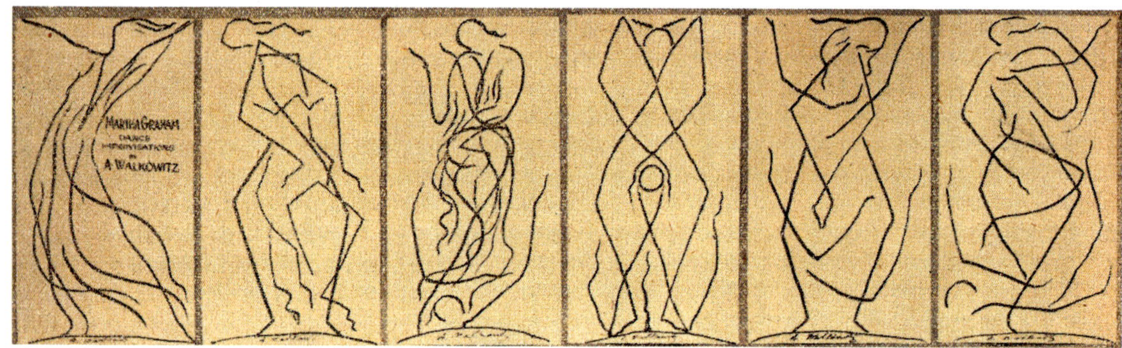


**Figure 24** Abraham Walkowitz, "Dance Improvisations," ink drawings of Martha Graham, 1930s.

Graham returned again and again to the Southwest, and its themes resonated in her work for many years. The flowering of her trips of the 1930s was *El Penitente,* a kind of play within a play featuring Graham dancing three aspects of the Marian character: first as a remote and unapproachable virgin, then as the Magdalene, and finally as a consoling Madonna. Her collaborator and future husband Erick Hawkins danced the part of the Flagellant (1940, fig. 25). Throughout the piece surged the intense emotional voltage generated by sin, penitence, and redemption. When the young Merce Cunningham took on the role of Christ, Graham, feeling that he looked too young for the part, commissioned the sculptor Isamu Noguchi to create a somber ritual mask and cloak for the Christ figure.

46

Noguchi, the young Japanese American sculptor, might have seemed an unconventional choice, but his design talents had already begun, some five years earlier, to leave an aesthetic imprint on Graham's productions. She had first collaborated with him on her solo piece *Frontier—An American Perspective on the Plains* (1935). *Frontier* invoked yet another powerful American place—the vastness of the American heartland and the determined efforts by newcomers to master its spaces. Before 1935 Graham had avoided sets, used only the simplest costumes, and strived to emulate the reductivist aesthetic of modernism. "Like the Modern painters and architects," she wrote, "we have stripped our medium of decorative unessentials. Just as fancy trimmings are no longer seen on buildings, so dancing is no longer padded."[46] So it was a departure for Graham when, for *Frontier*, she decided for the first time in her career to use a set, albeit a simple one. Noguchi's set differed from typical theater design in its spare, insistent shapes. From V-shaped ropes attached to the upper corners of the proscenium, Noguchi suspended a three-tiered pole fence, which served to join, in his words, "the total void of theater space to form and action." He described the sensitivity he and Graham shared for dance's habitation of sculptural space:

> I believe we had to find a dance theater with an emotionally charged space which, of course, is sculpture. It is the sculpture of space and it is not about objects. Martha moved in that sculptural space. It is correct to say that she was concerned with space rather than with painting. Painting, as a backdrop, is an assimilation of reality which sculpture overrides. Sculpture is reality itself. I conceive of sculpture as a permeation of space. I believe that's how Martha treated it.[47]

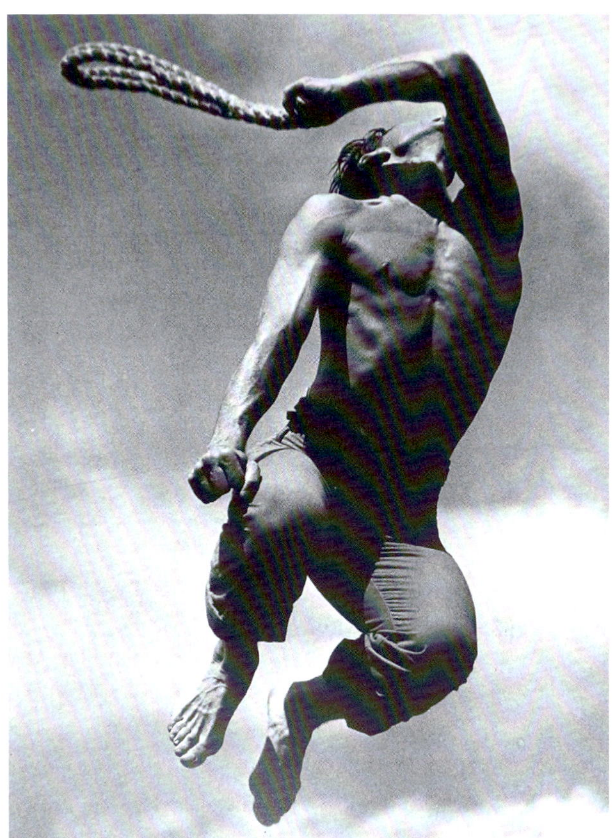

Figure 25 Barbara Morgan, *Erick Hawkins in El Penitente*, 1940, gelatin silver print. (University of New Mexico Art Museum, Gift of Van Deren Coke, 78.168; ©Barbara Morgan, The Barbara Morgan Archive)

What Graham learned from working with Noguchi is that visual artists, trained to think in spatial terms, know how to map the visual terrain dance covers. Noguchi went on to design Graham's *Appalachian Spring* (1944), another of her place-centered dances. By that time dancer and sculptor were deeply committed to enhancing the spectator's visual apprehension of relationships between forms and ideas in dance. In preparation for *Appalachian Spring*, Graham took Noguchi to the Museum of Modern Art to see Alberto Giacometti's sculpture *The Palace at 4 a.m.* (1932–33), in order to show him her idea for use of space in the new dance. Although the Giacometti work does not concern American space per se, its construction—wooden rods defining the outlines of a house—possessed a structural openness, a visual and physical permeability, that gave Graham and Noguchi an idea for the frontier house they needed. From that starting point, Noguchi recalled, he attempted "through the elimination of all non-essentials, to arrive at an essence of the stark pioneer spirit, that essence which flows out to permeate the stage. It is empty but full at the same time. It is like Shaker furniture."[48] That simultaneous vacancy and plenitude he evoked with such homely touches as a porch with rocking chair and, again, a fence to mark the foreground border of the homestead. Spare, plain, Noguchi's rough homestead fixes the emotional beginning point for some uniquely American characters, with Graham dancing the role of the young bride setting out on life's journey. Danced to music she had commissioned from Aaron Copland, *Appalachian Spring* became Graham's most popular production, another classic collaboration of visual art, music, and dance. In all, Noguchi would design twenty-two productions for Graham, at times creating designs so powerful, as in the case of her *Seraphic Dialogue* (1955), they would cause her to modify the expressive potential of her own work to harmonize with his. They found common cause in bringing her work to its fullest emotional pitch: his surrealist-inspired sets were exquisitely attuned to her psychological ballets, with their literary, often tragedic overtones.

Graham's aesthetic linkage of dance with modernist painting, architecture, and sculpture endeared her to other like-minded visual artists. Sculptor William Zorach (1887–1966) became interested in dance during summers spent with the Provincetown Players, for whom he painted scenery, acted, and produced plays. "I have always been interested in the dance," wrote Zorach. "From the beginning I felt that, in order to handle sculptural form and have it function rhythmically, one had to sense the correlation of form in one's own body."[49] As he pondered how to invest his sculpture with that rhythmic power, Zorach was asked by New York art dealer Edith Halpert to come up with some designs for the foyer and downstairs lounge of the new Radio City Music Hall. The result was his *Spirit of the Dance* (1934; fig. 26), a work strongly suggestive of the way a 1931 *New York Times* review by dance critic John Martin described Graham's choreography: "In arranging [her] movements into form, Miss Graham has developed a style that has much in common with modern painting and sculpture. It is economical of means, though no longer scanty, and eliminates all but the very essentials. It is strong of accent, and consequently distorted."[50] Zorach's *Spirit of the Dance*, at once monumental and modern, projects a strength and a riveting severity akin to Graham's own: angular, attenuated, making compositional use of solid

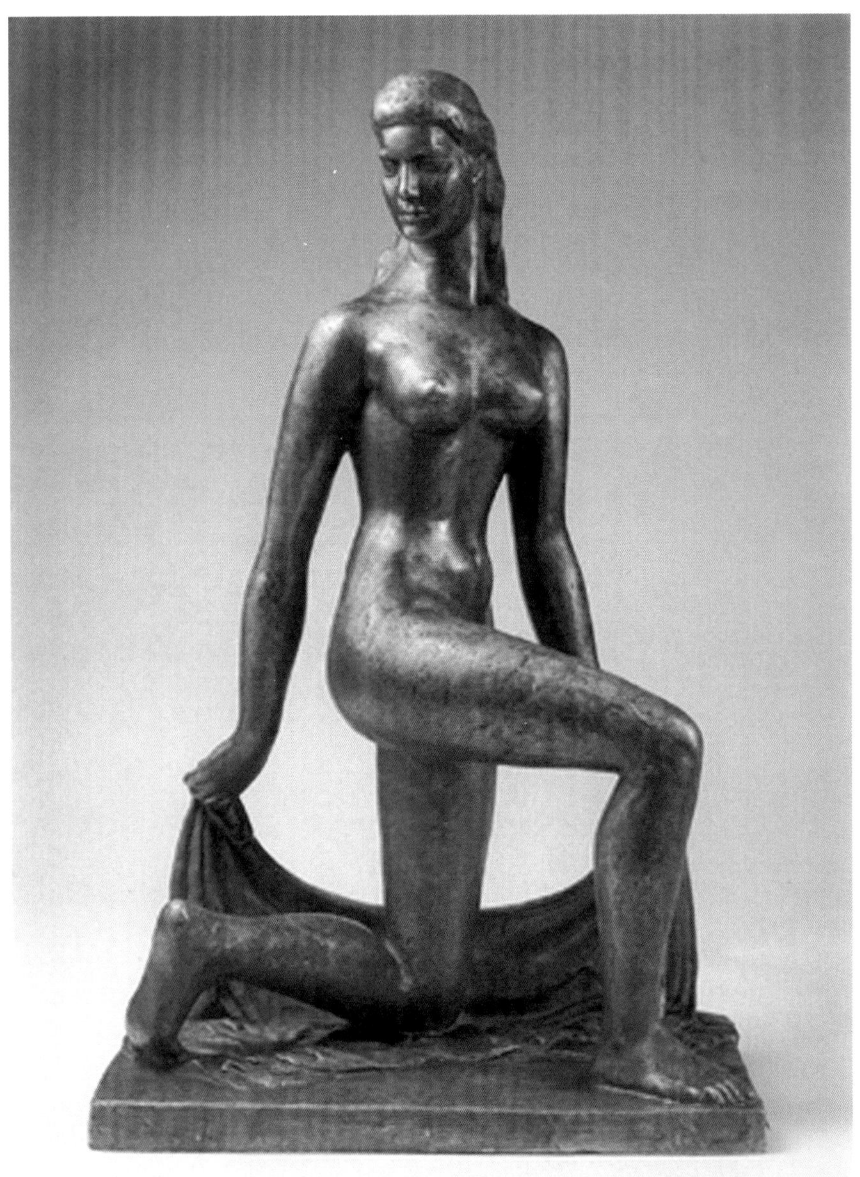

**Figure 26** William Zorach, *Spirit of the Dance*, 1934, cast aluminum, h. 25 ½ inches. (courtesy Tom Veilleux Gallery, Portland, ME)

forms adjacent to calculated negative spaces. Firmly grounded in its rhythmic balance of horizontals and verticals, of curving and straight lines, it exudes a classical, iconic simplicity. Graham would have known this well-publicized sculpture, cast in aluminum at a height of seventy-two inches for Radio City, and with other editions in bronze. Zorach concluded that he and the dancer shared a particular aesthetic reciprocity: "I remember Martha Graham telling me that she used to study my sculpture for the expressive gestures she found in it. And I used to study her dance for the same reason."[51]

Graham would soon stimulate the work of another of America's major sculptors, David Smith (1906–65), who took up dance subjects at key moments during his early career. His drawings and sculptures alluding to Graham seem to serve aims both formal and expressive. Trained first as a painter, Smith began making constructions in 1931, and the following year he became the first American artist to take up welding techniques. Created in rented space in the Terminal Iron Works factory in Brooklyn, Smith's metal sculptures of the 1930s show his sophisticated assimilation of European styles, incorporating both geometric and figurative elements. An early piece titled *Dancer* (1935; fig. 27) demonstrates his awareness of the metal sculptures of Julio Gonzales and Alberto

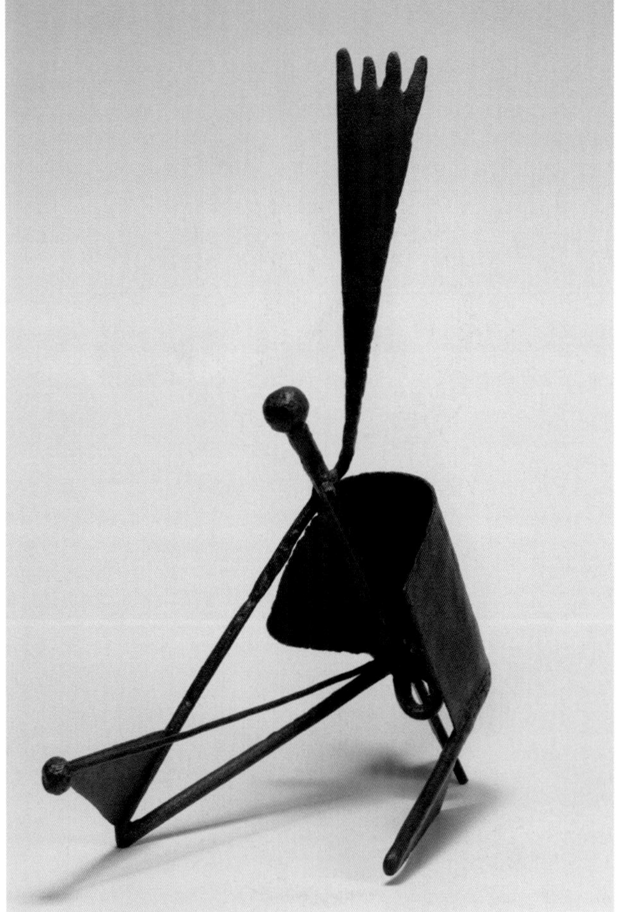

Figure 27 David Smith, *Dancer*, 1935, iron, 21 × 8¾ × 17⅜ inches. (private collection; art © Estate of David Smith/Licensed by VAGA, New York, New York)

Giacometti, but it suggests as well the way Graham's huge gestures claimed the space around her. Deborah Jowitt has suggested that Smith's wife, Dorothy Dehner, who studied with Graham, had likely taken him to see Graham's dances in the late 1920s. "What must have drawn Smith to Graham," writes Jowitt, "was the forceful lines and counter tensions that her body imprinted on space."[52] Barbara Morgan's photographs (collected in her 1941 book *Sixteen Dances in Photographs*) captured those gestures and tensions, prompting Smith to make drawings based on the photographs (*Martha Graham Series*, late 1930s/early 1940s, Estate of David Smith).

Then, pairing two attenuated dancers in a 1940 piece, *Dancers* (fig. 28), Smith began to open up space between their bodies, emphasizing wild, energetic movement at the peripheries while emptying out the central core of his composition, a deliberate challenge to traditional notions of sculpture. Subsequent pieces in the 1940s, such as his *Adagio* dancers (1945) and *Boaz Dancing School* (1945),[53] show Smith's inventive explorations of Cubist form and continued dematerialization of volumes. In the latter piece, spare metal rods suggest the outlines of a dance studio in the Surrealist, open-cage manner of Giacometti's *The Palace at 4 a.m.*, the piece at MOMA that had inspired Graham and Noguchi

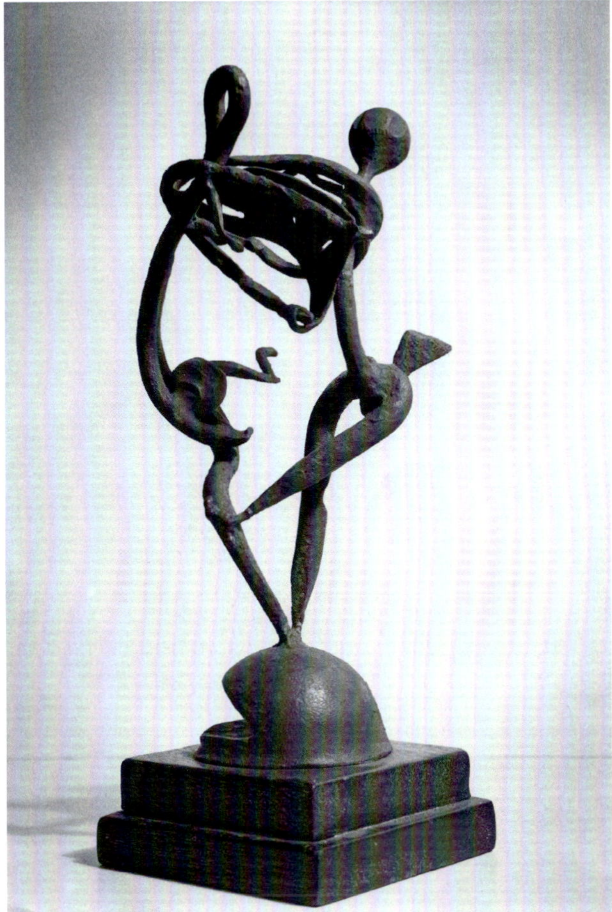

Figure 28 David Smith, *Dancers*, 1940, forged steel, 11 ½ × 5 ½ inches. (private collection; art © Estate of David Smith/Licensed by VAGA, New York, New York)

to incorporate some of its spare spatial framing for her *Appalachian Spring*. In later years Smith's sculptures became more monumental—sometimes painted, sometimes highly polished—but still attentive to the formal possibilities of space frames, and alternately engaging and resisting the active anthropomorphic references that earlier dancers, especially Martha Graham, had allowed him to study.

Yet another American sculptor of the period, Louise Nevelson (1899–1988) took inspiration from Graham's dances, and especially from the costumes and sets visual artists designed for those performances. Compared with Smith's work, Nevelson's reflects less overtly the kineticism and fluidity of dance, but she acknowledged her frequent preoccupation with the scale and presence of the human body moving through space. "Dance," said Nevelson, "made me realize that air is a solid through which I pass, not a void in which I exist."[54] A work on paper, *For Dance Design* (1937, Whitney Museum of American Art, New York) and her 1945 terra cotta series called *Moving-Static-Moving Figure* suggest the sculptor's focused explorations of dance movement. In a more general way Nevelson looked to Graham's dance sets as she evolved the sculptural concept of grouped gridded boxes that could be rearranged in space, some even functioning as walk-in environments for the viewer.

# 2

# African American Dance and Art
*A Confluence of Traditions from Minstrelsy to the Harlem Renaissance*

By the 1870s, when the West was still dancing out a complex interplay between myth and artistic representation, another cultural tradition, the American minstrel show, had reached its full flowering. Minstrelsy crystallized in the 1840s as combined performances of dance, songs, and jokes. Despite the paralyzing stereotypes of African Americans endemic in the heyday of American minstrelsy, talented performers, often appearing as the dancing and singing "Negro Boy" became important subjects in American art of the antebellum period. In paintings and especially in popular prints, the entertainers developed their own national audience and, like the live performances of traveling dancers who crisscrossed America, created common experiences for people otherwise unconnected.

Painter James Goodwyn Clonney (1812–67) included an African American dancer in his most ambitious painting, *Militia Training* (1841; fig. 29). Amid more than thirty figures, the dancing boy provides a focal point for many watchers in this lively genre scene. Clonney's dancer is African American, but in many works the "Negro boy dancing" was performed by white men in blackface, a character who became a stock clown in dance halls and circuses. For better or worse, prints and paintings of such subjects largely defined minstrel images for the American public. One such lithograph, *American Theatre Bowery New York (c. 1833),*[1] was likely the parent image for a later anonymous oil depicting an overflow crowd gathered on November 25, 1833, to watch a performance of the famous, original "Jim Crow" character created by blackface performer Thomas Dartmouth "Daddy" Rice (1808–60). In both print and painting (1833; fig. 30), the scene conveys at least as much about the audience as about the finer points of the performance. The occasion marks Rice's fifty-seventh performance "jumping" (dancing) and singing before some three thousand rowdy patrons in this sprawling middlebrow theater in lower Manhattan. Throughout the evening the action onstage had to compete with that in the audience. Rice created the character Jim Crow by appropriating the songs and dance of an elderly African American stablehand in Kentucky. For Rice, the character turned into pure gold, making him a celebrated and wealthy star of the eastern theatrical circuit. More durable than Rice's personal success was the term *Jim Crow,* which entered American speech as a stinging reference to segregationist codes perpetuated for decades after the Civil War.

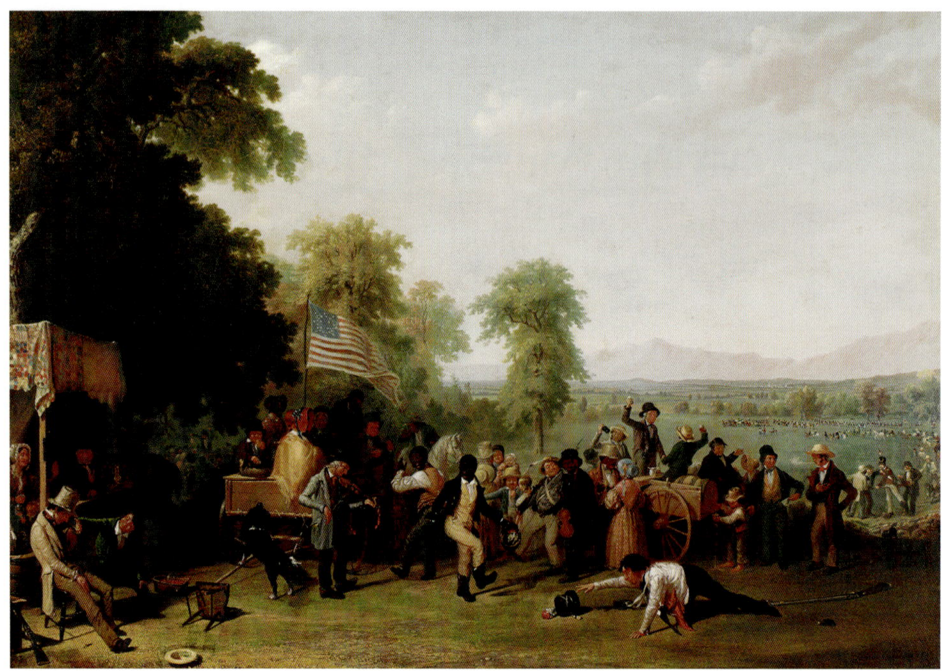

**Figure 29** James Goodwyn Clonney, *Militia Training*, 1841, oil on canvas 28 × 40 inches. (courtesy Pennsylvania Academy of the Fine Arts, Philadelphia, Bequest of Henry C. Carey, The Carey Collection, 1879.8.1)

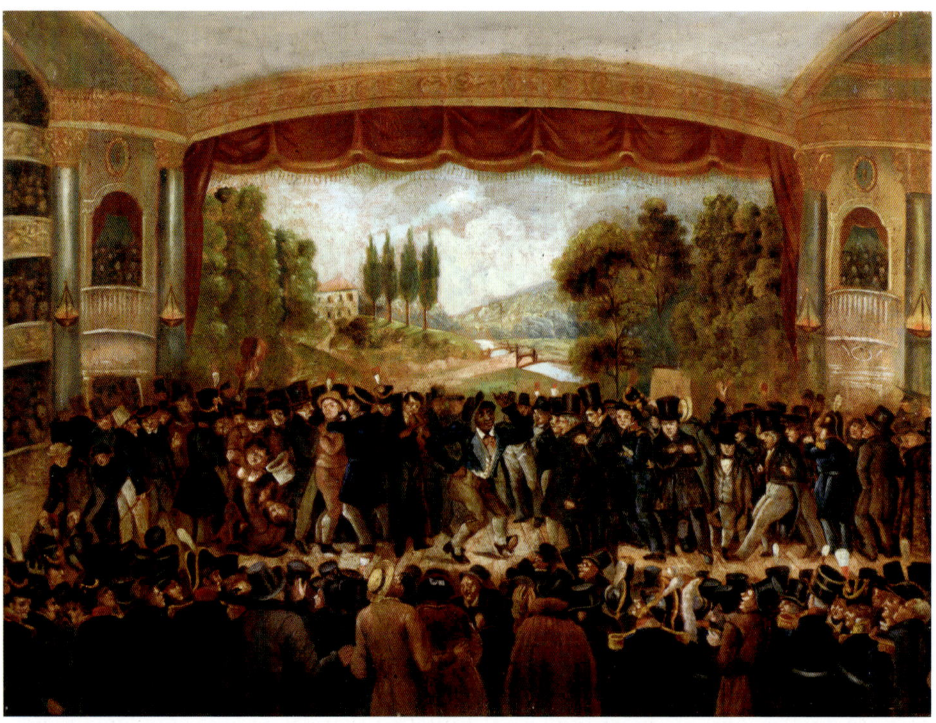

**Figure 30** Anonymous, *American Theatre, Bowery, New York*, 1833, oil on canvas, 22 × 30½ inches. (Museum of the City of New York, Gift of Carl F. Grieshaber, 32.483)

Daddy Rice's fame spread far beyond his live audiences through prints of his Jim Crow character.[2] In another (fig. 31) he is presented as the erstwhile dandy fallen on hard times: in flowing tie, ragged cutaway coat and waistcoat, patched trousers and worn-out shoes, Jim Crow dances in animated fashion, seemingly untroubled by his downtrodden appearance. On the banks of some tropical waterway, his companions are jungle denizens: crocodiles, frogs, and—most odious to modern viewers—simian types tricked out, like the dancer himself, in city finery. Such linkages, of African Americans (even blackface imposters) with jungle contexts, made them emblems of two denigrating cultural categories: first, they were closely allied to wild nature and the world of animals. Second, they were simultaneously exotic, that is fascinating in their difference, their cultural apartness from Anglo-American life. In this they belong to a lineage of African performers stretching back to the exotic blackamoors in a Rameau ballet opera. Images such as that of "Daddy" Rice were meant to amuse, underscoring the comedic elements of the minstrel show. And they no doubt did amuse consumers of these popular prints.

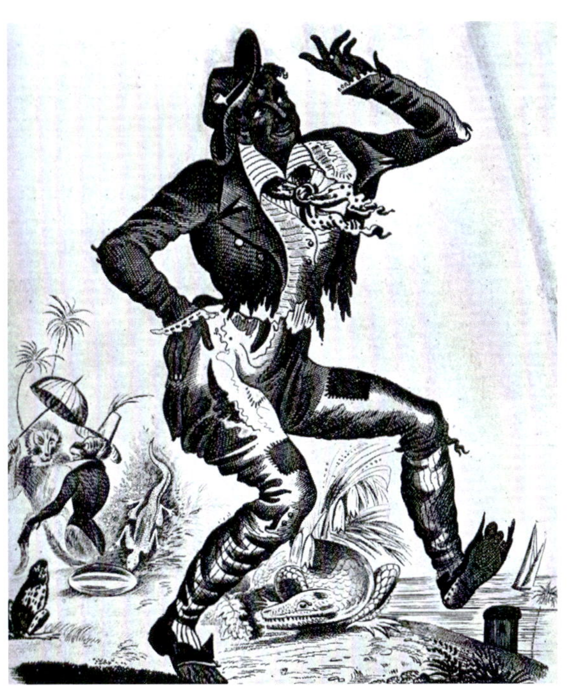

Figure 31 Anonymous, "Jim Crow" character created by blackface performer Thomas Dartmouth ("Daddy") Rice, n.d.

So pervasive were the stereotypes of African American dancers that they found their way into the prints of Winslow Homer (1836–1910), working during the Civil War as an artist-reporter embedded with the Union army. One of his earliest scenes of camp life, a wood engraving published in *Harper's Weekly,* is *A Bivouac Fire on the Potomac* (1861; fig. 32).[3] Homer was always at his best as a storyteller, and his wartime visual bulletins from the front conveyed narratives, both tragic and faithful, of what he saw. This engraving is an unusually

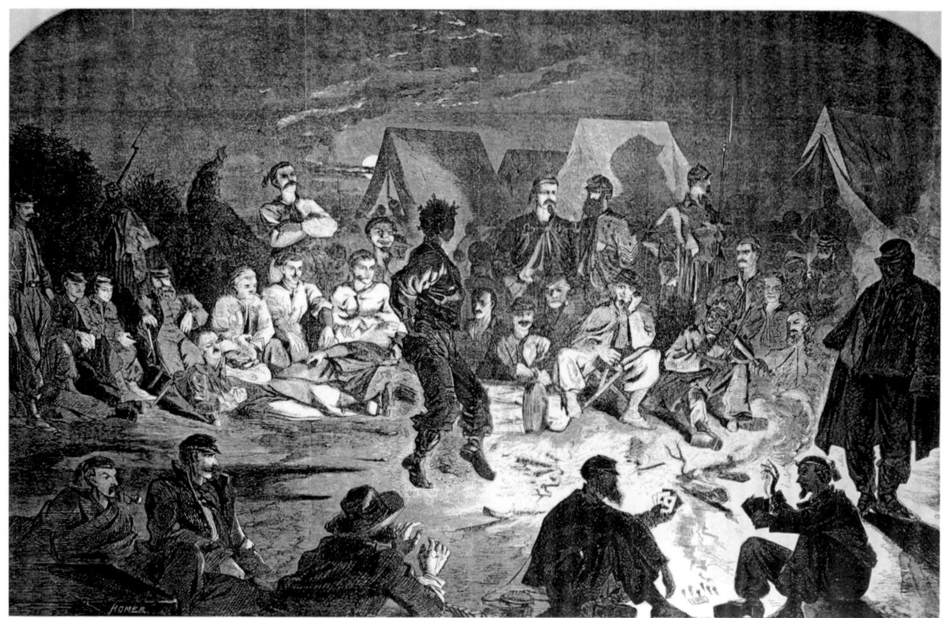

**Figure 32** Winslow Homer, *A Bivouac Fire on the Potomac*, wood engraving. (from *Harper's Weekly*, December 21, 1861)

lively image for the laconic Homer: around an evening campfire soldiers gather to watch an African American dancing to the music of a fiddler. The entertainment animates many of their fire-lit faces, caught in a rare moment of respite from the war's grisly daytime reality. The presence of the African Americans (sometimes escaped slaves) was not unusual in a Union camp. Many joined the ranks, some fighting on the battlefields, others assigned mostly menial tasks such as cooking and mule-driving. Later Homer would create complex, psychologically nuanced paintings of war's misery and boredom, but this early print, created for popular audiences eager for news from the front, conveys fact into art by means of existing stereotypes: with his tattered clothes and corkscrew curls, Homer's camp dancer reenacts the minstrel topos of Daddy Rice and his many fellow minstrel performers, the high-stepping black dancer entertaining a white audience.

Besides amusing American mass audiences, what the minstrel images did as well was to obscure the original contributions of African Americans to American music and dance. Much later, when the photographer Walker Evans (1903–75) hired on with the Farm Security Administration to help document the people and places of the South during the Great Depression of the 1930s, he came across old minstrel-show posters in Alabama towns. In the anonymously drawn *J. C. Lincoln's Sunny South Minstrels* (1936; fig. 33) the poster peels away from the surface of a brick wall, the process a ghostly reminder of the agonizingly slow eradication of black stereotypes in theatrical entertainment. But even as Evans's camera captured minstrelsy as a surviving anachronism in the 1930s, Thomas Hart Benton was painting a performance by a traveling minstrel troupe in the Midwest (1934; fig. 34). Painted during the year when Benton catapulted

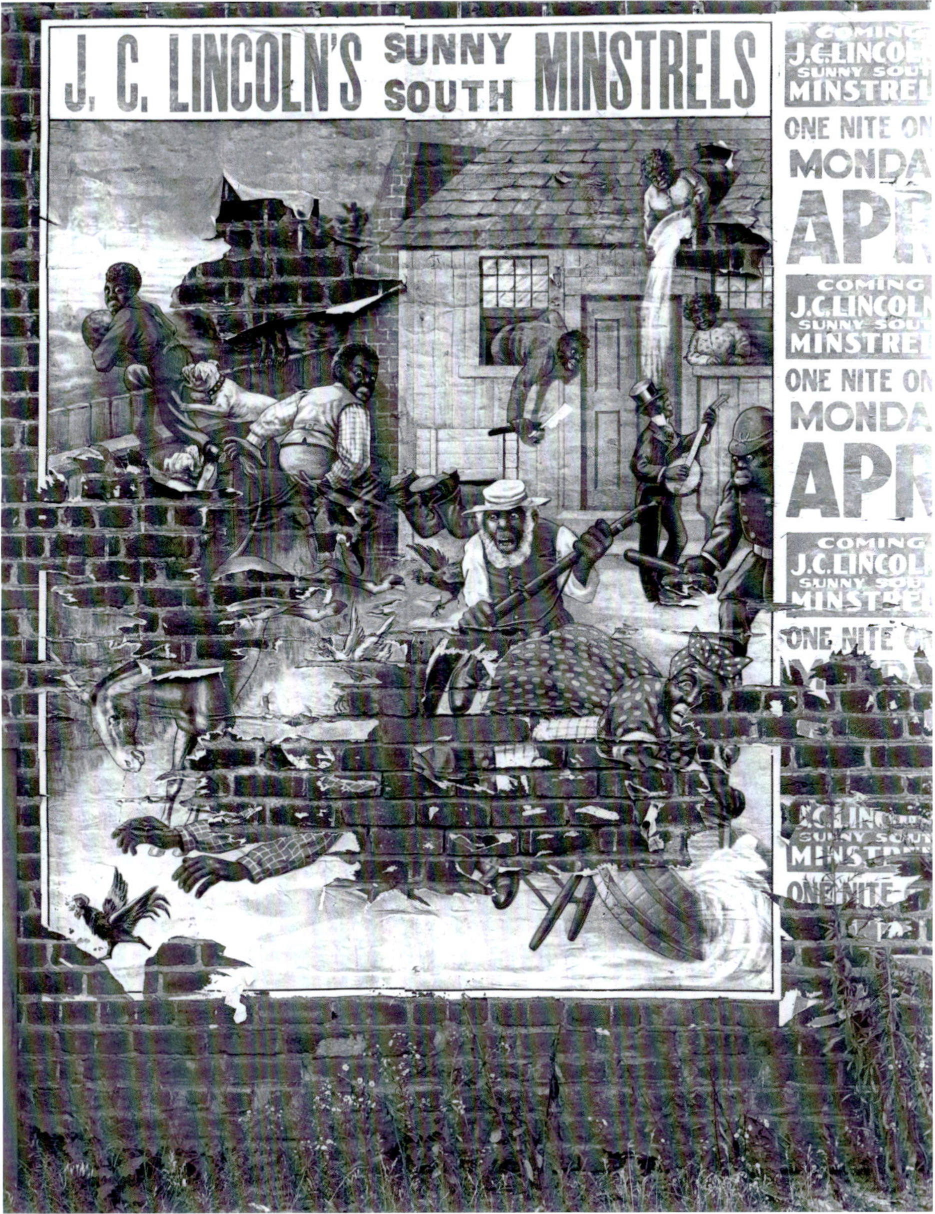


Figure 33 Walker Evans, photograph of poster of *J. C. Lincoln's Sunny South Minstrels*, 1936. (photo courtesy Library of Congress)

to national fame by popularizing (along with colleagues John Steuart Curry and Grant Wood) a "regional" American art, Benton chose subjects such as this to criticize what he perceived as the effete sophistication of eastern art culture. Although painted as if observed from life, one wonders if *Minstrel Show* portrays a memory from Benton's own Missouri boyhood, when such traveling troupes, featuring black (or blackface) dancers and musicians, often performed before audiences made up of rural whites. Here, against the simplest of

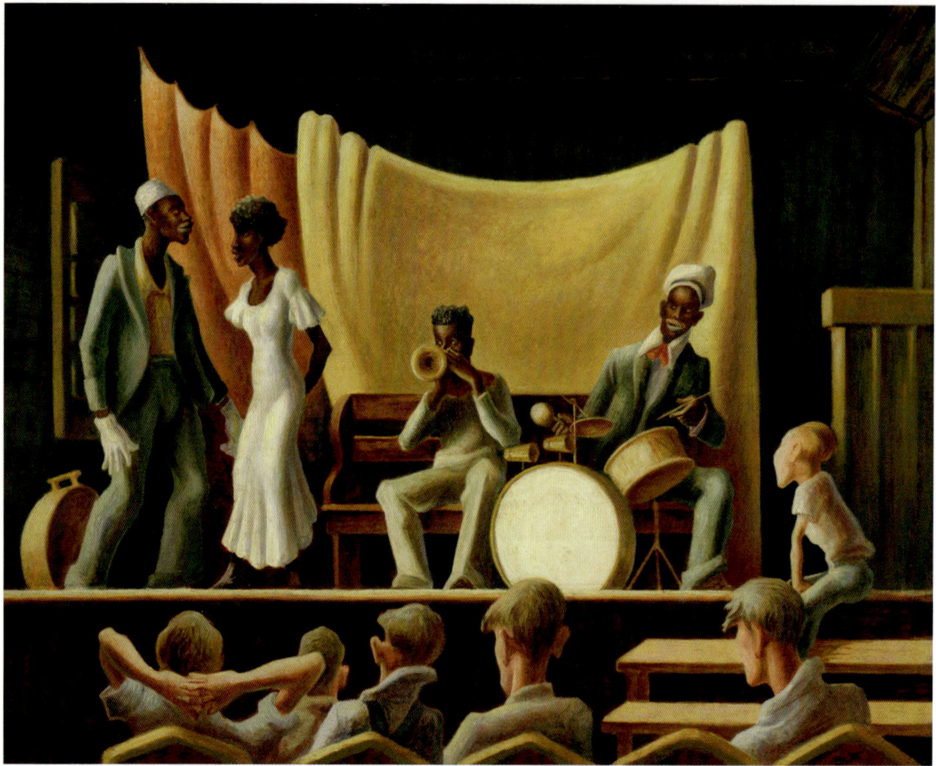

**Figure 34** Thomas Hart Benton, *Minstrel Show* 1934, tempera with oil on Masonite, 28 ⅜ × 35 ⅞ inches. (The Nelson-Atkins Museum, Kansas City, Missouri, Bequest of the artist, F75-21/13; photo: Jamison Miller; art © T. H. Benton and R. P. Benton Testamentary Trusts/UMB Bank Trustee/Licensed by VAGA, New York, New York)

temporary backdrops suspended from overhead wires, Benton's gently caricatured dancers have the rapt attention of their audience, especially the young lad at the right—perhaps a surrogate for Benton himself—who has climbed the stage steps for a close-up view.

However fondly he remembered it, by the time Benton painted his *Minstrel Show* the phenomenon was breathing its last gasp. Subject from its start to caricature both benign and malevolent, the minstrel tradition had been a feature of American life for nearly a century. And it had spawned some of America's greatest dancers, ranging from antebellum "dancing Negro boys" to transitional figures such as Josephine Baker, who would find ways to turn minstrel personae and "primitive" contexts to her own advantage.

Before continuing with the evolution of visual images grounded in the minstrel tradition, it would be useful here to look at two paintings—one of African American males, the other of European American females—that offer more complex and subtle variations on dance's role in postbellum American culture. Thomas Eakins (1844–1916) painted his watercolor *The Dancing Lesson [Negro Boy Dancing]* in 1878 (fig. 35). Unusual but not unique in his work, this dance subject is not a staged minstrel performance but—in a manner more like

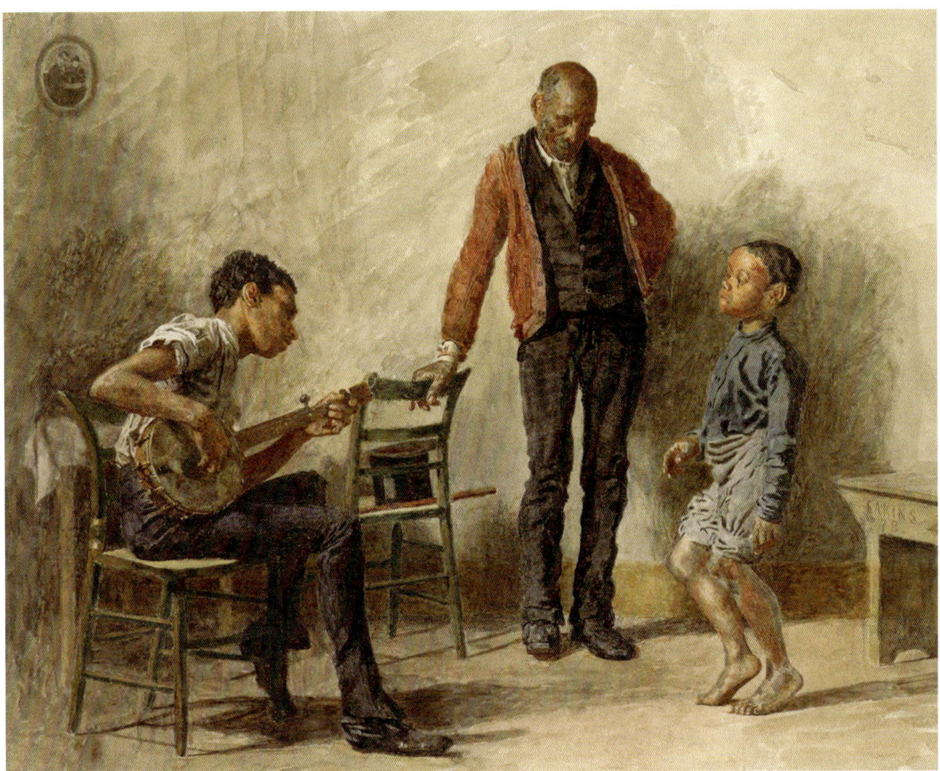

**Figure 35** Thomas Eakins, *The Dancing Lesson [Negro Boy Dancing]*, 1878, watercolor on off-white wove paper, 18 1/16 × 22 9/16 inches. (The Metropolitan Museum of Art, New York, Fletcher Fund, 1925, 25.97.1; image © The Metropolitan Museum of Art/Art Resource New York)

Eastman Johnson's—an informal, domestic scene.[4] Eakins's three figures are all African Americans, intelligently self-possessed. The young boy at the right practices a dance step to the tune strummed by a seated banjo player (at left), while an older man, who has placed his top hat and cane on the chair, watches his young protégé. The older man, perhaps the boy's grandfather, has likely just demonstrated the step to the barefoot youngster in this charming visual narrative. (One might almost imagine this as an episode from the dance training of the famous young dancer Juba, although no evidence supports such an interpretation.) As Eakins paints them, there is genuine connection, even tenderness, among the three males. But, unlike earlier images such as Johnson's, Eakins's *Dancing Lesson* may also be, in part, ideologically driven. Ideology, or at least a historical reference, enters by way of a small framed oval photograph in the composition's upper left where there hangs, as Martin Berger points out, a reproduction of a well-known 1864 Mathew Brady photograph of President Abraham Lincoln and his son Tad.[5] The parallels between the photograph and the African American family below it are clear: fatherly figures dominate in each scene, teaching their offspring, passing along knowledge to the next generation. But the whites transmit learning by way of the text Lincoln holds, while the blacks teach by way

59

of an oral/performance tradition. Beyond that, what Eakins's inclusion of the photograph also suggests is a continuing white patriarchal concern for African Americans, who are, in effect, the president's own symbolic children. Eakins, in juxtaposing these images, shows himself a painter of his own era, imbued with its history and symbolism. While abandoning the comic minstrel stereotype, he still looks at African Americans through their relationship to white culture.

American painter Cecilia Beaux (1855–1942) approached the subject of the dancing lesson from a distinctly different vantage point. While some of her early artistic training took place at the Pennsylvania Academy of the Fine Arts, the school where Thomas Eakins taught, she liked to say that his influence passed to her indirectly, through his pupils. Beaux admired Eakins's "deep steadfastness and sanity," qualities she tried to develop in her own portraits, which brought her renown in both the United States and Europe. Her sitters came from the fashionable world of New York and Philadelphia, mostly from families of her own privileged social class. Between 1898 and 1908 Beaux painted seven full-length double portraits, one of which is *The Dancing Lesson* (1898; fig. 36). Its subjects are Dorothea and Francesca Gilder, sisters painted from life in Beaux's temporary summer studio, an empty tobacco barn on the Gilders' farm in Tyringham, Massachusetts. The painting is a tour de force of fluid brushwork, paint texture and color—the artist at the height of her powers. Unusual in Beaux's oeuvre for its action, The Dancing Lesson also paints a lesson in female gentility, an older sister teaching her younger sibling how to move gracefully across a dance floor and, by implication, through life. These are proper young women, as we can judge from their gauzy, yet modest summer dresses. Like the males in Eakins's *Dancing Lesson,* they demonstrate that dance adds to the pleasures of life. But an important difference arises: while Eakins's young dancer may in fact be preparing for a stage career of dancing in top hat and cane, Beaux's young ladies are destined to entertain themselves in the sheltered world of genteel drawing rooms. However lively and individual, they are beautiful objects (like heroines out of the novels of Beaux's friend Henry James) who will never perform professionally, never need to earn their own keep. Their countenance is a secret smiling spirit of acceptance: with a kind of relaxed formality, their expressions and gestures acknowledge who they are and what their future holds. In strongly contrasting ways, dance was a protean signifier in the hands of both Beaux and Eakins. For each, dance pressed them to new technical achievements. And at the same time their varying contexts for dance situated their subjects within late nineteenth-century ideologies richly reflective of the era's race, gender, and class beliefs.

In the United States, inspired in part by dancers such as the legendary Juba (William Henry Lane, c. 1825–?), who was celebrated by Charles Dickens and applauded by audiences in both Europe and America, many other dancers of color took to theater stages. Over time, however, jobs for African American stage dancers grew scarce; most were filled by white minstrel-show performers in blackface, such as "Daddy Rice" and many others. Late in the nineteenth century the irony descended to a level of absurdity: racially segregated performances, where black dancers were not allowed to share the stage with whites, prevailed

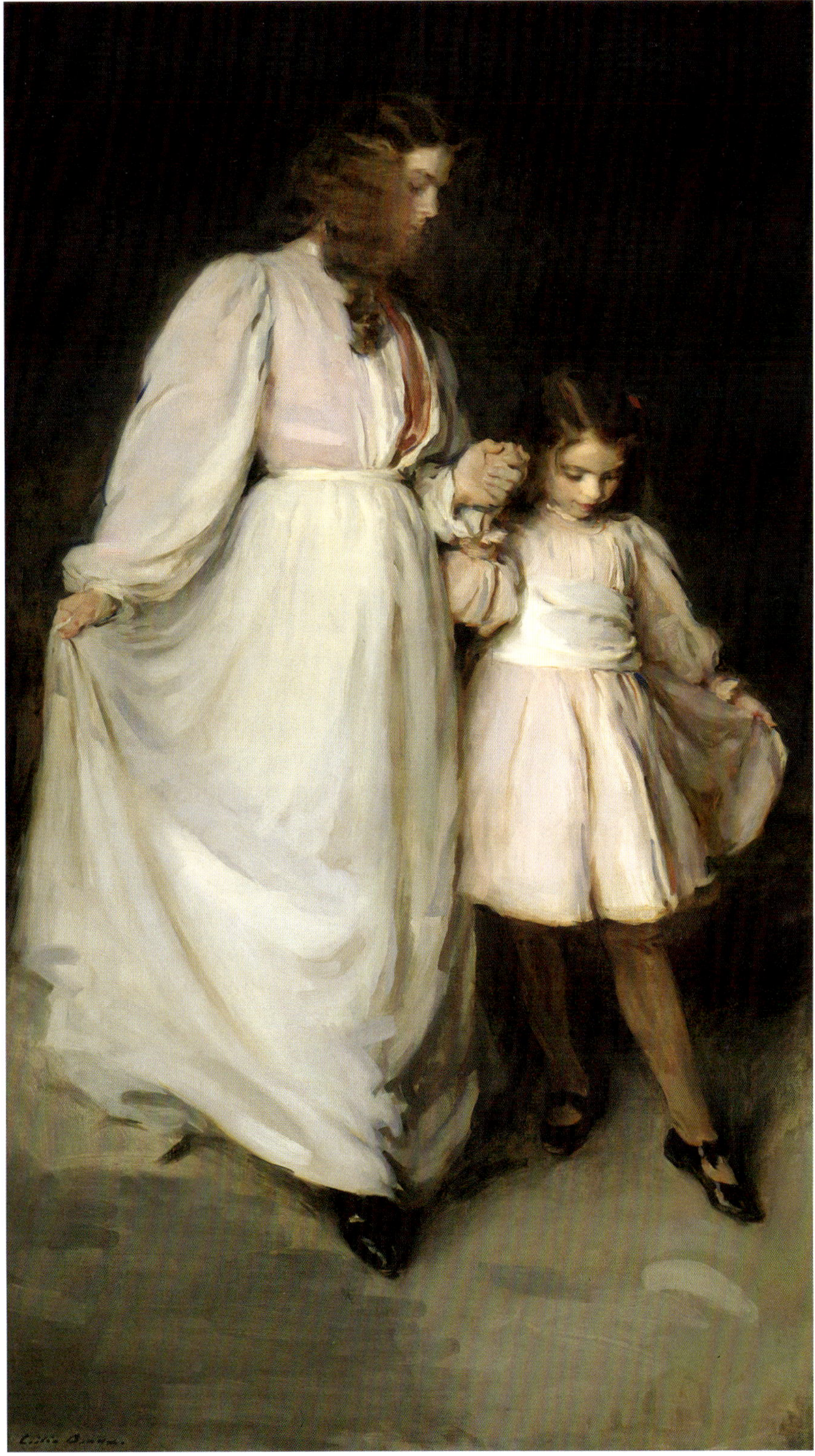

**Figure 36** Cecilia Beaux, *Dorothea and Francesca [The Dancing Lesson]*, 1898, oil on canvas, 80 ⅛ × 46 inches. (The Art Institute of Chicago, A. A. Munger Collection, 1921.109; photo © The Art Institute of Chicago)

for several decades. Still, instead of threatening the identity of African American music and dance, that separation forced a transition—from large-scale concert performance to more intimate social entertainment and varieties of social dance.

As reprehensible as theatrical segregation was, it did allow African Americans to concentrate on their own music in the dance halls of New Orleans, Saint Louis, and Chicago. In that emerging music, syncopated offbeats and rhythmic "breaks" became features of the dance as well as of instrumental performance. And the Cakewalk, a great exhibition dance, came into its own as an indigenous theatrical form. Like many dances, its origins were vague. Some sources described it as a dance contest derived from African harvest festivals (the winner of which "took the cake"); other accounts attribute the cakewalk's invention to slaves on southern plantations whose strutting movements were intended to mock the fancy manners of their white overseers. Whatever its genesis, the Cakewalk became a staple of blackface minstrel shows, part of high-strutting finale "walk-arounds." One such "walk-around" was described in a *New York Herald* feature from Juba's day as a comic display featuring "the lean, the fat, the tall, the short, the hunchbacked and the wooden-legged, all mixed in and hard at it." Those unfortunate characterizations found their visual counterparts in some popular images of the Cakewalk, such as Thomas Worth's Reconstruction-era watercolor reproduced by Currier & Ives (*De Cake Walk: For Beauty, Grace and Style; de Winner Takes de Cake* [1884, Collection of Museum of the City of New York]). Part of a series of "Darktown Comics" produced by Currier & Ives, the racist implications of *De Cake Walk* are clear: while advertised as "good-natured" and "free from coarseness or vulgarity," images of the African American residents of the fictitious "Darktown"—in this case the garishly dressed female cake-walkers—are in fact held up for ridicule before an audience of white consumers.

Later, as minstrelsy declined and Reconstruction's venomous caricatures faded into tired clichés, the Cakewalk made a triumphant return to American stages everywhere. It became an American craze, a kind of domestic counterpart to the unbridled European cancan. While popular imagery from sheet-music covers perpetuated a segregated "Darktown" legacy (*Darktown Strutters Ball*, 1917), the Cakewalk had by that time transcended racial stereotypes to become something else: a dance promenade of decided gentility, as in an anonymous American watercolor from about 1890 (Museum of Modern Art, New York). Here the handsome African American performers are the epitome of gilded-age style, not "Darktown" style. Outfitted in fashionable top hats, canes, fans, and gloves, these cake walkers have been painted within a delicate Victorian-style setting, preserved as if on an ornate greeting card of the era. They show the evolution of the Cakewalk into a competitive couple dance, each team judged by its fast steps, high kicks, leaps, and intricate turns—all of which made it thrilling to watch, whether by ordinary dance-hall observers or by visual artists. So engaging was the Cakewalk that it inspired countless expressions, easily crossing boundaries between the "high" and the "low" in the visual and performing arts. In 1910, for example, Claude Debussy wrote "Golliwogg's Cakewalk," one of three popular cakewalks he composed for piano.[6] From minstrel shows this extraordinary dance had migrated to performance venues before mixed-race audiences

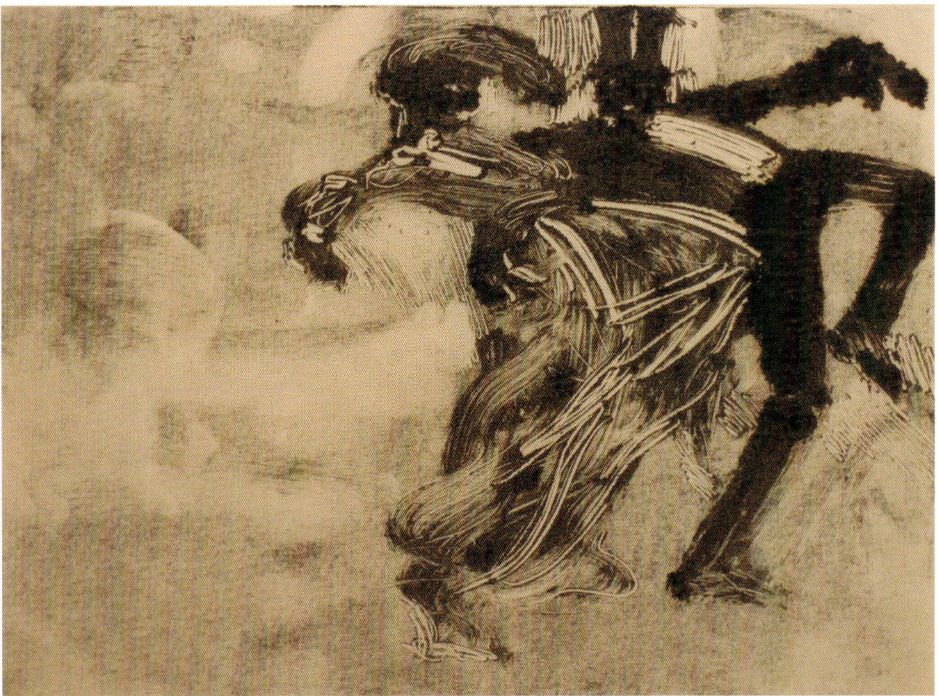

**Figure 37** George B. Luks, *Cake Walk*, 1907, monotype on paper, 5 × 7 inches. (Delaware Art Museum, Gift of Helen Farr Sloan, 1978, 1978–45)

in vaudeville and eventually into film, leaving a lasting legacy in American musical comedy.[7]

American visual artists found the infectious energy of the Cakewalk irresistible. George Luks, who had recently painted the immigrant experience in his *Spielers,* looked again through the versatile lens of dance at another aspect of America. In his monotype *Cake Walk* (1907; fig. 37) Luks captured the flashy footwork of professional performers. His high-stepping couple moves with such unstoppable energy they nearly escape the composition. Luks understood how to release the cake walk's exuberance for the viewer: he seems to anticipate— and resolve in advance—the incipient conflict between abstraction and representation in painting. He makes pure aesthetic sensation transcend subject matter, engaging the viewer in a response that is not merely perceptual but vividly physical, even visceral.

Theresa Bernstein (1890–2002), another urban realist associated with the Ashcan school, shared with Luks a desire to paint life as she observed it in city streets and public gathering places, especially those where music and dance were performed. Her *The Cakewalk—New Orleans* (c. 1948–50; fig. 38) appears to date from a time when Cakewalk performances had all but disappeared from the American scene, except for occasional reenactments in places such as New Orleans. In any case, her Cakewalk, like that of Luks made decades earlier, is essentially about the energy of the dance. Everything moves in this composition, even the cake held aloft by the central female dancer. Throughout, Bernstein's

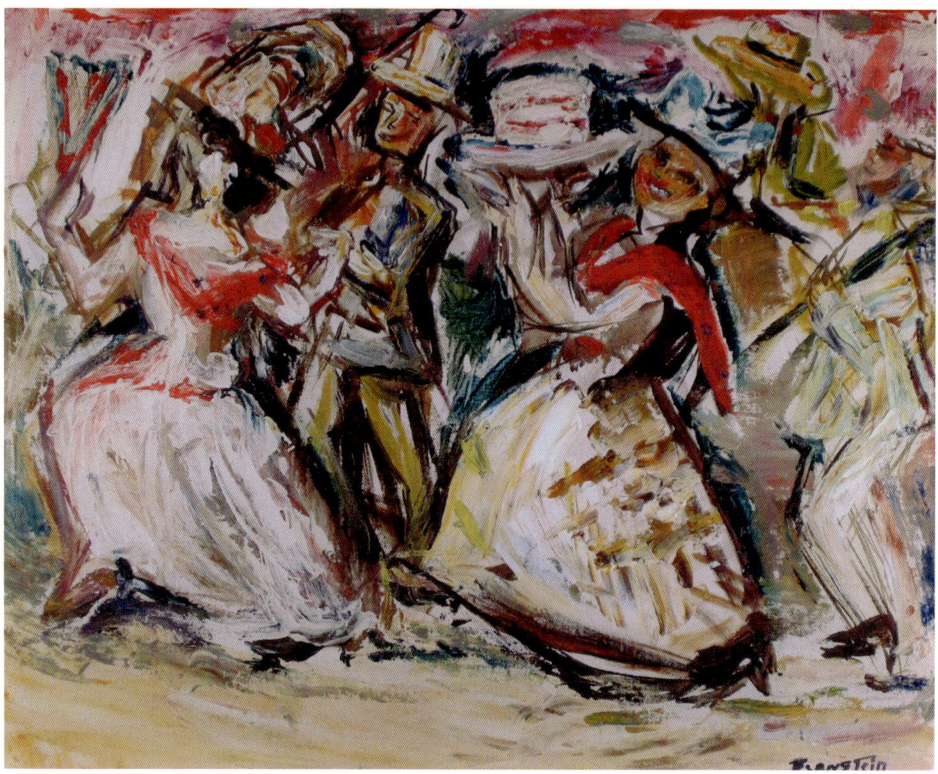

**Figure 38** Theresa Bernstein, *The Cakewalk—New Orleans*, c. 1948–50, oil on canvas, 20 × 24 inches. (collection George H. Ward, Milford, Connecticut)

bold, angular line and her vivid accents of black, red, blue, and gold, applied like thick strokes of cake frosting, pulse with the rhythm of the room. "My approach to painting is direct," Bernstein said. "I try to keep my expressions in touch with life and to enlarge upon these works with a technique that will best express the motive."[8] In that effort—matching her technique to the frenetic energy of the Cakewalk—Bernstein succeeds admirably.

## Seeking Roots: Dance and the Harlem Renaissance

After the turn of the twentieth century African American artists faced the challenge of moving beyond lingering racial stereotypes embedded in a Jim Crow culture that still disenfranchised and oppressed them.[9] Poet Langston Hughes lamented,

> I swear to the Lord
> I still can't see
> Why Democracy means
> Everybody but me.

64

Still, if social equality eluded African Americans in Hughes's day, they could draw on artistic expressions of all kinds to promote a nascent black consciousness. Hughes's poem "Dream Variation" muses on a black identity that borrows its energy from dance, using light/dark metaphors taken directly from nature:

> To fling my arms wide
> In some place of the sun,
> To whirl and to dance
> Till the white day is done.
> Then rest at cool evening
> Beneath a tall tree
> While night comes on gently,
>     Dark like me—
> That is my dream!

For Hughes and many others, dance and ritual became keys to opening many varieties of black consciousness, expressed by African American artists with infinite subtlety throughout the range of cultural production. While African American dancers and artists had long found common aesthetic roots in tragedy, oppression, and injustice, after World War I growing numbers of them were ready to move beyond a cultural history fixed and defined by the West. What they found often fortified an emerging critique of colonialism in art. Notions of the "primitive," if they remained part of that emergent history at all, would be increasingly complex and self-determined.

While some theorists, notably Alain Locke, would continue to argue for a "pure" form of black aesthetics, some Black artists looked to Africa and Egypt for cultural forms that could help to revive a creative cultural force. Writers such as W. E. B. DuBois (1868–1919) heightened interest in Pan-Africanism early in the century. In his book *The Negro* (1915) DuBois called Africa "at once the most romantic and most tragic of continents. Its very names reveal its mystery and wide reaching influence. It is the 'Ethiopia' of the Greeks, the 'Kush' and 'Punt' of the Egyptians, and the Arabian 'Land of the Blacks.'"[10] Howard Carter's 1922 discovery (and subsequent publication) of the treasures of Tutankhamun's tomb propelled Egyptology to a new level of popularity, as well as scientific interest. Building on information derived from travel literature, from archaeology (and enhanced access to Egyptian antiquities in museum collections), African American artists delved into Pan-African themes, particularly the relationship between Egypt and Ethiopia, as a mine of visual sources.

DuBois believed, for example, that ritual was a key to understanding links between generations, even epochs, in Africa. Might tribal dance also be a means to discover bridges between African and Western realities? Many historic rituals had been destroyed for American blacks through slavery and oppression. But some black choreographers and visual artists attempted to reconstruct or create new forms of movement ritual. One of them was Aaron Douglas (1899–1979), the first African American painter to engage with both African art and modernism. In such works as *Aspects of Negro Life: The Negro in an African Setting,*

Douglas began to investigate, in serial fashion, the legacy of ritual, especially ritual dance. In a splendid study for the first panel of this WPA/FAP-sponsored mural at a public library in Harlem, Douglas painted an African couple dancing to the beat of drums (1934; fig. 39). Around them, concentric circles of light reinforce the rhythm of the dance, while a sculptured figure floats above them, suggesting the presence of spirits in their culture. While referencing the horizontal hand gesture familiar in older Egyptian art, Douglas's figures owe something as well to the active sense of life and movement introduced in the swelling, curvilinear forms of New Kingdom painted reliefs. Familiar from Akhenaton-era sculpture are Douglas's sleek, swept-back head and headdress profiles, combined with sharp angularities of bent limbs, the latter an old-new idiom as readily observable in Egyptian art as in the Cubist bodies Douglas saw in modern French paintings at Philadelphia's Barnes Foundation.[11]

Douglas worked at the Barnes Foundation on scholarship, sketching the African masks and Cubist paintings to which Albert Barnes gave equal prominence

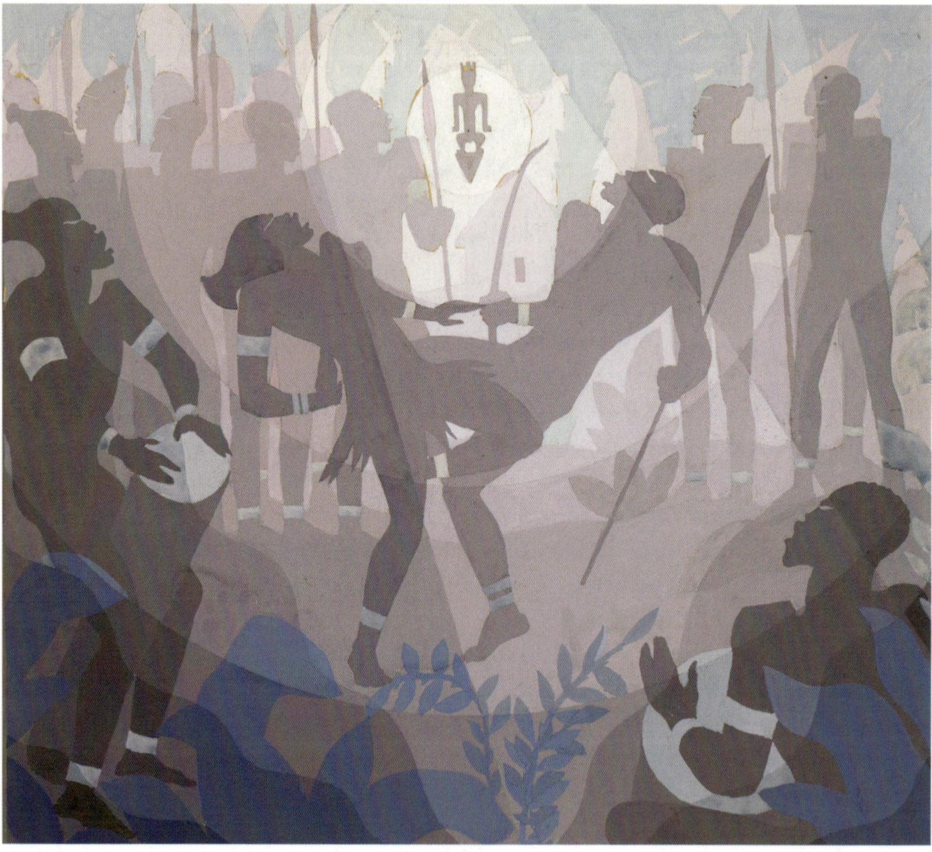

**Figure 39** Aaron Douglas, *Study for Aspects of Negro Life: The Negro in an African Setting*, 1934, gouache with touches of graphite on illustration board, 37 ¹/₁₀ × 40 ³/₅ inches. (Art Institute of Chicago, Solomon Byron Smith and Margaret Fisher funds, 1990.416; photo © The Art Institute of Chicago)

in his collection. Encouraged by Barnes to seek a modern "primitivism," Douglas was exposed to the twin benefits and limitations of the view that African art of the past could help modern African American artists to forge a platform upon which they could build a new racial self.

In short, the study of Africa and Egypt provided an expanded scope for understanding who and what the "New Negro" might represent. Sculptor Meta Vaux Warrick Fuller (1877–1968) took a Pan-Africanist approach in her work, acknowledging in it a hereditary union between black Africa and black America. Born into a middle-class Philadelphia family who encouraged her interest in art, Warrick studied at the Pennsylvania School of Industrial Art, and then won a scholarship for study in Paris. Upon her arrival there in 1899 she became friends with the American black expatriate painter Henry O. Tanner, and subsequently with Auguste Rodin, both of whom encouraged her work. She also met W. E. B. Du Bois in Paris, and through him broadened her understanding of nationhood and the colonial experience in the United States and abroad. By 1902 she was exhibiting at S. Bing's famous gallery for modern art and design, L'Art Nouveau. Under Rodin's influence, she showed a number of dance subjects at the gallery, including *Oriental Dancer* and *Danseuse* (both now unlocated). Given the dance activity in Paris in those years, and especially given Rodin's attention to such American dancers as Loïe Fuller and Isadora Duncan, one wonders whether Warrick might have been depicting those American dancers in Paris.

Following Warrick's 1909 marriage to Liberian-born psychologist Dr. Solomon Fuller, the couple settled permanently in Framingham, Massachusetts. Although she was not officially connected to the Harlem Renaissance and never lived in that area, Warrick made art that forecast some of its themes. Her best-known work is *Ethiopia Awakening* (1914, formerly, Schomburg Center for Research in Black Culture, New York Public Library), which anticipates by a decade the New Negro, proclaimed in 1925 by Alain Locke as a model of black society. It is an image of a beautiful black woman whose head and torso emerge from the wrappings of a mummy, a clear metaphor for the African American experience of reaching forth from bondage to freedom. Despite her frequent use of solemn, even macabre, black subject matter (*The Talking Skull*, 1937, Museum of Afro-American History, Boston), Warrick explored other areas as well, sometimes returning to subjects of the dance to make African American statements in visual form. Her *Bacchante* (1930, collection of Solomon Fuller, Bourne, Massachusetts) expresses the liberating ecstasies of dance, a subject discussed at length in part 2. Here, as often in Warrick's work, the subject serves as yet another metaphor of the black American experience.

African American sculptor Richmond Barthé (1901–89) achieved renown for his bronze dancers. They, like the dance subjects of Douglas and Warrick, link Western aesthetics, sometimes even modern dance of the 1930s, with tribal dance. Trained at the Art Institute of Chicago in the early 1920s, Barthé developed a skilled naturalism into which he incorporated aspects of African sculptural form. Understanding that dance and ritual are closely related in African art, Barthé's figures often demonstrate a connection, by means of posture and physical movement, to African ceremonial art. Barthé's *Kalombwan* (1934; fig. 40), and his *African Dancer* (1932–33, Whitney Museum of American Art, New York) demonstrate such affinities for African art very clearly in their characteristic bent-knee and bent-armed stance. At the 1933 annual exhibition of the Whitney Museum, *African Dancer* generated both critical and popular interest for its convincing portrayal of the lyrical dancing body.

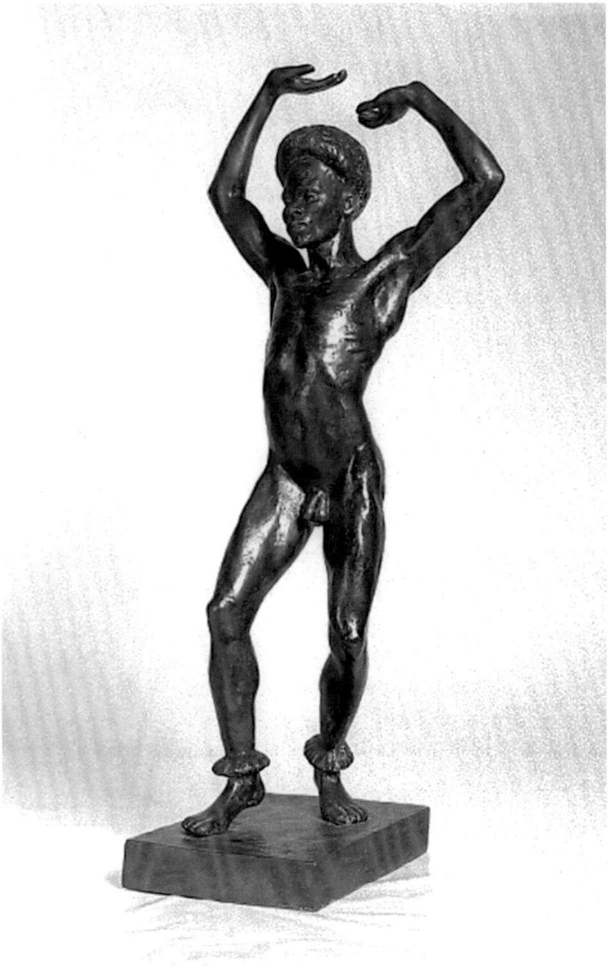

Barthé's sculpted dancers also warrant comparison with similar prototypes from the ancestral continent where, as early as the seventeenth century, Western visitors had noted the postures of African dance: "The most desirous of dancing are the women, who dance without men, and but one alone, with crooked knees and bended bodies they foot it nimbly."[12] Despite their naturalism and idealization, Barthé's dancers show decided connections with that postural tradition, as well as with a Yoruba sculpture made in Africa only a few years before his. Olowe of Ise (d. 1938) carved a covered divination bowl made to hold ceremonial objects, atop which four women, their knees slightly bent, link arms in a ritual circle dance. It is an African dance posture consciously assisting communion with the divine, perhaps the destiny-revealing god Olodumare (c. 1925; fig. 41). Separated by vast cultural distances, Olowe's dancers are nonetheless kin to Barthé's African dancers. Taken out of ritual context and anchored firmly within a Western sculptural tradition, Barthé here speaks in an African-derived visual dialect of the powerful relational language of dance.

Barthé went on to demonstrate his versatility with dance subjects by representing yet another kind: the vernacular dance of his own era. According to Carl Van Vechten, a close observer of the Harlem Renaissance, in 1928 the new dance known as the Lindy Hop (named after the famed American aviator who

**Figure 40** Richmond Barthé, *Kalombwan*, 1934, bronze, 30⅜ × 12 inches. (collection Hampton University Museum, Richmond Barthé Trust)

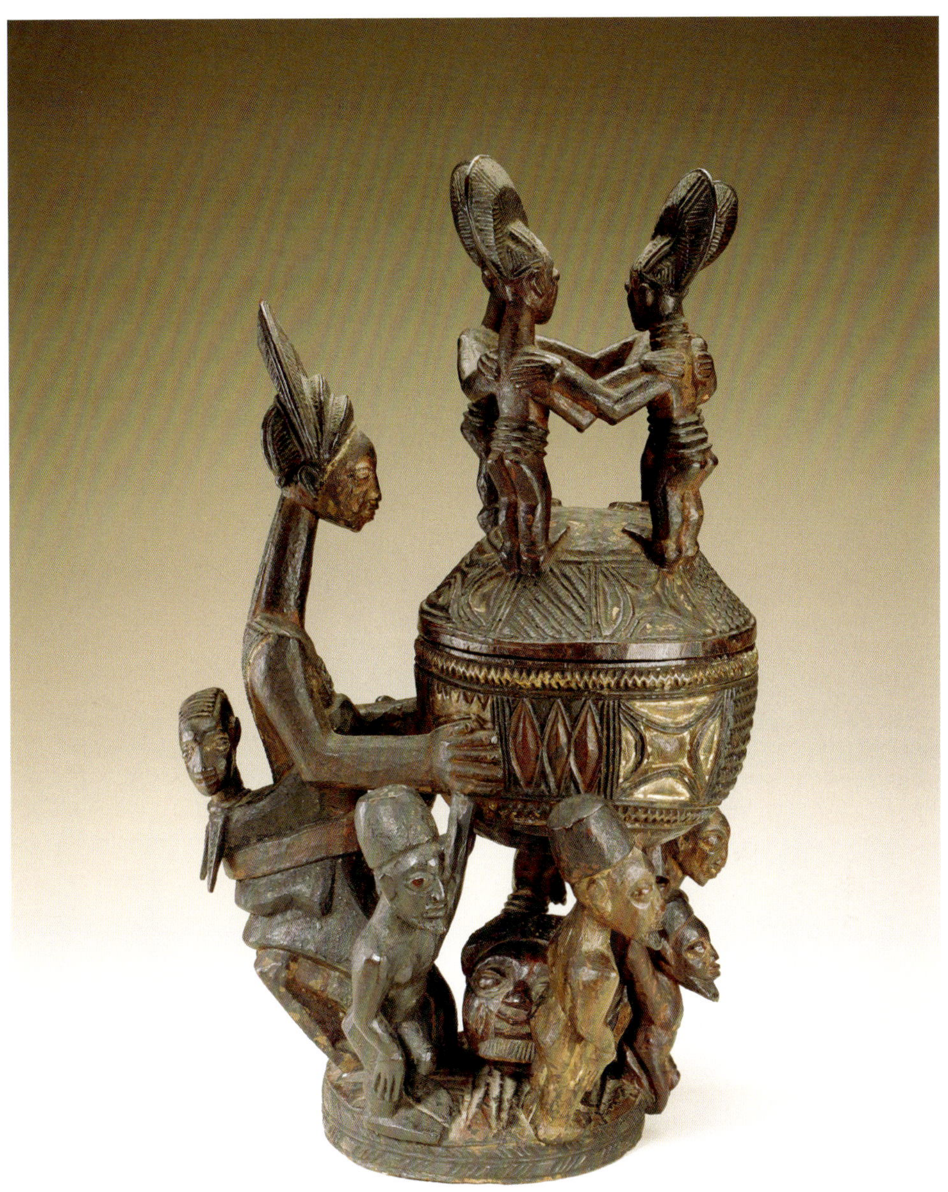

**Figure 41** Olowe of Ise (Yoruba peoples, Nigeria), *Bowl with Figures* (carved divination bowl), c. 1925, wood, pigment, 25 ¹/₁₆ × 13 ⁵/₁₆ × 15 ³/₈ inches. (National Museum of African Art, Smithsonian Institution, Bequest of William A. McCarty-Cooper, 95-10-1; photo: Franko Khoury)

had recently "hopped" the Atlantic) was officially introduced at the Manhattan Casino. On that occasion, as described by Van Vechten, the new dance appeared to be "a certain dislocation of the rhythm of the Fox Trot, followed by leaps and quivers, hops and jumps, eccentric flinging about of arms and legs, and contortions of the torso."[13] An artist of lesser experience might have hesitated to take on such a catalog of moves, but Barthé had grown into a confident interpreter of dance. His *Lindy Hoppers* (1939; fig. 42) execute a daring dip as their bodies press close together in this new and visually exciting dance. The sheer materiality of Barthé's bronze dancers, their obdurate weight and solidity, testify to the almost physical power sculptural objects can exert over their beholders, a power sometimes lost or lessened in the more transient seductions of painting.

At first glance, the paintings of African American artist William H. Johnson (1901–70) might be taken for naive, expressive "folk" compositions, but a closer

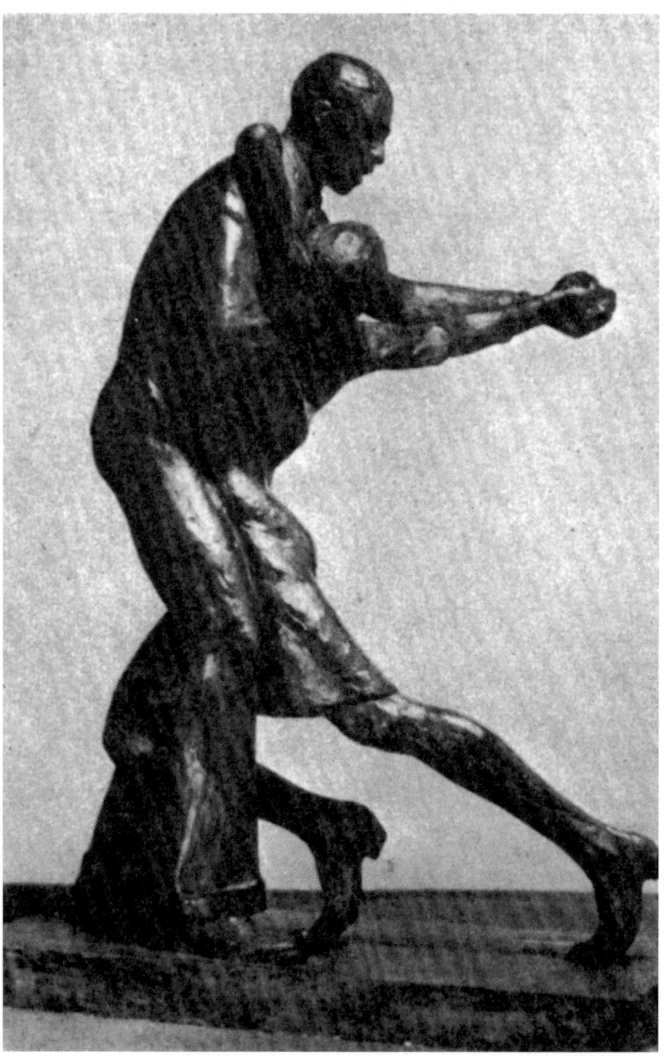

**Figure 42**
Richmond Barthé,
*Lindy Hoppers*, 1939,
bronze, n. dim. (Current
location unknown;
photo courtesy National
Archives, Washington,
D.C.)

look at this artist reveals them (and him) to be much more complex. Born in South Carolina, Johnson moved at seventeen to New York, where he put himself through the National Academy of Design, learning an essentially academic realist style. Upon graduation he headed for Europe, where he remained for most of the next fifteen years. In Paris, deeply affected by the expressionist work of Chaim Soutine, Edvard Munch, and Vincent Van Gogh, Johnson discarded his realism for a deliberate stylistic primitivism. As war clouds gathered in 1938, Johnson returned to the United States, where he settled in Harlem and found employment with the murals division of the WPA. Harlem's lively street life soon engaged the painter, who stripped down his palette, simplified and flattened his forms, and focused on aspects of African American life, both historic and contemporary. Johnson's reach was broad: his stated intent was "to give, in simple and stark form, the story of the Negro as he has existed."[14] Johnson's style of self-declared primitivism bewildered some viewers, who saw in it a troubling throwback to old "plantation" art and "colonialist" literature, such as seen in the sheet-music covers discussed above. The residue of old attitudes plagued this (indeed all) debate about primitivism: was Johnson buying into the old, always-dubious proposition that "primitive" art showed humanity at an earlier stage of development, or even at a lower evolutionary rung? Johnson defended his reductive style in terms of his own artistic agenda—a personal response to something cumulative in the larger African American experience: "My aim," he said, "is to express in a natural way what I feel, what is in me, both rhythmically and spiritually, all that which in time has been saved up in my family of primitiveness and tradition, and which is now concentrated in me."[15] In his painting *Jitterbugs II* (c. 1941; fig. 43), Johnson uses the subject of dance to convey the vibrant rhythmic and spiritual dynamic of black experience. In pose, Johnson's *Jitterbugs* seem based on the slightly earlier prototype of Barthé's sculpture *Lindy Hoppers* (fig. 42), but the difference in medium conveys a different emotional pitch. While Barthé's couple merge dramatically into a single sweeping C-curve, Johnson's couple—with their angular, energetic dance movements, bright colors, and bold patterns—express a post-Depression mood of swing culture, slang, and exuberance.

Archibald J. Motley, Jr. (1891–1981) was the first visual artist to study black nightlife in the cities. He challenged prevailing stereotypes, portraying his subjects as individuals, not types, and allowed them to move and socialize freely in his paintings of urban life. They dance, drink, and enjoy themselves in environments bathed in artificial or natural light and often suffused with the infectious energy of jazz. In *Nightlife* (1943; fig. 44), Motley takes viewers inside a club in Chicago's Bronzeville neighborhood, home to more than 90 percent of the city's black population in the 1930s. In *Nightlife,* the artist paints his figures as clear-cut elemental shapes, highly diverse in their appearances and reflective, as Motley said, "of a great variety of Negro characters" he identified among Chicago's African Americans.[16]

James VanDerZee (1886–1983) represents yet another aspect of dance in the Harlem Renaissance: his hundreds of photographs portrayed the urban personality of the New Negro. Perhaps best known today of all his Harlem

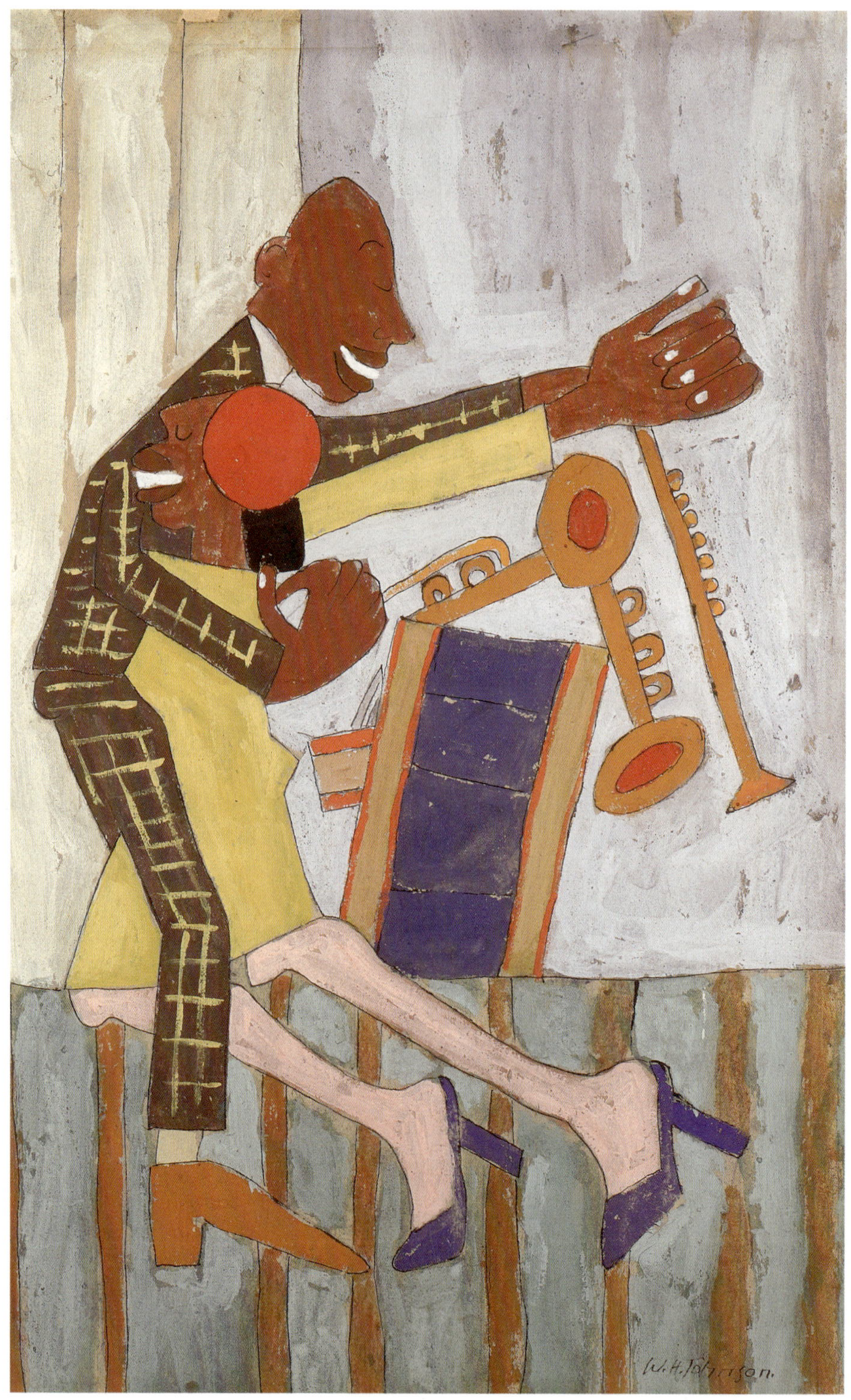

**Figure 43** William H. Johnson, *Jitterbugs II*, c. 1941, tempera, pen, ink, pencil on paper, 18 × 12 3/16 inches. (Smithsonian American Art Museum, Gift of the Harmon Foundation, 1967.59.1047R-V)

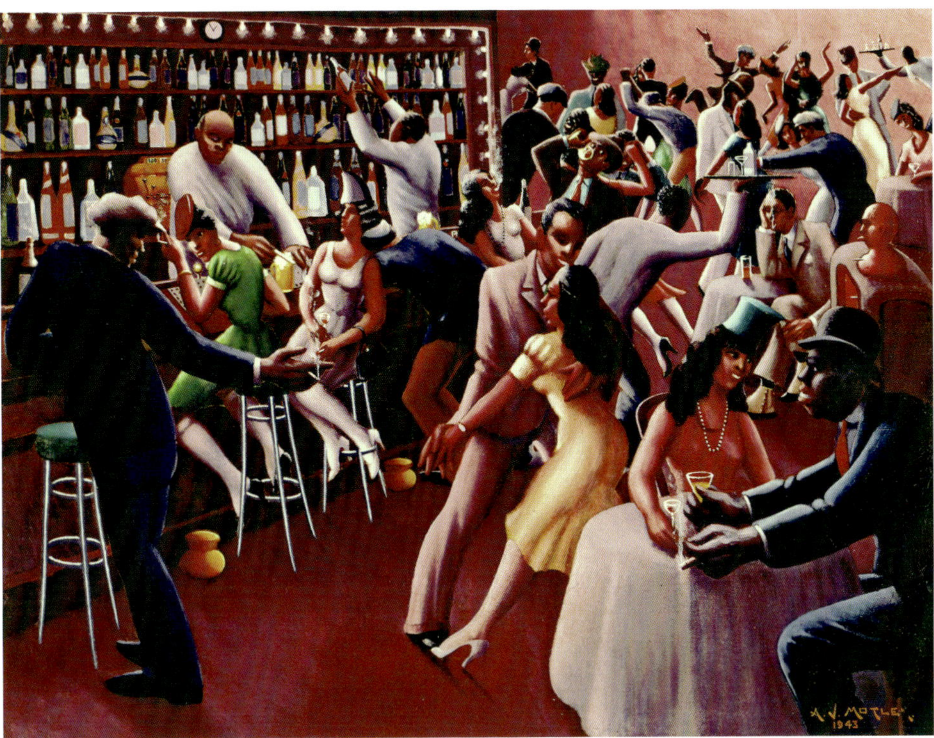

**Figure 44** Archibald J. Motley Jr., *Nightlife*, 1943, oil on canvas, 36 × 47⅘ inches. (Art Institute of Chicago, Restricted gift of Mr. and Mrs. Marshall Field, Jack and Sandra Guthman, Ben W. Heineman, Ruth Horwich, Lewis and Susan Manilow, Beatrice C. Mayer, Charles A. Meyer, John D. Nichols, Mr. and Mrs. E. B. Smith Jr.; James W. Alsdorf Memorial Fund, Goodman Endowment, 1992.89; photo © The Art Institute of Chicago)

contemporaries, VanDerZee was a painter and musician as well as photographer of celebrities, families, ceremonies, interiors, and street scenes. Dance formed such an important part of the social life and entertainment of Harlem in the 1920s and 1930s that VanDerZee used it to define a number of his sitters. In his studio VanDerZee photographed performers in their costumes, as in *Dancer, Harlem* (1925), resplendent in feathers, spangles, and harem pants. She is vaguely exotic, slightly sensual, and proud of who she is. By contrast, VanDerZee's *Tap Dancer* (1935) is an exuberant young female performer who shows off the bows and frills befitting her youth. Vastly different from each other, both dancers display the dignity that became a hallmark of VanDerZee's portraits. A third dance subject, *Dancing School* (1928; fig. 45), departs from their formal poses and staged backgrounds to capture five lively girls in a dance studio. Two moppets in the foreground—already stage veterans with their top hats and canes—pose coyly, while the three girls in the background, perhaps less accustomed to the camera, are caught candidly in mid-step. The effect is charming, a blending of the constructed artifice and authentic pride typical of VanDerZee's photographs.

In the collection assembled by Albert Barnes of Philadelphia there is a remarkable example of African American dance viewed by a white artist, Charles

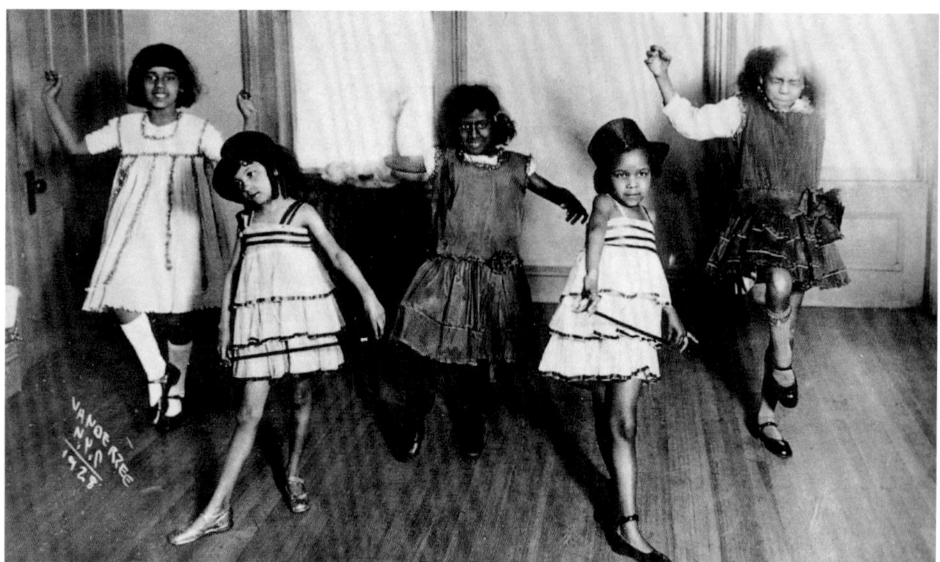

Figure 45 James VanDerZee, *Dancing School*, 1928, gelatin silver print, 5 ½ × 9 ¹⁵⁄₁₆ inches. (private collection)

Demuth (1883–1935). Barnes collected many watercolors by Demuth, ranging from his exquisite floral still lifes to his circus subjects. Of extraordinary vitality are his *Negro Dancing (At Marshall's)* (1917, Barnes Foundation Collection, Merion, Pennsylvania) and his *In Vaudeville [Dancer with Chorus]* (1918; fig. 46). Both are paintings of spectral intensity. In each, the tap dancer seems to float above the floor, head lowered, elbows raised symmetrically like a set of great wings. Demuth catches that nearly aerial aspect of some tap dancers, whose solo improvisations share as much with drumming, or gymnastics, as they do with floor-bound tap. The painter creates a stylized body for expressive purposes, pushing the dancer's salient character almost, but not quite, to the point of caricature.

In these anonymous dancers, observed in New York nightclubs, Demuth communicated an uncanny essence, something like the capture of a single, telling gesture beloved of poster designers. In those pre-Prohibition days the Marshall, a black club located under the Sixth Avenue El on West Fifty-third Street, was a favorite destination for Demuth and his artist friends, including Marcel Duchamp and Marsden Hartley. There and in Harlem clubs they formed part of a racially integrated clientele gathered to watch some of the most gifted black vaudeville performers of the day. Demuth's biographer describes one such remarkable scene: in his watercolor *Negro Jazz Band* (1916, private collection) the artist made a first-hand visual record of the celebrated "Florence Dunbar in an Irene Castle dress . . . dancing 'The Seven Veils' while singing 'Fatima Brown.'"[17]

Another artist who, like Demuth, could concentrate a black dancer's focused energy into a startling, graphically simplified image was Winold Reiss (1888–1953). Reiss, a German American painter who mentored Aaron Douglas, is best known for his portraits of Native Americans, yet he also made fine portraits of

African Americans. Reiss's ink drawing *Interpretation of Harlem Jazz I*
(c. 1925; fig. 47) forms a fascinating
comparison with Demuth's work.
Made the same year that Art Deco
was given its debut in Paris, Reiss's
drawing incorporates some of that
style's streamlined, linear elements.
Along with a female dance partner
dressed in syncopated black and
white stripes, Reiss includes musical instruments, a bottle, and elements of African design—in the
form of mask elements. Clearly he
seeks to express a synoptic view of
the Harlem jazz experience, rhythmically and graphically charged at
full bore.

The energy and rhythm of
American jazz would permeate the
art of Stuart Davis (1892–1964) for
decades. Davis started his artistic
career as a second-generation Ashcan
painter. These younger artists, who
also included George Bellows,
Edward Hopper, and Rockwell Kent,
shared the radical-realist spirit of the

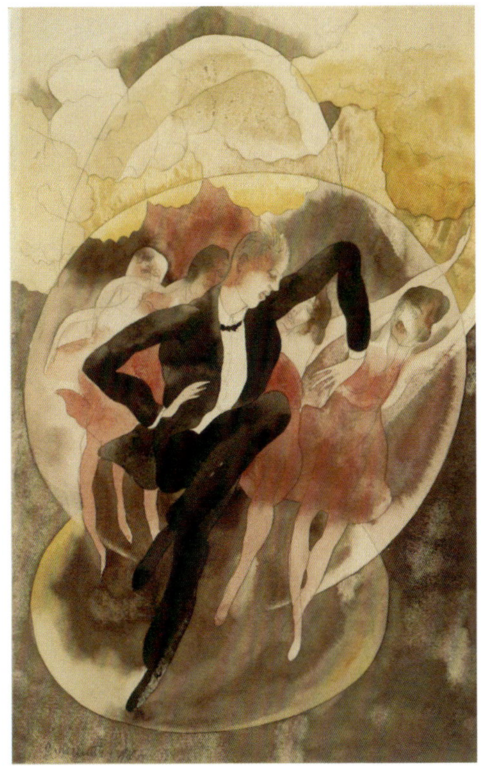

Figure 46 Charles Demuth, *In Vaudeville
[Dancer with Chorus]*, 1918, watercolor and
graphite on off-white wove paper, 13 × 8 ⅛
inches. (A. E. Gallatin Collection, Philadelphia
Museum of Art, 1952-61-18)

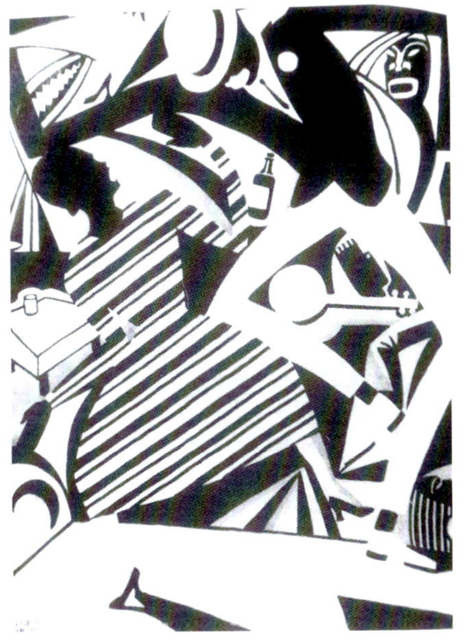

Figure 47 Winold Reiss,
*Interpretation of Harlem Jazz I*,
c. 1925, ink on paper, 19 ½
× 14 ½ inches. (from *Survey
Graphic* Magazine, 1925)

Eight, absorbing and extending the anarchic attitude that changed American art early in the century. Davis studied with Robert Henri between 1909 and 1911, adopting from him a love of themes from ordinary urban life. And, befriended by John Sloan, the younger Davis plunged into the politically charged Ashcan sphere and joined their efforts to break the hold of the conservative National Academy of Design on American art. After only three months of work in oil, Davis exhibited five canvases in the important 1910 Exhibition of Independent Artists. Sloan, who was art editor of the radical *The Masses*, invited Davis to contribute to the periodical. His illustrations, cartoons, and covers appeared often, inspired by the energetic European precedents of Daumier or Toulouse-Lautrec. Such artistic beginnings imbued Davis with a deeply felt aesthetic pluralism and a refusal to draw sharp distinctions between high and "low" art.

Pursuing themes drawn from urban experience, Davis often visited saloons and dance halls in the New York area, places where the pulse of the city beat strongest. He took a special fancy to the bands who played in the seamier clubs of Hoboken and Harlem. Davis made drawings of a number of these jazz-bar joints, such as *Negro Dance Hall* (1912–13, private collection). In that work he casts some of the then-prevalent stereotypes of African Americans as free and sensuous in their dance. On the floor in the background the woman dancer's pose—knees bent, buttocks thrust back—contributes to that sexually charged view of African Americans. When Davis's works in this vein were published in *The Masses*, a reader complained that they "depress[ed] the negroes themselves and confirmed the whites in their contemptuous and scornful attitude."[18] Max Eastman of the magazine staff defended Davis, saying that such criticism completely misconstrued Davis's intent, which was solely for art itself. One wonders how widespread such criticism was, and whether Davis downplayed such stereotyping thereafter. Whatever the cause, he began to focus more closely on investigating physical "facts" so as to establish objective order in his work. But that did not preclude his continuing interest in dance subjects. In fact, he would find some of that desired order precisely within jazz dance rhythms. In the Armory Show of 1913 one of the five works Davis showed was a watercolor called *Dance* (now unlocated). Besides his own, the artist saw a number of other dance-related subjects at the Armory: Picabia's *Dances at the Spring* (1912, Philadelphia Museum of Art); Matisse's *Nasturtiums with the Painting "Dance"* (1912, Metropolitan Museum of Art, New York) and, most notably, Van Gogh's *Bal à Arles [Dancehall at Arles]* (1888; fig. 48).[19] All three of these important European works incorporated non-naturalistic color and shape patterning, two formal directions Davis was already considering. He then painted a new work, *The Back Room, Bar House, Newark* (1913; fig. 49), incorporating some of Van Gogh's juicy impasto and color: Prussian blues, greens, and oranges dabbed on heavily. The figures in Davis's *Back Room, Bar House* wear impassive masks for faces, the dancers reflecting little joy in the music generated by the piano player and drummer. Davis's mood here is of general despair and fatigue, the same found in Van Gogh's slightly earlier *Potato Eaters* (1885, private collection). More directly from the Dutch painter's *Bal à Arles* are the globes of light, which reappear in Davis's work as a single overhead lamp and the highlighted barrel ends stacked on shelves along the left wall. Davis, as has often been noted, was swept away by the European innovations he encountered at the Armory Show. He later recalled,

> I was enormously excited by the show, and responded particularly to Gauguin, van Gogh, and Matisse, because broad generalizations of form and the non-imitative use of color were already practices within my own experience. I also sensed an objective order in these works which I felt was lacking in my own. It gave me the same kind of excitement I got from the numerical precision of the Negro piano players. . . . [A]nd I resolved that I would quite definitely have to become a "modern" artist.[20]

Becoming a modern artist, for Davis, involved a dramatic change of outlook and the willingness to experiment with the formal departures the Europeans had made. Following the Armory Show he would try out—besides Van Gogh's juicy impasto—Matisse's serene color planes and the Cubist restructuring of form. But, besides learning from other art, Davis realized that being modern involved incorporating contemporary American experience—technology, transportation, and, not least, the rhythms of jazz. Davis believed that jazz captured the special

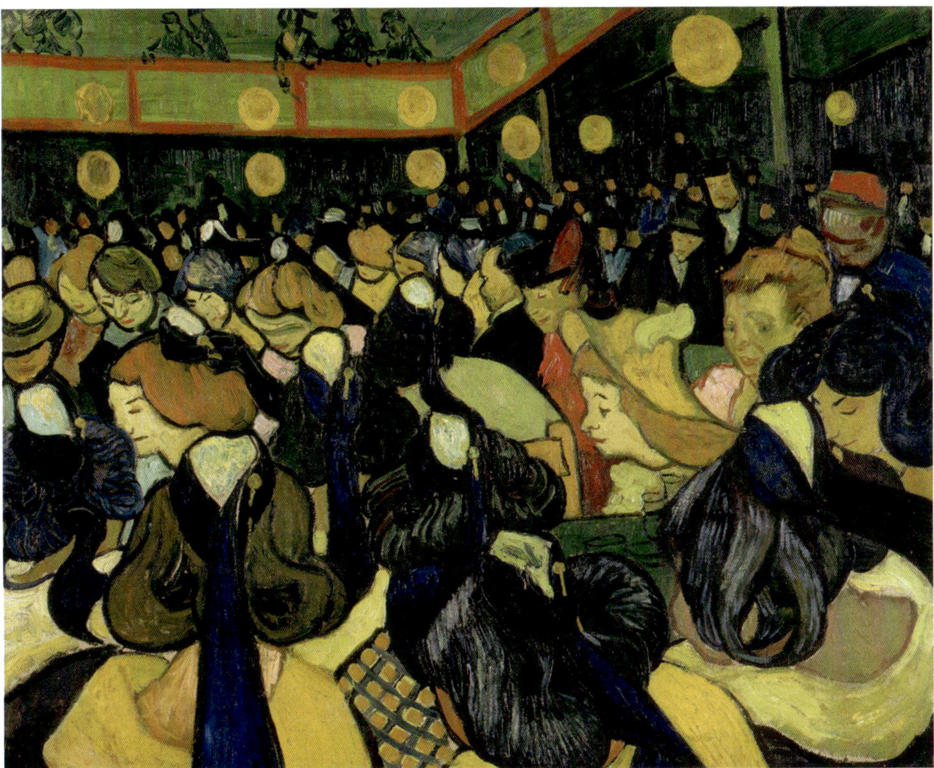

**Figure 48** Vincent Van Gogh, *Bal à Arles [Dancehall at Arles]*, 1888, oil on canvas, 25 ½ × 31 ⁹⁄₁₀ inches. (Musée d'Orsay, Paris; image © Réunion des Musées Nationaux/Art Resource, New York)

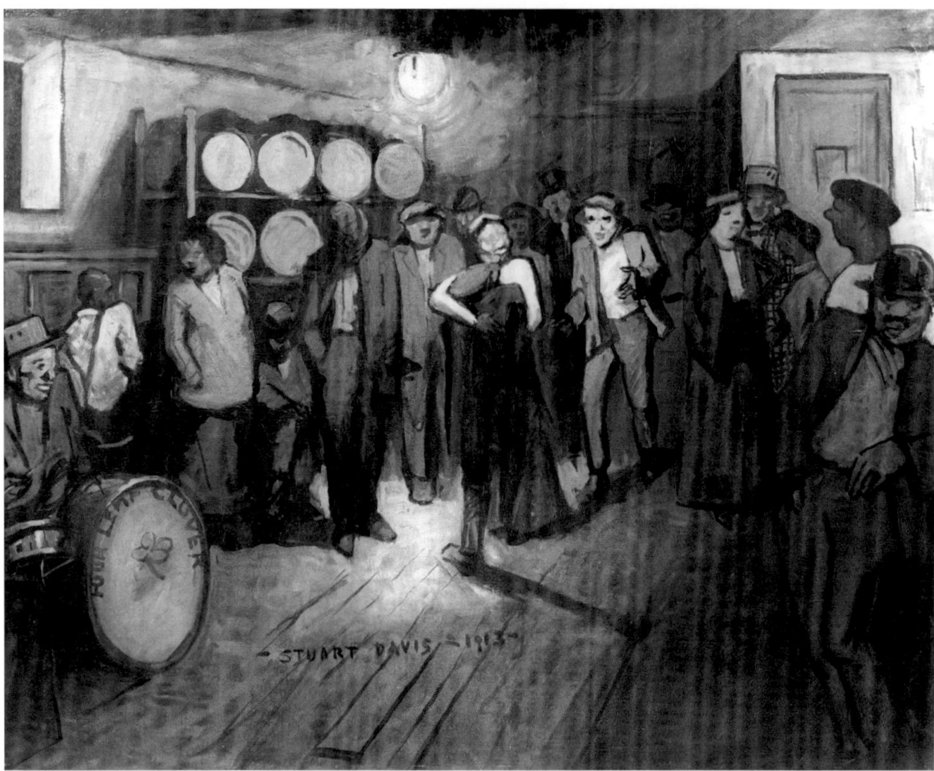


**Figure 49** Stuart Davis, *The Back Room, Bar House, Newark*, 1913, oil on canvas, 30¼ × 37½ inches. (Whitney Museum of American Art, Gift of Mr. and Mrs. Arthur G. Altschul, 69.114; art © Estate of Stuart Davis/Licensed by VAGA, New York, New York; photo: Geoffrey Clements)

tempo and flavor of American life; it was also organic and, as he said of abstract art, "changes, moves and grows like any other living organism."[21] For Davis, then, jazz—with its roots in the American South—represented the first native expression of the modern in both art and life, supplying the structural underpinnings of his own nascent modern style. Davis's challenge was to reconcile native imagery with modernist method. The road to that synthesis was a winding one, veering into and out of foreign influences and propelled often by the rhythms of the dance.

A trip to Cuba afforded Davis the chance to transpose his beloved urban subject matter into an exotic new color key. The island was close and inexpensive, warm and lushly vegetated. Americans were being encouraged to come and spend their tourist dollars in what was touted as "the most advanced, the most progressive, the most sanitary and the wealthiest republic in the tropics." Davis had few tourist dollars to spend, but he ventured south to Cuba in December 1919 for a two-month stay. In the company of his artist friend Glenn Coleman, the twenty-seven-year-old Davis wandered through the plazas and streets of Havana, soaking up the color and lively activity of the capital. It was an opportunity to engage with new, picturesque city subjects: horse-drawn carriages, the harbor, the Parque Central, balconied houses with serpentine iron grillwork, barnyard animals roaming the streets. These were exotic variants on the city themes Davis already knew well. In a city where climate and custom encourage it, much activity in Havana takes place on the streets. There Davis painted dancers, strollers, pairs in conversation, streetwalkers, burlesque performers— an array of characters sprinkled across some two dozen watercolors. They are organized into rhythmic patterns based on flattened shapes and intensified color. Lavenders, pinks, and transparent blues contrast with clear greens and yellows, creating bold surprises of color. Echoes of Matisse and Gauguin, and evidence of Davis searching for order in his compositions appear everywhere. Among the most successful of these watercolors are *Havana* (1920, private collection) and *Dancers on Havana Street* (1920; fig. 50). In both, Davis sets up a rhythmic structure by superimposing varying wall colors (perhaps visible "facts" in this color-drenched Latin city), complex rooflines, and sky activity. In the former work five dancers, anonymous pink figures, cavort like frenetic paper dolls on the cathedral steps. Abrupt perspectival shifts in both paintings add to the energy, but it is the dancers who provide the work's urgent vitality. In *Dancers on Havana Street* two languid onlookers survey the scene from doorway and balcony while the animated dancers—flat shapes in red, mustard, and black— sway in a spirited tableau vivant punctuated by a fat brown piglet in the foreground. Except for a mysterious tall black figure, perhaps a costumed performer to whom the other dancers seem to relate, the identity of the dancers is unimportant; it is the complex movement of colored shapes against flat planes that interested Davis. And the startling effects of dazzling sunlight or deepest shade. Dance is here the brightest thread in the artist's Cuban tapestry, his metaphor for a lively engagement with life, color and the intoxication of rhythmic movement.

Back in New York Davis continued his exploration of the tempo of American life, listening to, as he recalled, "Earl Hines' hot piano and Negro jazz music in general." Even while struggling with the rigors of Cubist form as part of his modernist quest, he worked with familiar subject matter, elevating the popular, the social, and the commonplace. Asked what abstract art was, Davis turned to the concept of the autonomous existence of a painting. "The generative idea of abstract art is alive. It changes, moves and grows like any other living organism."[22] Movement, crystallized in Davis's thought by music and dance, often supplied the life he wanted to infuse into his paintings.

In 1928, still chewing on questions about the influence of European art on Americans, Davis went abroad again. It would be his only trip to Europe, more than a year spent painting and absorbing Paris. Fresh from an intense, focused period during which he produced his advanced Eggbeater series, Davis seemed to be taking the measure of his own modernism against that of the French, to whom Americans were still (and usually disparagingly) compared. In Paris he painted some historical buildings, modern commercial facades and signs. As in Cuba, he used planes of rhythmic architectural color, but they are surely invented rather than observed in the more sober French neighborhoods. And the Paris oils lack figures. They are more like stage sets from which the actors have departed. No street dances enliven Davis's Montparnasse, but that is not to say that Davis

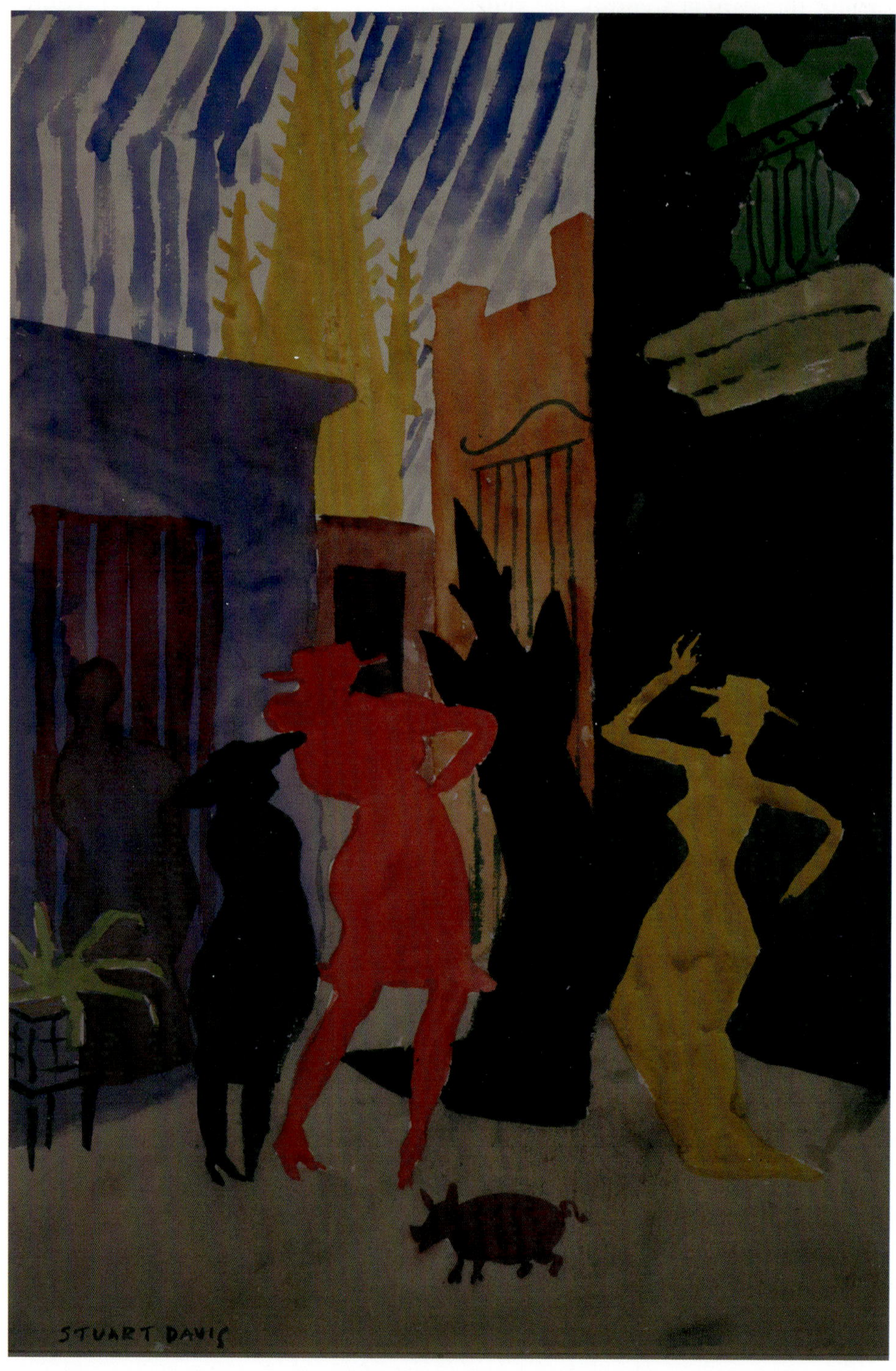


**Figure** 50 Stuart Davis, *Dancers on Havana Street* 1920, watercolor on paper, 23 × 15 ⅝ inches. (photo by Seth C. Jayson, formerly, Salander O'Reilly Galleries, New York; art © Estate of Stuart Davis/Licensed by VAGA, New York, New York)

avoided the café or cabaret scene. Perhaps as an antidote to the restrained formality of the Paris pictures, Davis and his wife immersed themselves in the Bohemian nightlife of the city. A young American art student named Ione Robinson wrote of her introduction, through Davis, to that scene:

> Last night . . . we went back to the Café Select and met an American painter named Steuart [*sic*] Davis and his wife [Bessie Chosak], who took us all to a place where they said we would see African sculpture in the flesh, the Bal Nègre. I was so frightened at what I saw. . . . Mr. Davis asked me to dance, but it didn't work very well as he was trying to dance like the Negroes, who were as wild as anything I have ever seen. Mrs. Davis was wearing a hat of jet beads that made her head shine in the colored lights, and the Negro women, who come from French Martinique, wore large, bright-colored bandanas tied high on their heads. . . . I felt so completely out of place that nothing anyone could say would make me stay at the Bal Nègre. Mr. Davis kept trying to persuade me that this was a wonderful experience, and the way to understand Negro sculpture, but I had had enough, and I finally got home.[23]

Obviously Davis and Robinson viewed the Bal Nègre with different intent. Unable to lose her self-consciousness in the unfamiliar, "wild" dance scene, she could not get past its foreign, uninhibited flavor. Davis's insistence, on the other hand, that dancing at the Bal Nègre was a kind of direct access to "African sculpture in the flesh," is itself highly revealing. What similarities did he see—color, anatomy, dance movements? And to what art might the dancers be linked? We will return to the Bal Nègre and its star Josephine Baker after a final look at Stuart Davis and a few white artists in Harlem.

Davis's decades-long admiration for the "numerical precision of the Negro piano players," begun in the Armory Show era, ripened into a passion for converting jazz syncopation into visual form. He liked to say, quoting Duke Ellington, that "it don't mean a thing if it ain't got that swing." By the late 1930s Davis was ready to try embedding edgy swing rhythms into a canvas of monumental proportions. Like Richmond Barthé, Davis was commissioned by a depression-era federal arts agency to create a new work for a New York–area public housing project. Burgoyne Diller (1906–65), head of the FAP, was determined to sponsor some abstract work as an alternative to the prevailing narrative paintings, and Davis took up the challenge. Davis's *Swing Landscape* (1938, Indiana University Art Museum, Bloomington), dispenses with literal references to dance, but insists, in its riot of color and pulsating forms, that even mundane objects like girders, cables, ladders, and buoys can jump and jive in an abstract visualization of Swing. New York's harbor was never so alive as in the jazz syncopations of Stuart Davis.

American Adolf Dehn (1895–1968), whose frequent forays into dance subjects began during most of a decade spent abroad in the 1920s, returned to New York in time to catch the energy of Harlem nightlife. On late-night prowls to the Savoy Ballroom, Connie's Inn, and the Cotton Club, Dehn and his companions

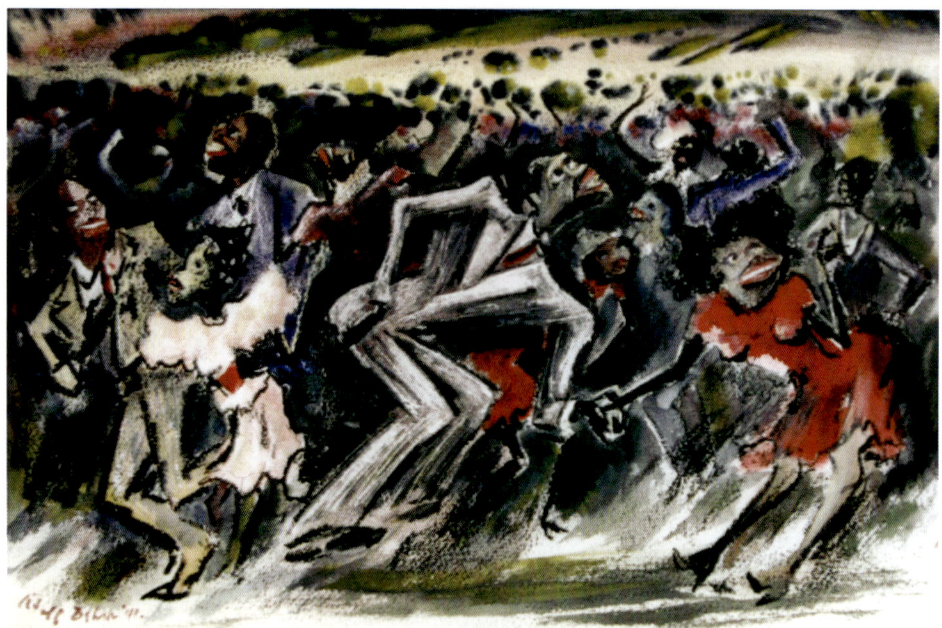

**Figure 51** Adolf Dehn, *Swinging at the Savoy*, 1941, watercolor, 12 ½ × 18 inches. (courtesy Dehn Quests)

(who included artists Reginald Marsh and Yasuo Kuniyoshi and the writer John Dos Passos) all recognized the currency of jazz as an idiom of modernity and exotica, and trekked regularly to Harlem in search of subjects for their art. Thrill-seeking was an acknowledged element on those nights, and for the sensitive among them it was not an untroubled activity. As Andrée Ruellan remembered, "We knew there was a sad, miserable side to Harlem and there was a touch of guilt in our slumming up there in the late evenings; but we were all sympathetic to the blacks, we knew the black artists and writers personally and frequently went with them to the Harlem clubs."[24]

From those 1929 and 1930 visits to Harlem, Dehn made many prints, including *Up in Harlem* (1932), in which mixed couples on the dance floor— both races drawn in caricature—express the free racial interaction that was part of Harlem's appeal. Even more evocative of the lively dance scene in Harlem is Dehn's *Swinging at the Savoy* (or *At the Savoy*) (1941; fig. 51). In the huge Savoy Ballroom, which occupied a whole city block at Lenox and 140th Street, two bands alternated, so the music never stopped. In this scene Dehn foregrounds the dancers, who are all African American. And like those black dancers he had recorded in Europe's capitals (discussed in chapter 10), Dehn gives his Harlem dancers a spasmodic visual phrasing that corresponds to the syncopated energies of jazz itself. While admittedly perpetuating essentialist stereotypes of the uninhibited, rhythmically endowed African American, Dehn did so with conscious admiration: for him, these Harlem denizens convey the ecstatic, jagged grace of reinvented ritual. Dehn saw jazz as an engine of American creativity, and as a reason for optimism about a distinctive cultural future. With Gilbert

Seldes, writing in *The Dial,* Dehn could agree that "jazz, for us, isn't a last fever-ish excitement, a spasm of energy before death. It is the normal development of our resources, the expected, and wonderful, arrival of America at a point of creative intensity."[25]

## Josephine Baker: Paris Creates an American Legend

One of the most celebrated of African American performers of her era was the legendary Josephine Baker (1906–75), the Saint Louis–born dancer and singer whose career began as a chorus girl with troupes in Philadelphia, Boston, and New York. On Broadway she danced in *Chocolate Dandies* and in the floor show at the Plantation Club. By 1925 Baker took Paris by storm as the lead dancer in La Revue Nègre at the Théâtre des Champs-Élysées. In the sold-out theater audience on opening night were a mix of the celebrated and the curious from Paris's literary, visual, art, and music hall world: Gertrude Stein, Fernand Léger, and Maurice Chevalier took their places among the two thousand mauve-colored velvet seats, while twenty excited students from L'Ecole des Beaux-Arts occupied the first row. As they entered the dance-steeped building, ticket-holders were reminded of an earlier American star: the Théâtre des Champs-Élysées had been embellished throughout with images of Isadora Duncan by Bourdelle and Maurice Denis. Josephine Baker was about to create a different kind of uproar, a visual spectacle aimed at a new generation. Artist Paul Colin recalled the contrast between the

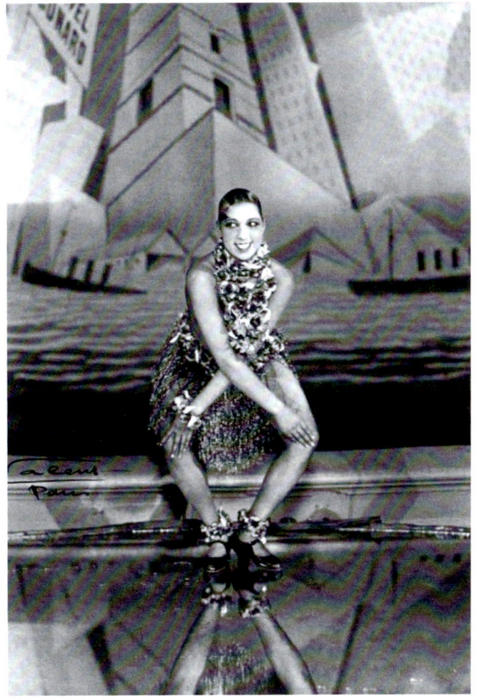

Figure 52 Anonymous, photograph of Josephine Baker dancing the Charleston, 1920s.

sedate theater decorations and the raucous African American revue: "The symbolic figures in Maurice Denis's frescoes, which crowned Auguste Perret's architecture, seemed to stiffen at the sight of this black tumult. Angels and muses flinched in indignation. Celestial harpists reacted in visible horror to the clattering sound of tap shoes. A generation separated violin melodies from the possessed uproar of clarinets and saxes. Harlem on the Champs-Elysées!"[26]

Baker's show, and the dance the French called "le Charleston" made her an instant sensation (fig. 52). Like many another popular dance, the origins of the Charleston are murky, but one frequent conjecture is that it originated among blacks living on a small island hear Charleston, South Carolina, where it was performed as early as 1903. From there it migrated north, showing up in Harlem stage shows by 1913 and hitting the big time when a male chorus line danced and sang James P. Johnson's "Charleston" in the Broadway musical *Runnin' Wild* in 1923. Whatever its origins, the Charleston and Josephine Baker seemed made for each other.

But Baker's appeal to the French was more complex and various. She came to symbolize both the exotic and the erotic on the Parisian stage; to French dance critic André Levinson she embodied "the black Venus that haunted Baudelaire." Her powerful physical presence, according to Levinson, echoed some of the formal strength incumbent in African sculpture: "Certain of Miss Baker's poses, back arched, haunches protruding, arms entwined and uplifted in a phallic symbol, had the compelling potency of the finest examples of Negro sculpture. The plastic sense of a race of sculptors came to life and the frenzy of African Eros swept over the audience."[27]

Baker was an entrancing conundrum for French audiences: On one hand, her dance was called sensual and hot-blooded, drawing attention to her own sexualized body through its vague associations with African stereotypes. As an entertainer in search of notoriety, she turned that symbolic capital to her own advantage, carefully exploiting her blackness and exoticism. Baker took to parading with a live cheetah along Parisian boulevards, causing onlookers to wonder (in the decidedly racist vein of the day) which "animal"—Baker or the leashed cheetah—was more wonderfully "savage." Other Parisian critics fastened onto the animal metaphor, comparing her to a snake, a kangaroo, or a giraffe, all of which Baker turned to positive publicity purposes. For photographers she posed knowingly with her cheetah, but marveled privately that "The white imagination is sure something when it comes to blacks."[28] Despite the feathered and fringed primitivizing of the Revue Nègre, it, and Baker herself, came to represent in French minds the rich vitality and exotic beauty of African American culture and specifically of the body of the black dancer.[29]

At the same time, the troupe employed an economy of artistic means: "[T]hese Negroes," remarked artist Paul Colin, "made use of elementary means to achieve astonishing results in which the purest, because the most instinctive, artistic feeling comes through free of all constraints. . . . The same thing makes for the interest and disconcerting beauty of the famous Douanier [Henri] Rousseau's paintings."[30] Sharing an aesthetic with a beloved French painter couldn't hurt. Seeming at once modern and tribal, Baker played up both aspects of herself. As Wanda Corn explains, "Onstage [Baker] often dressed as a jungle creature—one famous costume consisted of a low-slung belt of dangling bananas—while off-stage she fashioned herself as an ultramodern, with streamlined dress, slicked-down hair, and makeup applied so perfectly that it looked as if it had been applied by machine."[31] The machine reference applied to Baker is an apt one. She stood exactly at the convergence of two ideas crucial to jazz dance: the modern mechanized body, and the notion of the "primitive." As Norman Bryson writes, "the release of energy in the dance of Josephine Baker is controlled by presenting Baker as the object of an insistent voyeurism, and at the same time as ethnically other: the fascinations and threats posed by her 'primitive' movements, which nevertheless are also the quintessential movements of the machine age, are contained by reimposing upon them the combined authority of the masculine, colonial gaze."[32]

Visual artists were not slow to recognize Baker's allure, and many emphasized her free and unfettered persona. Baker became a favorite subject for many European and American artists. Among the American artists who saw her perform were Adolf Dehn, whose later devotion to Harlem and jazz were primed by sketching Baker in Paris and Berlin during the 1920s. Another artist whose long sojourns in Paris during the 1920s brought him into close contact with the world of theater and dance was Jan Matulka (1890–1972). A Bohemian-born painter who immigrated to America in 1907, Matulka's art studies and early career took place in New York. But for years he also kept a studio in Paris, where he consorted with French modernists and devotedly attended performances of Diaghilev's Ballets Russes, making many drawings of them. He also collected African art, a passion he shared with other American artists in Paris such as Patrick Henry Bruce, John Graham, and John Storrs. Exhibiting both in Paris and New York in those years, Matulka kept abreast of modernist tendencies in visual art and music, to which he listened in live performance and in recordings.

Even had he wanted to, Matulka could scarcely have ignored Josephine Baker's sensational *tumulte noir*, the spectacle on everyone's lips during the late 1920s in Paris. Either she or a dancer in her troupe seems the likely inspiration for *Dancing Woman with Parasol,* painted by Matulka in 1929 (fig. 53). A staple of Baker's *Revue Nègre* was a wild dance performed as a caricature of the famous French actress Jane Marnac (1886–1976) best known for her role in *Pluie* (Rain).[33] In Baker's revue the *faux* Marnac performs a brash parasol dance in the rain, clad in vivid colors and waving an umbrella with abandon. Matulka's *Dancing Woman with Parasol* may well be a remembered view of such a performance. But it is, at the same time, considerably more complex and interesting in its iconography. During this same period in the late twenties, Matulka executed a number of evocative still lifes, often combining such objects as a phonograph, African masks, shells, and musical instruments. One of these is his *Arrangement with Phonograph, Mask, and Shell* (c. 1930; fig. 54), a lively design made up of bright linear patterns, oblique perspective lines, and long, swinging curves delineating edges and connecting the objects to one another. While the phonograph grinds out mechanical music, the richly patterned African mask opposite it looks on impassively. *In Dancing Woman with Parasol* Matulka has used a similar mask and affixed it to the body of a high-kicking dancer—a body constructed of the same sweeping lines and patterned disklike forms of the phonograph and mandolin in the still life.[34] The music thus *becomes* the dance, personified in the living, gesticulating form of the black dancer. Perhaps she is Baker herself, perhaps some surrogate. But in the end the parasol dancer's identity does not matter much, for in his witty, complex transfer of forms Matulka has succeeded with his real project: using the fused energies of music and dance to transform still life into exuberant life, a metamorphosis that brings unexpected vitality to a frankly decorative series of paintings.

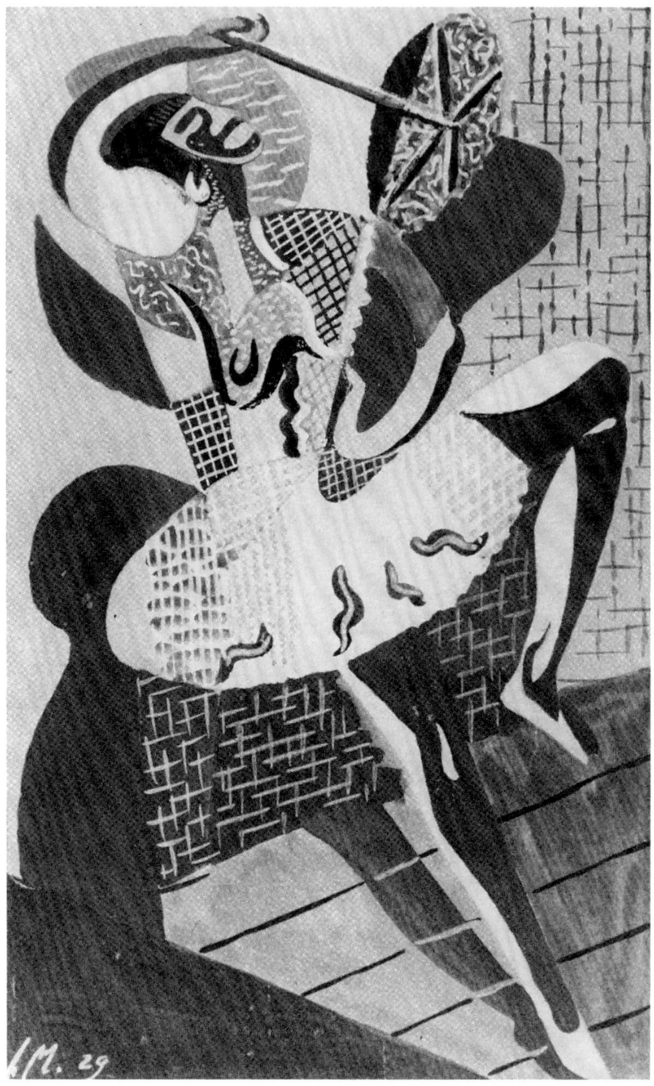

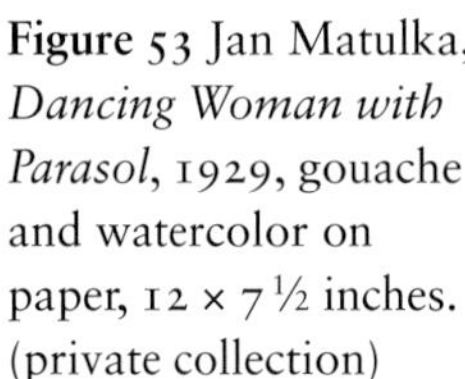

**Figure 53** Jan Matulka, *Dancing Woman with Parasol*, 1929, gouache and watercolor on paper, 12 × 7 ½ inches. (private collection)

In sculpture, Alexander Calder (1898–1976), whom Matulka knew in Paris, made several versions of the unstoppable Baker in wire. One, appropriately, resides in Paris (*Josephine Baker* 1926–27, Musée National D'Art Moderne, Centre Georges-Pompidou, Paris), the city that took Baker to its heart and made her an international star. Calder's sculptural trajectory brought him almost inevitably to dance. His inventiveness, sense of balance, and whimsical expressiveness emerge from several aspects of his training and temperament: schooled in engineering, he was comfortable with new tools and materials, but equally conversant with Dada's levity and the role of fantasy in art. Early experiments by Duchamp, Gabo, and Moholy-Nagy had employed hand-cranked or motorized sculptural movement. In the 1920s Calder created his famous miniature circus, whose acrobats and performers, shaped by the sculptor in wood and wire, moved in witty and unforeseen ways. Dancing characters in the circus include

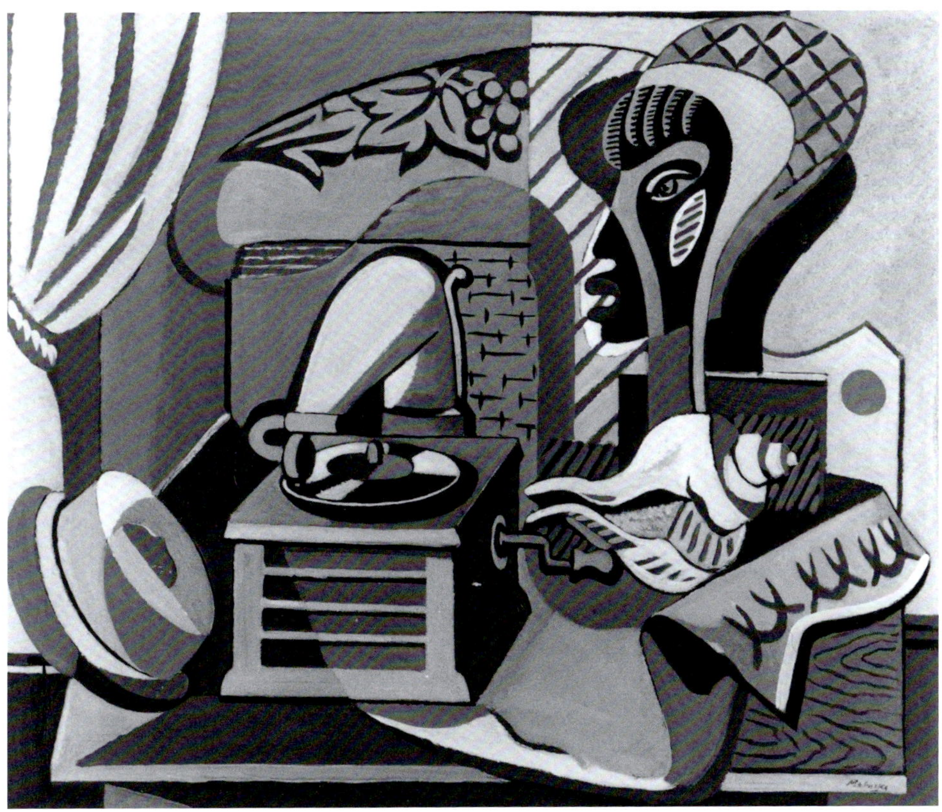

Figure 54 Jan Matulka, *Arrangement with Phonograph, Mask, and Shell*, c. 1930, oil on canvas, 30 ⅜ × 35 ¼ inches. (Smithsonian American Art Museum, Museum Purchase, 1978.158)

*Fanny, the Belly Dancer from Calder's Circus* (1926–31, Whitney Museum of American Art, New York); and *Exotic Dancer from Calder's Circus* (1926–31, Whitney Museum of American Art, New York).

Taken by the bold style and energy of the frenetic Baker, whom the French called La Bakaire, Calder outlined her in iron wire, the perfect material to suggest her wiry energy (1927; fig. 55). Calder's Baker, with her animated head and waving sticklike appendages, resembles some electrically charged X-ray. At strategic points—her pelvis and breasts, the sculptor affixed coils of wire, like erotic concentrations that suggest the coiled energy she generated onstage. Audiences may have confused Baker's lineage as African rather than African American, but as one of her biographers, Phyllis Rose, points out, "Some of the principles of her dancing, as well as her posture and moves, stem from an African tradition which was in part preserved in America." Dance theorist Anthea Kraut, writing more recently, finds Baker's choreography compelling both for its origins and for its inventive aesthetic: "[W]ith its polycentric, polyrhythmic, and angular qualities, Baker's dancing manifested a number of African-derived aesthetic imperatives."[35] Those are precisely the qualities that generated not one, but four, wire portraits by Calder, sculptures that perfectly capture Baker's onstage angularity, constant movement (particularly in the waving appendages), and multiple

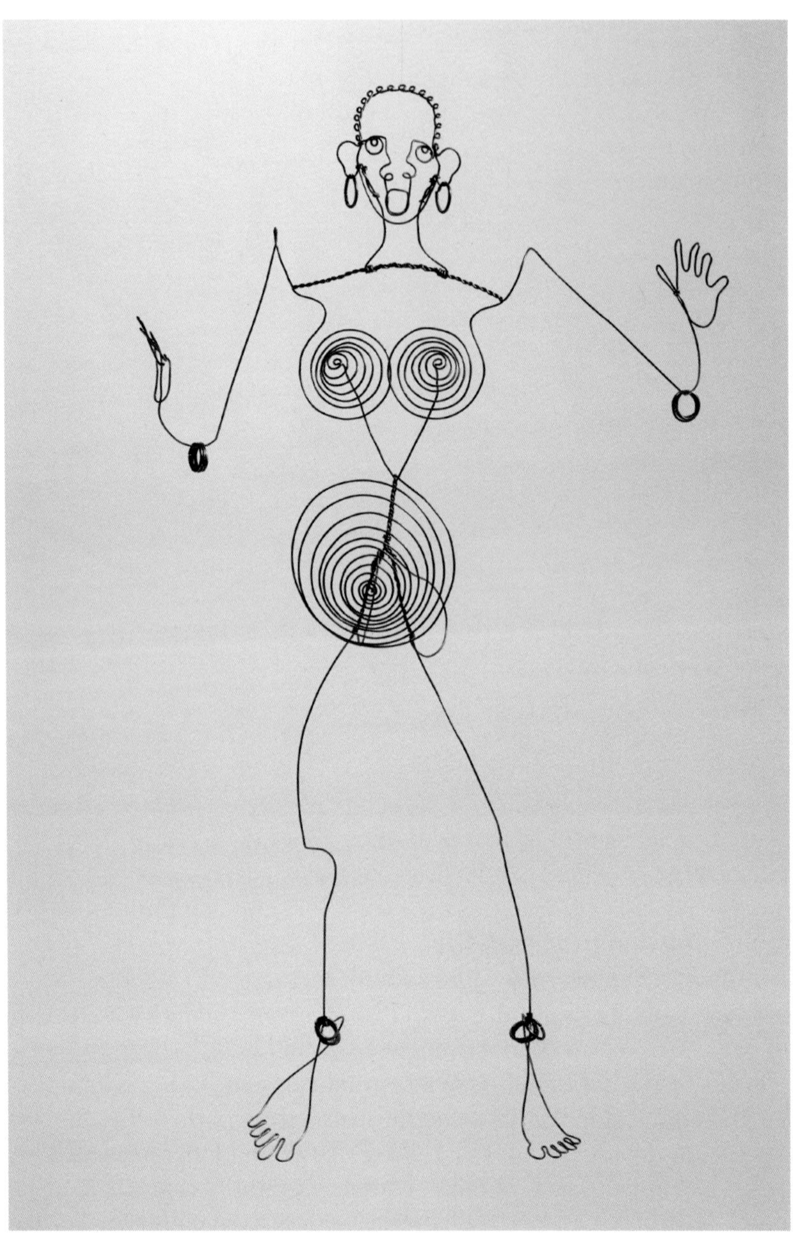

Figure 55 Alexander Calder, *Josephine Baker*, 1927, iron wire construction, 39 × 22 ⅜ × 9 ¾ inches. (Museum of Modern Art, New York, Gift of the artist, 841.1966; image © The Museum of Modern Art/Licensed by SCALA/Art Resource, New York)

accent points. Calder has caught her eclectic stage persona perfectly: she is at once fragile and frenetic, transparent and tough. Truthful in their spontaneity and gesture, his wire portraits succeed as symbolic, abstract portraits of the celebrated black dancer.

The incomparable Baker was eventually given iconic status in the world of French art when Henri Matisse, late in his life, used her as inspiration for his large gouache cut-out *La Negresse* (1952–53, National Gallery of Art, Washington, D.C.), completing the apotheosis of the dancer into high-art circles.[36] Down the decades, Baker's laughter resonates.

We have just looked at some ways in which American dance participated in a reinvention of its national heritage, gradually emerging from its long indenture to transplanted European customs and beliefs. Looking back, it is clear that nineteenth-century dance, and its representations in art, functioned as powerful, if sporadic components of America's early efforts to define itself. Still, while dance's expression in the visual arts helped to lay a foundation for our self-comprehension as a people, that process still was incomplete at the start of the twentieth century. As a nation of immigrants, Americans had yet to fully confront the classic American dilemma of nativism. Cultural critics just before World War I argued that the United States had failed to find, encourage, or allow the growth of a vital, independent culture. In fact, their argument went, Americans willingly maintained European American culture on their own shores, preventing the development of a deeply rooted culture of their own. "Briefly," writes Matthew Baigell, "the American character was considered frayed, fragmented, and buried beneath generations of psychological and sexual repression. People lacked a sense of organic culture and also lived in profound isolation from each other."[37]

Some thought that the arts, especially dance, could play a key role in opening, deepening, and unifying American culture. Josephine Baker, seen as part of a cultural explosion created by black Americans early in the twentieth century, represents not just a powerful force in exporting American dance culture; she also signified an emerging confrontation with aspects of the American past, especially the perceived "generations of psychological and sexual repression" Baigell points out. Encouraging such confrontations within the American character was a continuing interchange of dancers, with European dancers energizing American artists even as American dancers abroad inspired new visual imagery there. Part 2 deals with the ways dance and art loosened traditional American constraints on the overt expression of pleasure and passion in the arts.

# Part Two

# Dance and the Legacies of Romanticism in American Art

American visual artists have given much attention to the physicality of dance itself, its sensuous appeal, and consequent broad potential for both formal and emotional interpretation. The dancing body fascinates the visual artist because it can never be entirely grasped: just as soon as the artist approaches and attempts to fix an image, that body is somewhere else. This enticing elusiveness is allied to a whole range of Romantic impulses in American art, now recognized as a visual heritage of great complexity, modernity, and expressive power. On one hand, Romanticism was a celebration of nature in its vast, poetic diversity—a living, active context within which all kinds of dance subjects could unfold. In this sense, the role of nature becomes a metaphor, abetted by dream, memory, and imagination, for the subjective mood in American consciousness. Often, as we will see in the works of artists discussed in the following chapters, form and metaphor dance out epic struggles with imaginative endeavor and moral aspiration. By invoking poetic consciousness from the Romantic past, often through the refiguration of earlier works, American artists carried forward an abundance of meanings, condensing within their work the drama and concerns of their predecessors.

Yet there are other ways, more sensual ways, through which Romanticism flavored dance subjects for visual artists. Beyond its historic uses in religious ceremonies and balletic court entertainments, dance—due to its inherent physical appeal—has lent itself to erotic practices by both sexes throughout known history. The dancing body, enhanced by states of dress or undress, calls up *desire* in many forms. And beyond immediate experience, dance—at least in the imagination—has seemed to embody the living, pulsing eroticism of the world, wedding the fantasy of a free, desiring self to a living subject that represents the temporary possession of unattainable desire. We will look at the ways in which American dance has been allied with the poetic or subjective appetites to produce pleasure and meaning for all kinds of audiences, whether in a studio, on a public dance floor, or in a theater. As if the aesthetic role of pleasure still needed defending, art historian Helen Gardner noted as late as 1973, "People think of pleasure as a low word, but all art exists to give pleasure."[1] Visual artists have long seen the ways in which dance mediates complex notions of pleasure. And it is no secret that much great art, whether ancient or modern, has been created to serve a clear, if sometimes incidental, erotic purpose.

If human emotion expresses itself most spontaneously in bodily gesture, then dance—whose vehicle is ever the human body—may indeed have the longest lineage of the arts. And visual artists, from cave painting forward in time, have looked closely at those physical gestures in an attempt to recreate the individual mood, or perhaps the collective ritual power, of the dancing they witnessed. Modern dance historians have widely discounted the old belief that dance arose out of ecstasy, whether the ecstasy of worship, of grief, or of love itself. Still, against the tide of that skepticism, factions within the dance and visual arts communities have always wanted to find dance's origins in emotions akin to the ecstatic. Lucian, the Greek satirist and orator of the second century, declared that the dance is as old as Love, the oldest of the gods. Nearly two millennia later, Russian art theorist Wassily Kandinsky held out for the Lucian view: "The origin of dancing is probably purely sexual," wrote Kandinsky. "In folk dances we still see this element plainly. The later development of dancing as a religious ceremony joins itself to the preceding [sexual] element and the two together take artistic form and emerge as the ballet."[2] Writing shortly after the turn of the twentieth century, Kandinsky claimed no special expertise in the history of dance, nor did he draw a significant distinction between dancers and choreographers. The point in citing Kandinsky is this: he was, in his day, a strong advocate for the modern reengagement of ritual and visual art, and his was a powerful voice attended to by many visual artists on both sides of the Atlantic. Kandinsky's desire was to discover through all the arts— whether expressed in color, sound, or gesture—the most direct possible expression of emotion. In that effort his outlook remains essentially Romantic and recapitulates neoprimitivist attitudes of many like-minded Americans discussed below.

Another line of inquiry into the Romantic legacy of dance in America, pursued in chapter 4, leads us to consider the many ways American artists looked at imported dances and dancers from distant lands to supplement home-grown productions. Of special interest, first to American artists traveling abroad and later to artists at home, were the fiery dances of Spain, which captured the imagination of dozens of painters and sculptors, including John Singer Sargent, Mary Cassatt, and Robert Henri. "Exotic" Eastern subjects, especially the many incarnations of the dance of Salomé, riveted certain painters and sculptors, while others followed the lead of James McNeill Whistler in addressing Japanese and other Asian dance forms. Those dances of the East, while of importance to dance history, are largely beyond the scope of this book and have been given only brief attention.

Still other European sources opened American sensibilities to new experiences of the physical body: artists, dancers, and writers took inspiration from such dances as the high-kicking cancan, at once shocking and acrobatic, and already interpreted by European artists to great formal and expressive effect. After the turn of the century, Henri Matisse's dance subjects showed American artists new possibilities for finding meaning and decorative appeal in the archaic circle dance. And, as will be seen in chapter 5, a veritable tidal wave of Romantically tinged dance imagery was spawned by the 1916 arrival of the Ballets Russes in New York. This major dance company would further open American eyes to dance and engage cultural sensibilities in unforeseen ways. The Ballets Russes was one of a number of new creative models for dancers and visual artists, models that addressed fertile, multiple pasts, both real and invented. From those cultural diggings emerged important alternative ways of reconsidering the body, the passionate life of the senses, and the longing for authenticity of expression.

Early in the twentieth century the emergent disciplines of psychology and sociology had begun to revolutionize thinking about human behavior, both individually and collectively.[3] As Matthew Baigell has pointed out, the liberation so often sought by artists and dancers in the early twentieth century was based on their perception of American culture as repressed and inherently hypocritical.[4] For many moderns, visual representations of dance afforded new access to an interior life of the uncensored, the irrational, the libidinal. A revitalized dance, they argued, not only fought against old constrictions, but would simultaneously serve higher social purposes by freeing individualized expression of movement and—perhaps most importantly—enhancing democracy by restoring our bodies to us. Choreographer Doris Humphrey looked back on the founding years of modern dance in those liberating terms:

> Dance, and dance drama, persistently robust after thousands of years of snubbing by asceticism, scholasticism, and puritanism, can make profound revelations of that which[,] significant in the relations of human beings, can restore the dignity of the body, which prurience and hypocrisy have damaged, can recall the lost joys of people moving together rhythmically for high purposes, can improve the education of the young, can, to a much larger extent than it does, restore vitality to the theater, can contribute a moral stimulus to the furtherance of more courageous, coordinated, and cultured behavior.[5]

Such high-blown expectations for dance would not be easily achieved, either on stage or in American art exhibitions. Still, as we look at the multiple legacies of Romanticism we glimpse in dance subjects the ways American visual artists found validation for a life more open to sensory experience and to sensuality in general. This section, then, looks at the ways in which American artists, beginning in the nineteenth century and continuing into the twentieth, joined dance to a Romantic search for passion and for the production of pleasure. In fact, I will argue that dance has enabled American artists, historically constrained by a widespread antipathy to the expression of physical pleasures in the visual arts, to wedge open a door to that forbidden realm.

# 3

# Revisiting Arcadia
## *America's Longing for the Natural, the Pagan, and the Passionate*

One means of liberating the American senses was seen to emanate from the conscious revival of "pagan" ideas, which gained widespread attention late in the nineteenth century. For purposes of this study, paganism involves the simultaneous rejection of external religions or moral restrictions and the cultivation of natural drives.[1] In the early years of the Common Era a pagan was often the same as a heathen (that is, pre- or non-Christian, or polytheistic), but in an even older sense a heathen is merely one who resides on the heath, the land. In other words, a pagan is thus a country-dweller in close touch with arcadian nature. By whichever path, the pagan doubles back to nature and to an earthy acceptance of life in all its sensual aspects. In the late nineteenth century such desires erupted anew in all the arts, proving that pagan themes, besides being remarkably durable, were also wonderfully adaptable.

Americans were keenly aware that European writers, artists, and dancers regularly fused pagan abandon with the energies of dance, sometimes to evoke an imagined state of preliterate innocence, sometimes en route to the invention of calculated personal mythologies. Before she achieved fame as one of her era's most penetrating chroniclers, the French writer Colette (1873–1954) left her music critic husband in 1906 to dance in gold tights through provincial music halls into the salons of Paris. As dancer and writer, Colette mixed innocence and urban cynicism in her musings on nature and love. She believed that the body, capable of its own kind of thought, exercised its natural prerogatives through dance. "When my body thinks," she wrote in *Retreat from Love*, "all my flesh has a soul." Colette's *Dialogue de bêtes* (1904), a paean to rural life and animals, marked a sharp departure from her usual urban themes, reflecting a rising pagan temper of the times. French Poet Francis Jammes, something of a faux-naif in the manner of Henri Rousseau, had already declared in a 1897 literary manifesto that "all things are worth describing so long as they are *natural*."[2] In the plastic arts, the term *natural* was also capturing the attention of the sculptor Auguste Rodin, who sought to express in his work "the latent heroism of all natural movement."[3]

What emerges strongly in these European expressions is a powerful revisualization of nature, outfitted with a new, joyous pagan affirmation. Well underway was the new literary movement of Naturism, exemplified in Maurice LeBlond's "Essay on Naturism" (1895) in which he contrasted this rediscovery of natural life with spiritual escapism: "As for ourselves, the Beyond does not move us; we profess a gigantic and radiant pantheism."[4] And novelist Charles-Louis Philippe wrote in a 1897 letter: "What we need now are barbarians. . . . One must have a vision of natural life. . . . Today begins the era of passion."[5] And passion's visible incarnation, as often as not, was in dance.

Such sentiments drifted across the Atlantic, meeting in American artistic expressions some of the same desire for the pagan, the natural, and the passionate. Encouraged often by literary models, visual artists bodied forth in painting or sculpture the uninhibited range of motion called up by images of the Dionysian Bacchanal. In his last novel *The Marble Faun* (1860), Nathaniel Hawthorne summoned an artist's memory of an ancient arcadian or golden age when his characters dance in a sun-dappled glade: "As they followed one another in a wild ring of mirth, it seemed the realization of one of those bas-reliefs where a dance of nymphs, satyrs, or bacchanals is twined around the circle of an antique vase." Into that scene of gaiety Hawthorne inserts a contemporary American observer, who rapidly deflates the euphoria: "The sole exception to the geniality of the moment . . . was a countryman of our own, who sneered at the spectacle, and declined to compromise his dignity by making part of it."[6]

Such themes were taken up by noted visual artists, including the American Mary Cassatt (1844–1926). Following early art studies in Philadelphia and Europe, Cassatt settled in Paris, where she lived most of her life. From there, she made significant journeys to other European destinations, there absorbing the lessons of the Old Masters, reworking their subjects and techniques in her own manner. Cassatt knew Hawthorne's *Marble Faun* and shared its interest in exploring American perceptions of Europe's differences and the evolution of its cultural traditions. While in Parma, Italy, in 1872 she painted *Bacchante* (1872; fig. 56), a subject with clear undertones of the kind of frenetic pagan-inspired dance described in Hawthorne's novel. With her ivy headdress and cymbals, she strikes a rhythmic note so animated that—while her lower body is hidden— her feet are surely engaged in a fevered dance. But this Bacchante is also modern, dressed in a Romany carnival costume reminiscent of Courbet or Manet, both of whom Cassatt admired. Dance, as a part of festivals both old and new, allowed Cassatt to reinvent a classical subject, working within her perennial goal of maintaining connection with tradition while innovating from it.

Cassatt's simultaneous preoccupation with the ancient and the modern also engaged Symbolist Albert Pinkham Ryder (1847–1917), whose work inspired many later modernists. Ryder explored the theme of pagan nature in his *Dancing Dryads* (by 1879; fig. 57) in which three pale wood nymphs circle a satyr. *Dancing Dryads* was exhibited in 1881, accompanied by the following poetic lines by Ryder: "In the morning, ashen-hued / Came nymphs dancing through the wood."[7] Dance in such works served several iconographic purposes, not least of which was as a component in the nostalgic elegy for a disappearing American Eden. As Elizabeth Kendall writes, "Dance was . . . part of [America's] pastoral longings, part of that impulse to find a freer, simpler relation to the physical world in the midst of the overwhelming rush to industrialize."[8]

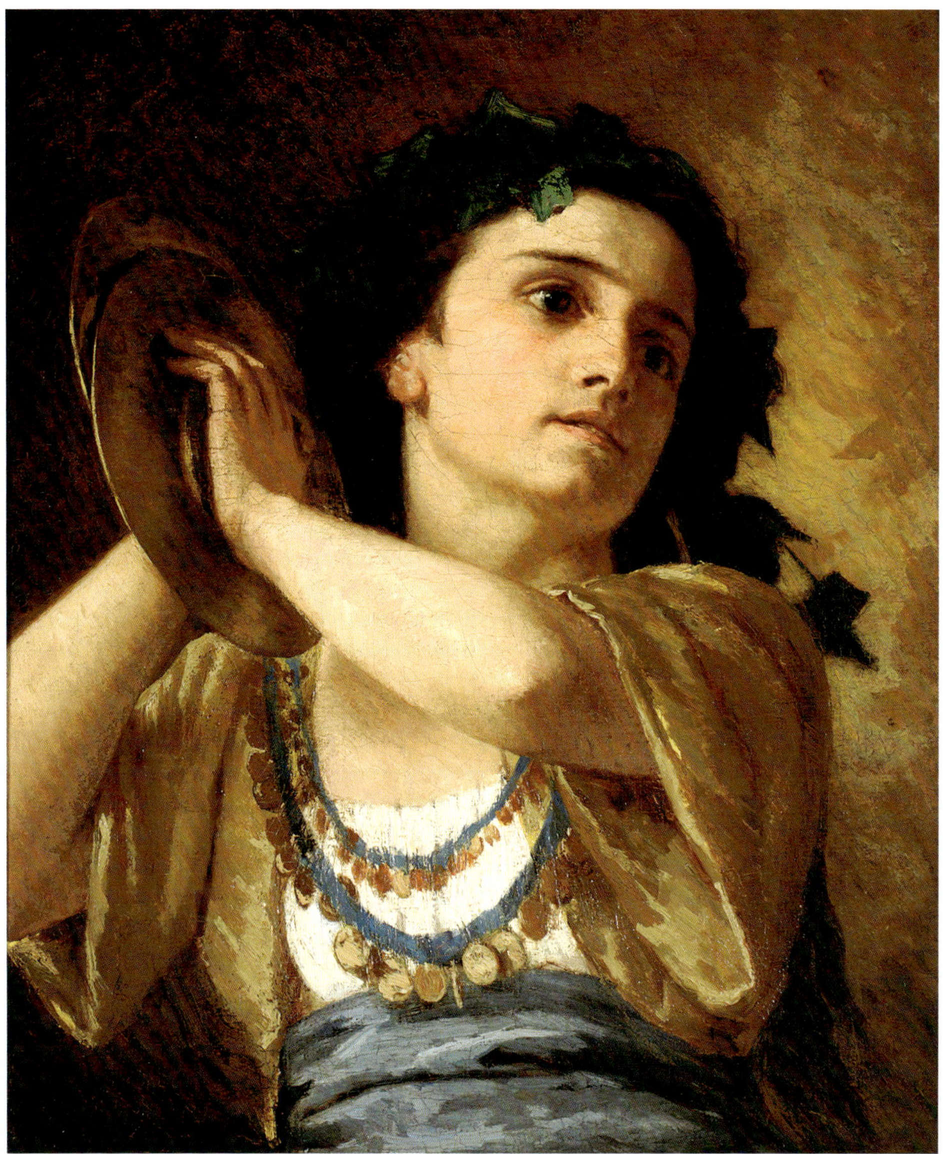

**Figure 56** Mary Cassatt, *Bacchante*, 1872, oil on canvas, 24 × 19 ¹⁵⁄₁₆ inches. (courtesy Pennsylvania Academy of the Fine Arts, Philadelphia, Gift of John Frederick Lewis, 1932.13.1)

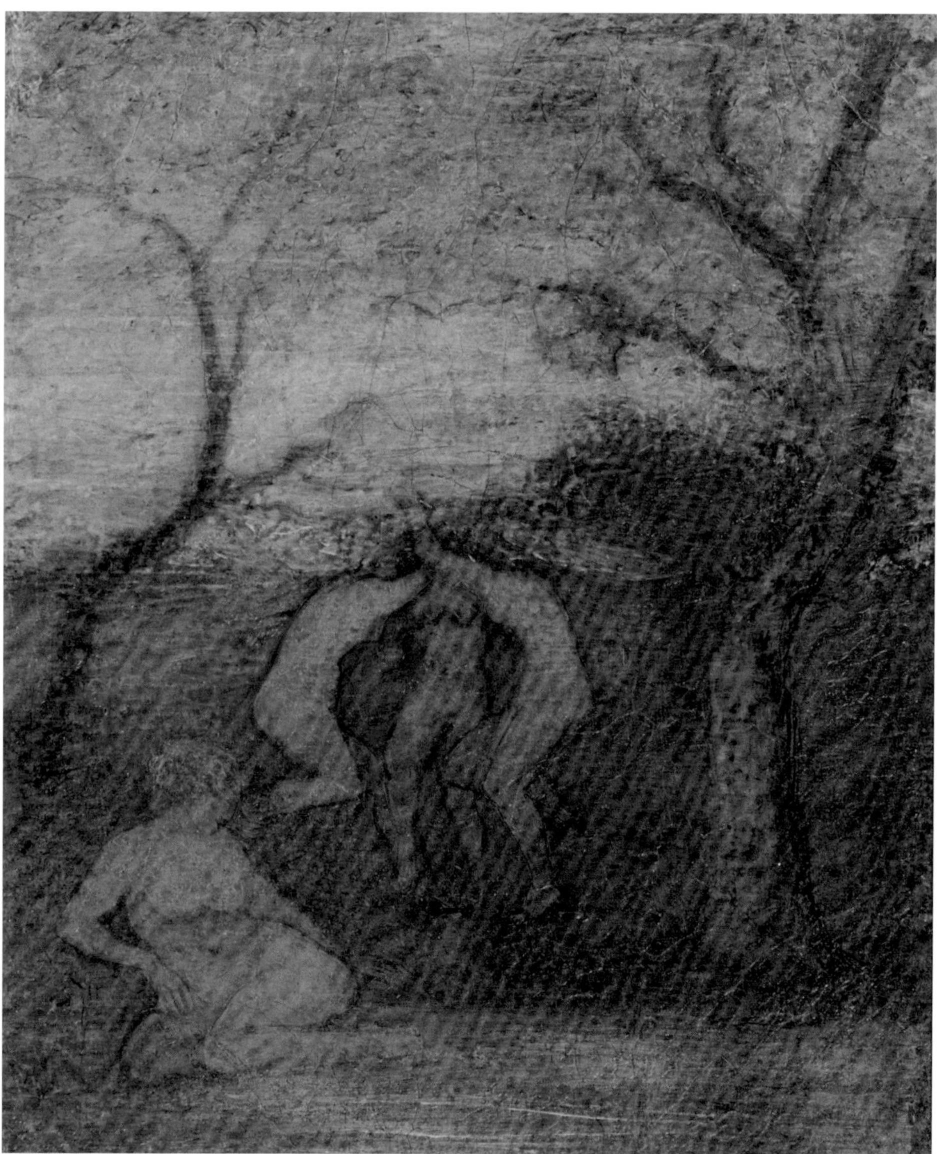

**Figure 57** Albert Pinkham Ryder, *Dancing Dryads*, by 1879, oil on canvas, 9 × 7 ⅛ inches. (Smithsonian American Art Museum, Gift of John Gellatly, 1929.6.93)

That "simpler relation" sent many painters, sculptors, and photographers tramping through forests and marshes in search of "natural" settings in which to pose their dancing figures. Performing rituals of pagan reenchantment, those figures dance human reconnection to magic nature. Rooted in pagan spectacles and holidays, those ancient bonds had been undercut by Judeo-Christian belief, which folded nature-based sacraments into a new monotheistic religion and sought to set the conscious, thinking self apart from nature. But dance, as a surviving residue of an ancient metaphysics of desire, reminds us that our bodies, at least, remain linked to older, indelible metanarratives of nature. Still surviving at the end of the nineteenth century was the venerable, powerful art historical convention of pastoral settings in which dances of psychic and sensual renewal were performed.

As Charles Eldredge has shown, American painter Charles W. Stetson (1858–1911) often explored fin-de-siècle themes of pagan sensuality and bestiality through dance subjects. For his day, Stetson's *A Pagan Procession* (1892; fig. 58) and his sketch for the *Invitation to Dance* (1899, unlocated) were both slightly subversive, allowing the artist to address Darwinian concerns about humanity's evolutionary connections with lower animals while alluding simultaneously to religious rites and to the sensual life denied to proper Victorians. In *A Pagan Procession* Stetson's iconography, seemingly self-invented, depicts an imaginary religious procession with bacchantes in the foreground playing the lyre, tambourine, and ram's horn. They join hands at the center with a somber, receding column of monklike figures who carry banners or crosslike forms. Although the painting's precise meaning remains mysterious, Stetson's true subjects are dance and color, seen in the intense blueness of the sky and the jewellike tones of the bacchantes' garments.

Nobody expressed American longings for the natural, the passionate, and the pagan better than two cultural heroes who bridged the nineteenth and twentieth centuries. One was Walt Whitman, who helped to redraw the map of America's senses, connecting neopagan sensations from the romantic poetry

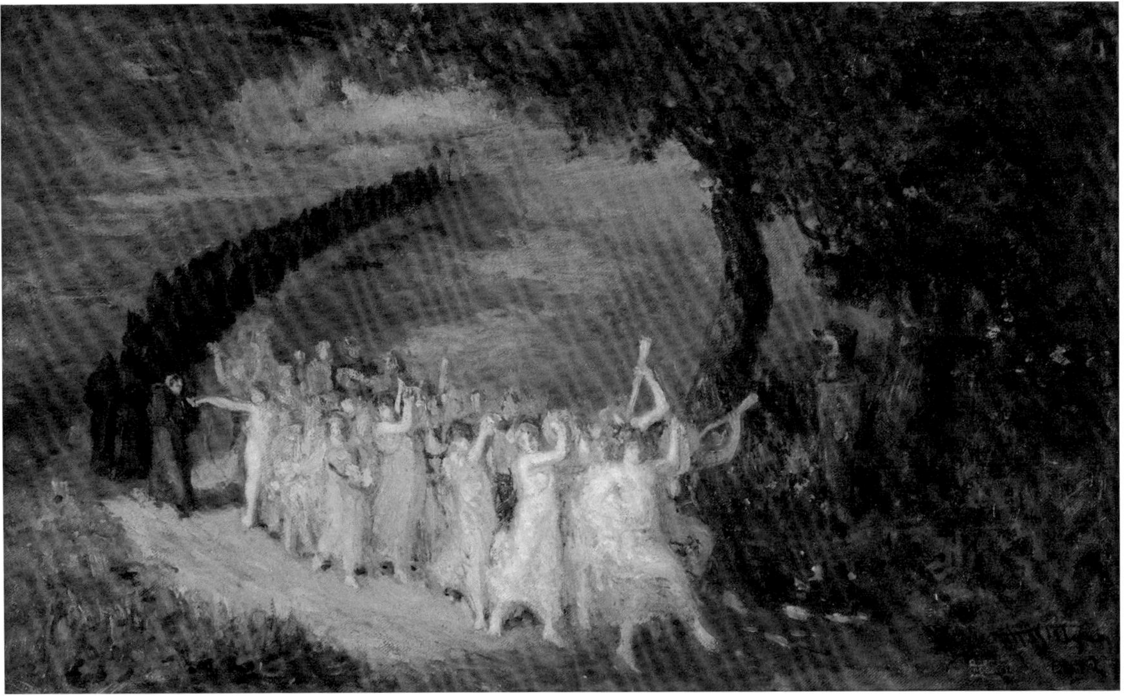

**Figure 58** Charles W. Stetson, *A Pagan Procession*, 1892, oil on canvas, 12 × 20 inches. (Museum of Art, Rhode Island School of Design, Providence, Bequest of Isaac C. Bates, 3/970)

of Keats, Shelley, and Burns to the American landscape. Whitman's nature poetry is famously ripe with a kind of pagan love of the land and of the body. "I believe in the flesh and the appetites," he wrote in *Song of Myself*. Both Whitman and his admirer D. H. Lawrence believed in the power of sensuality and the liberation of desire. Later, Lawrence would write specifically of the ways dance and ecstasy interweave in a poetics of desire. His notorious Lady Chatterley slips into dance in a moment of release:

> [She] ran out with a wild little laugh, holding up her breasts to the heavy rain and spreading her arms, and running blurred in the rain with the eurythmic dance-movements she had learned so long ago in Dresden.[9]

The writings of Whitman and Lawrence spawned a legion of literary and visual works celebrating the physical and the reunion of the human with the natural world.[10] The nude, and especially the dancing nude, communicated the joy and liberation of that union, often overlaid with an erotic charge. Dance historian Curt Sachs noted that the early twentieth century saw an American desire to "exchange stereotyped movement for something genuinely of the soul. . . . [Our generation] cries out . . . for nature and passion."[11]

Within its capacious embrace, dance had already shown its ability to weave nature idylls into the poetic and dreamlike imagery of the Symbolists. Their opposition to materialist and rationalist values sought expression in literature and painting that explored nonmaterial realms of imagination, emotion, and dream. It was, in the words of Charles Eldredge, "a personal, subjective and not infrequently visionary aesthetic which ran counter to the prevailing naturalism and materialism of late nineteenth-century culture."[12] Symbolism's ability to express the subjective *Idea* through outward forms was perfectly suited to dance because dance, according to Symbolist poet Stéphane Mallarmé, could make arcane fantasies visible: "Dance is the visual embodiment of the Idea," he insisted. "The dancers' bodies appear only as rhythm on which everything depends for him who understands."[13] What the poet did not specifically say about his own writing—but is eminently relevant here—is that he favored the haunting, repetitive phrase over concrete elucidation, the former a characteristic deeply embedded in much dance.

Through dance subjects, American artists and writers absorbed many Symbolist ideas from European sources. The influence of American expatriate Whistler, of Pierre Puvis de Chavannes, and of Paul Gauguin appeared in American art as early as the 1890s. And the visionary work of Odilon Redon (1840–1916) used subjects of dance and dancers to great effect; seldom was dance so appealing in its potential for fantasy and the allure of decadence. In a burst of seventy-five paintings and drawings at the Armory Show of 1913, Redon's work would be made known beyond an existing circle of American artist-admirers.

Armory show organizer Arthur B. Davies combined an interest in mythology with blatantly erotic overtones in his own art. Davies's *Clothed in Dominion* (c. 1912; fig. 59) is a friezelike choreographic presentation of male nudes apparently

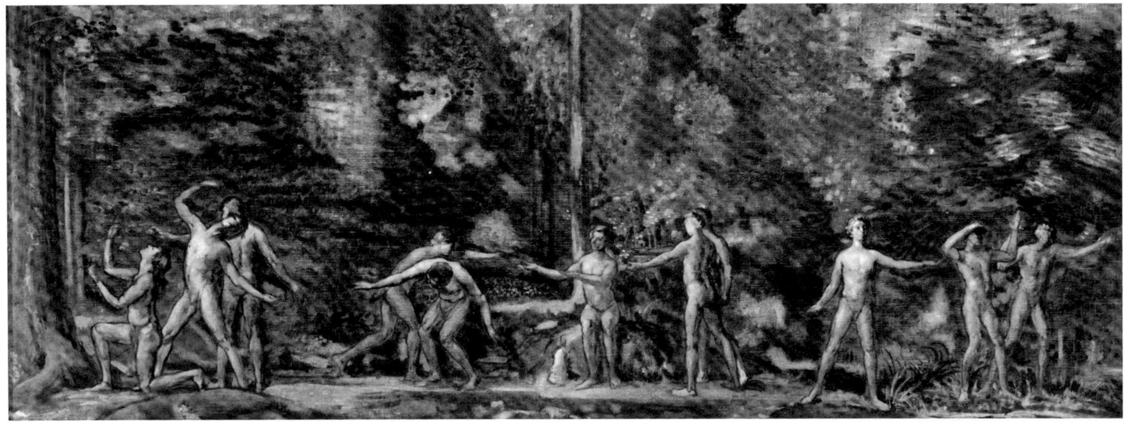

**Figure 59** Arthur B. Davies, *Clothed in Dominion*, c. 1912, oil on canvas, 24 ⅜ × 60 ½ inches. (Museum of Art, Rhode Island School of Design, Providence, Bequest of Miss Lizzie P. Bliss, 31.336)

engaged in a kind of spring ritual involving flowing water in a lush forest interior. Likely formal sources for Davies's alfresco male tableau have been located in the stylized poses of both Cézanne and Puvis de Chavannes,[14] but I would like to posit an earlier prototype in the famous Renaissance engraving *Battle of the Ten Nudes* (c. 1465) by Antonio Pollaiuolo, a work owned in Davies's day by the eminent collector Joseph Pulitzer.[15] Although Davies's nudes purport to dance rather than to fight, the poses are similar. Additionally, both artists carefully outlined their figures and used a single body type, seen from numerous points of view and frozen in taut gestures. Here is the irony of the comparison: both artists employed dancelike movement to explore divergent male appetites—in Pollaiuolo's case for virility and violence, in Davies's Symbolist era, for a dream of male sensuality.

Davies was an avid reader of James Frazer's *The Golden Bough* (1890), one of the systematic studies of folk tales, paganism, and premodern myth that proliferated late in the nineteenth century. There he read of Zeus's transformation of Dionysus into a goat to escape the wrath of Hera. Davies, using animals he photographed on a neighbor's farm, recast the Dionysian tale in his painting *Wild He-Goats Dance* (1920; fig. 60). Davies's own two sons are the boys in the composition. Boys and animals cavort in uninhibited fashion, taking on the randy characters of Pan, fauns, and satyrs, their pagan context perhaps lending a varnish of euphemism to artist's own famously wayward libido. Certainly the goats' designated participation in *dance*, rather than in mere barnyard or sylvan animal revelry, underscores that association with male desire. Davies's style in *Wild He-Goats Dance* contributes to the expression of a compositional unity. By grouping faceted forms into broad areas of dark and light within a shallow, shifting space, the artist moves decisively in the direction of Cubism.

Pagan themes involving dance, as an aspect of a larger cultural primitivism, were sometimes folded into a reformist cultural agenda. Gertrude Vanderbilt Whitney, a dancer as well as a sculptor, exhibited her sculpture *Paganism*

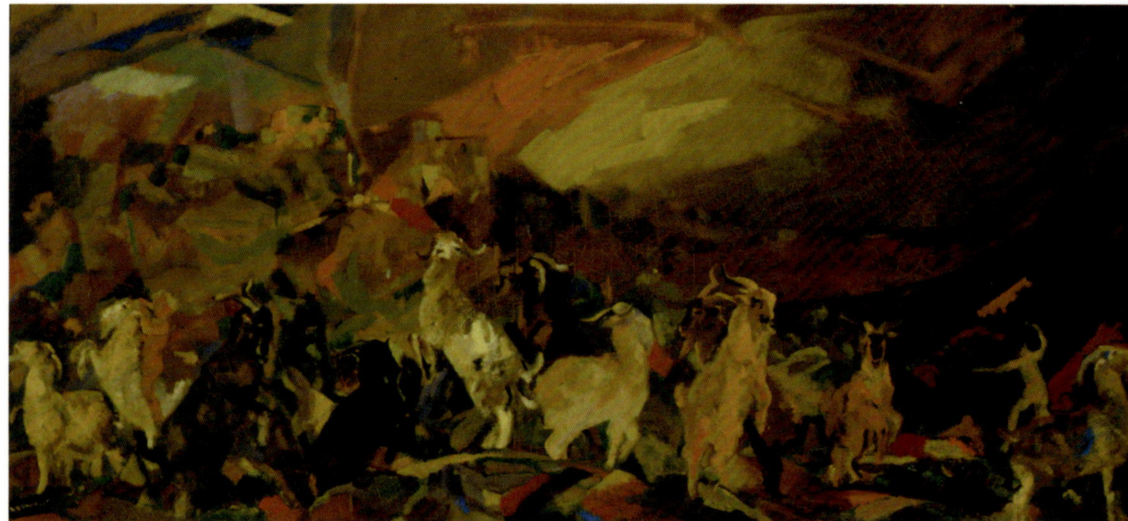

**Figure 60** Arthur B. Davies, *Wild He-Goats Dance*, 1920, oil on canvas, 18 × 40 inches. (Maier Museum of Art at Randolph College, Lynchburg, Virginia, Gift of Mrs. A. Conger Goodyear, 1952)

*Immortal* at the National Academy of Design, where it won a distinguished rating in 1910. It was exhibited again in the Armory Show. Whitney was, in the words of Elizabeth Kendall, "one of the first American women to wear a Poiret gown, to take up sculpture, to patronize native painters, and to dance, à la Orientale."[16] Her languid elegance prevails in Robert Henri's reclining portrait (1916, Whitney Museum of American Art, New York), while in John Singer Sargent's portrait drawing Whitney appears as a vibrant dancer, arms outstretched, head uplifted (c. 1913; fig. 61). Pagan themes, high society, and serious sculpture met in the person of Gertrude Whitney.

Marguerite Thompson Zorach (1887–1968) explored pagan dance subjects in a distinctive medium, tapestry paintings. Her colorful and complex *The Dance* (after 1916; fig. 62) is an outdoor revel of sheer exuberance. It features some twenty-eight figures, six of them musicians grouped within a central circle surrounded by eleven dancing couples who cavort amid birds and flowers in an arcadian outer ring. Trained as painters, Zorach and her husband, William, experimented with Cubist ideas, designed vivid expressionist theater sets for the famous Provincetown Players, and participated in important New York exhibitions such as the Armory Show and the 1916 Forum Show. When their children were born in 1915 and 1917, Marguerite found her studio time limited and turned instead to needlework, a medium she could pursue despite frequent interruptions. Building her complex compositions from smaller increments, Zorach continued to think like a painter, using stitches like brushstrokes to texture, tone, and animate her surfaces. Her silk and wool threads yielded colors of extraordinary brilliance, becoming true paintings in embroidery. With its inventive dance poses and erotic couplings, *The Dance* expresses the true spirit of erotic, pagan nature. In the bohemian circle in which the Zorachs moved,

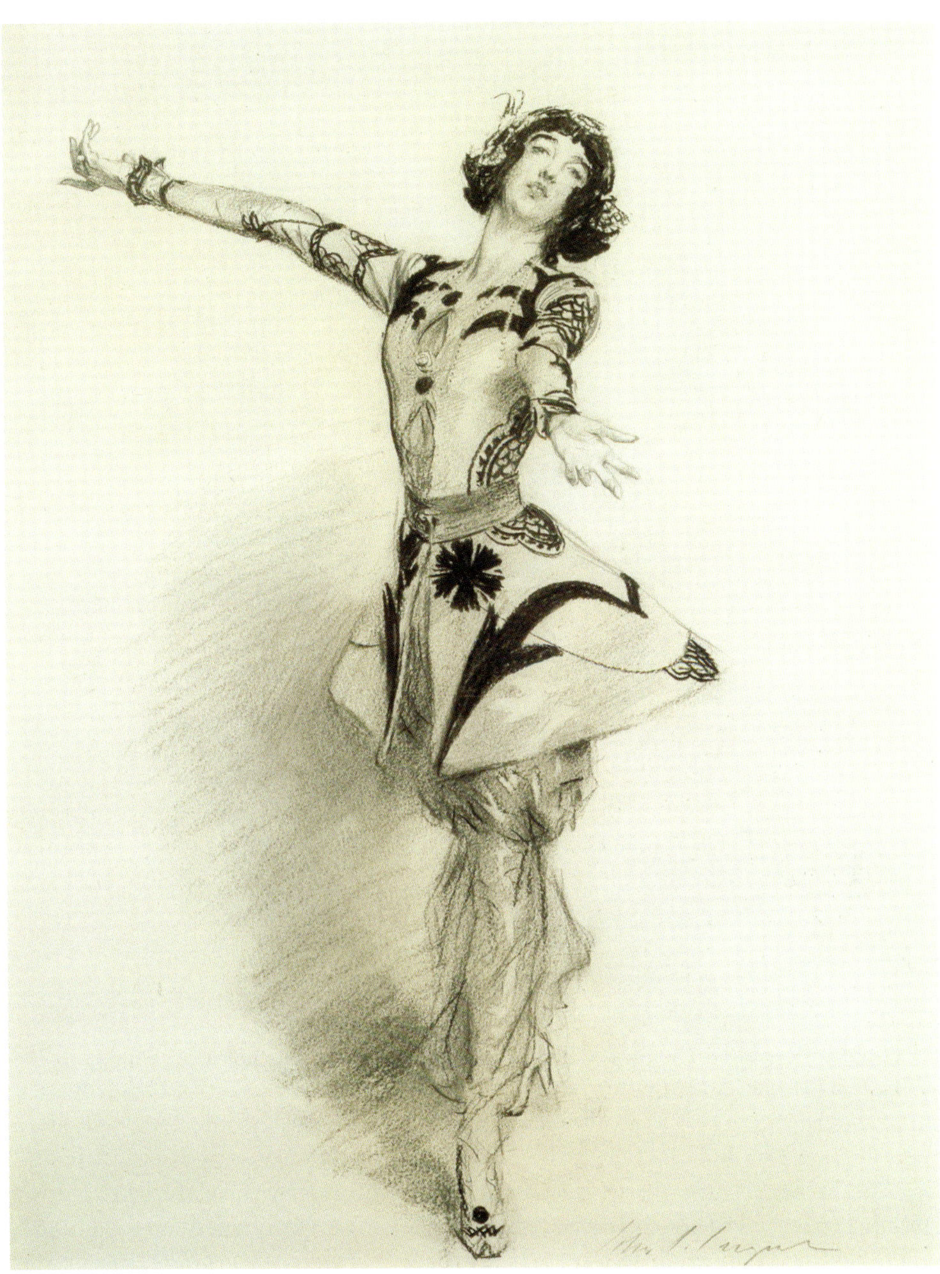



**Figure 61** John Singer Sargent, *Gertrude Vanderbilt Whitney*, c. 1913, charcoal and graphite pencil on paper, 24⅝ × 19⅝ inches. (Whitney Museum of American Art, New York, Gift of Flora Miller Biddle, Pamela T. LeBoutillier, Whitney Tower, and Leverett S. Miller, 92.22)

the idea of pagan revelry was broadly interpreted, far beyond a mere rejection of orthodoxies, to describe a general pursuit of hedonism in New York's Greenwich Village, and her tapestry painting bridges the gulf between Paganism's ancient and modern allusions.[17]

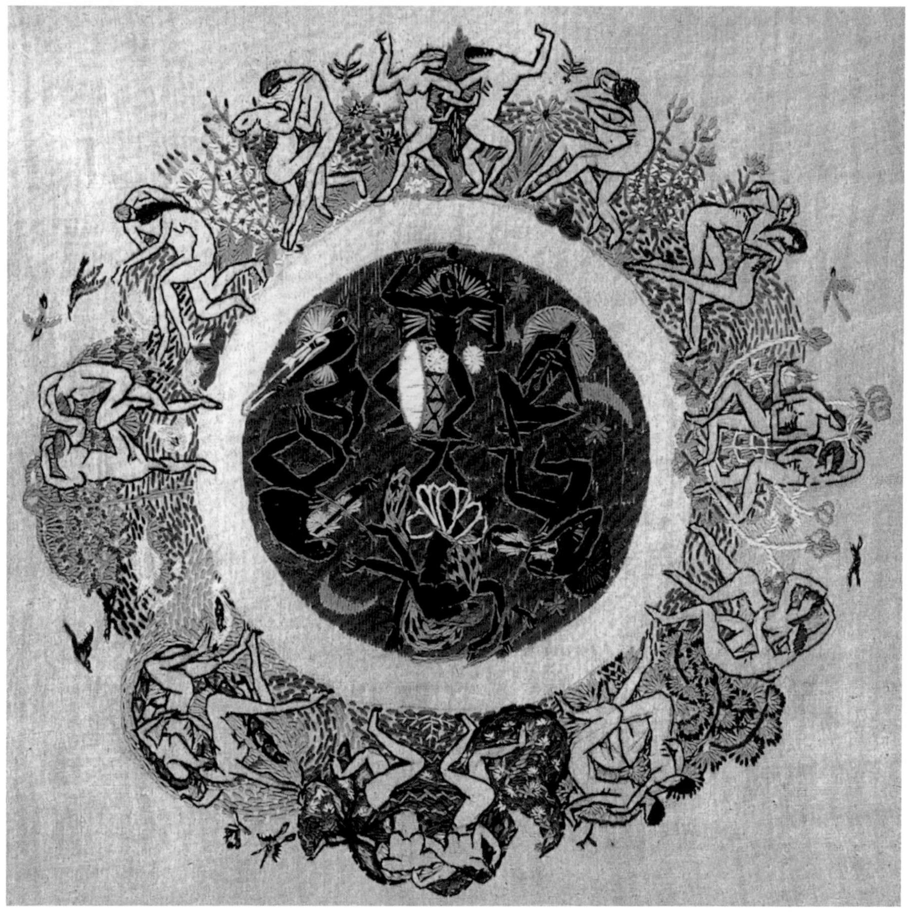

Figure 62 Marguerite Thompson Zorach, *The Dance*, after 1916, tapestry painting, n. dim. (Smithsonian American Art Museum)

Meanwhile, on the West Coast, a bacchante subject by the California painter Arthur F. Mathews (1860–1945), reflects a Tonalist style, characterized by softly defined areas of color closely related in intensity. In *Dancing Ladies* (1917; fig. 63), Mathews clusters a tight circle of seven dancers, who nearly burst through the picture frame as they reach out, leap, whirl, and bend in exuberant individual motion. Lest their wild, disparate poses threaten the effect of a pervasive natural harmony (akin to Mallarmé's "rhythm on which everything depends"), Mathews tames and unifies his composition by carefully positioning each of his dancers' heads along the same horizontal plane, subtly introducing an allusion to classical repose amid the Dionysian frenzy of castanets, cymbals, and pipes.

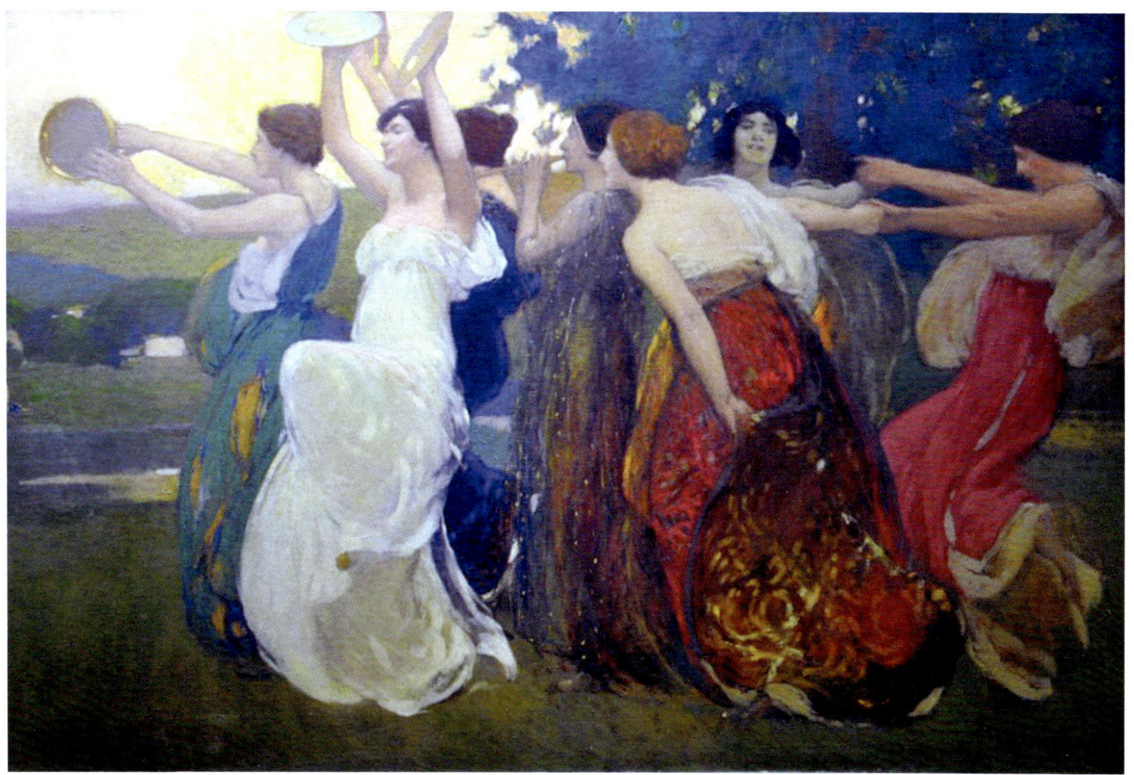

**Figure 63** Arthur F. Mathews, *Dancing Ladies*, 1917, oil on canvas, 34 × 52 inches. (Garzoli Gallery, San Rafael, California)

If many American artists pursued the type of the erotically charged, barely clothed dancer as a type of vestigial pagan, for some American artists it was enough just to place their dancers outdoors, where the nude in nature revived old, imagined idylls of individual liberation. The dancing nude went a step beyond, to suggest the ecstasy of release through rhythmic physical movement. Not surprisingly, there were those who saw, with Matisse, its communal, ritualistic possibilities. Beginning in the 1930s John Marin, best known for his semi-abstract landscapes, would find new ways of expressing the liberating power of nature by introducing the female nude, either as bather or dancer, into his oeuvre. His first forays into this new subject were conventional—reclining bathers by the seashore—but they soon overcame inertia to rise and dance on the waves or even in the sky. By 1936 Marin's seaside nudes were disporting themselves on the sand. Donna Cassidy writes that, like Matisse's, "Marin's nudes similarly express the emotional freedom of an arcadian, primitive world. . . . His choice of this pagan, mythological subject suggests his intention to construct a lost paradise in such works as *Dance by the Sea* [1942; fig. 64], just as Matisse had done in *Joy of Life*."[18]

Like many other early American modernists, Marin—admittedly naively—shared the beliefs of neoprimitivists such as Lawrence, who argued for spiritual and social regeneration through self-expression and communion with nature.

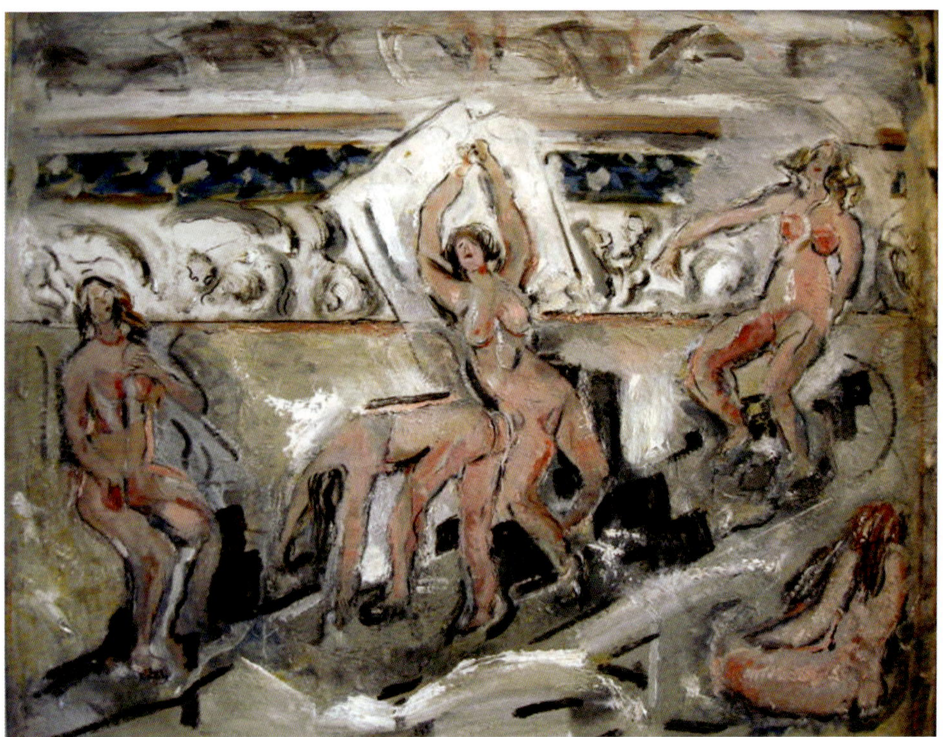

Figure 64 John Marin, *Dance by the Sea*, 1942, oil on canvas, 25 × 30 inches. (© 2010, Estate of John Marin/Artists Rights Society [ARS] New York)

For Marin, dance was a vehicle on the direct road to such regeneration, and Native American dance was his first model for uncorrupted, intuitive movement in tune with the seasons and rhythms of the universe. While spending summers in New Mexico in 1929 and 1930, he first saw through Native Americans how humanity might engage in meaningful ritual practice to reconnect with nature. From there, modern dance would be an important next step in Marin's reeducation. He was deeply impressed with the emotional potential of dance, especially as reinvigorated by Isadora Duncan, Angna Enters, and his Maine neighbor Lilian Seligmann, who was his first dancing subject in 1935. Marin's dancing nudes never displaced landscape as his chief subject, but they provided him with something vital: new ways to open up the figure–landscape relationship. Among other things, they lend approximate scale to the landscape, placing the figure in physical relation to an image that is—in its entirety—much larger than we are. But Marin abridges the landscape surrounding his dancers; with their buxom contours they hold their own against and within it in assertive fashion. Seen thus, Marin's dancing nudes were formally liberating, but they represent far more than that in his work. Like his Native American dancers, they gave him entry into an antipuritanical world peopled by "natural" beings. On the seashore Marin introduced a fugitive erotic undertow; his dancers there engage without inhibition in the delights of the sensuous world.

For many creative Americans in the late nineteenth and early twentieth centuries, a recovery of pagan nature unlocked perceptual doors and ushered in a new poetics of movement. In some cases, encounters with new places and cultures opened new spiritual passageways. Martha Graham (1894–1991), following her family's move to Southern California at the age of fourteen, recalled that the area's Asian and Spanish influences, combined with its fine weather, moved her "in the direction of paganism, though years were to pass before I was fully emancipated."[19] For Graham and for countless others, dance helped to unlock an enhanced sensory understanding of the world.

<h1>4</h1>

# Romantic Imports
*American Art's Love Affair with*
*European Dance*

## Spanish Dance and the Romantic Ballet

The cultural influences, Asian and Spanish, that nudged Martha Graham toward paganism must both be considered within the eclectic American cultural mix shared by dancers and visual artists. In California, Graham would have encountered Spanish influence in centuries-old architectural forms, but also in Spanish dance, which had by then engaged Americans for decades and was, at the time Graham settled in California, approaching its zenith of popularity in the United States.

American artists and dancers dug deeply to uncover the ancient roots of Spanish dance, which had been celebrated since the early days of the Roman Empire, when dancers from Cadiz caused a sensation in the Imperial capital, attracting enough notice to be recorded in Roman texts. Through the Iberian peninsula passed Phoenicians, Greeks, Romans, Celts, Moors, and Romany (Gypsies), all of whom danced and some of whom surely added to the evolving tradition of Spanish dance. Some dance historians, for example, have argued that Spanish dancers may have inherited certain movements and poses from late Greek Tanagra figurines: sideways movement, gestures of arms and hands, backward tilt of head and body, even the use of castanets—all these were found in both Greek and Spanish dance.

Whatever its precise origins, Spanish dance was much modified by the intervening movements of peoples. Like its language, Spanish dance grew into a living hybrid, so important culturally that it appeared, for example, in many paintings by Goya. Disseminated perhaps by British and French soldiers returning home from the Peninsular War of 1808–14, Spanish dance reached Paris. From there the fame of Spanish dance and its theatrical performers—of whatever nationality—radiated outward. As Walter Sorell has written, "In general, it can be said that Spanish dancing is a mixture of Eastern and Western dance with a dash of exoticism added for good rhythmic measure . . . There are several aspects of Spanish dance which overlap and manifest the essence of folk as well as theatrical dancing."[1] Through its disarming frankness, inherent drama, and theatricality, Spanish dance had definitely moved from folk art to theatrical experience. On stage, visual artists found in Spanish dance a heritage perhaps best preserved in the truth of gesture itself.

Meanwhile, Spanish themes continued to infuse European music, as in Georges Bizet's opera *Carmen* (1875), which electrified audiences with its earthy love triangle entangling a fiery Andalusian gypsy with an army officer and a toreador. Such Andalusian characters had already appeared in the dance-themed paintings of Delacroix and Manet, among others. Most of those images were taken from the classical Spanish dance style known as the *escuela bolera* which evolved, like ballet, from European court dance and regional dance. Manet's *Spanish Ballet* (1862, Phillips Collection, Washington, D.C.) features a troupe performing in costume, one of whose dancers closely resembles the famous Lola de Valence, whom Manet also painted individually (*Lola de Valence*, 1861–62, Louvre, Paris).[2]

As the nineteenth century unfolded, a new lexicon of steps and body positions evolved. Modern Spanish dance differs from ballet in its disdain for fixed positions, its high-held torsos, free-floating arms, undulating hips, and curled arabesque hand gestures. In his bronzes *Spanish Dance* and *Dancer with Tambourine* (various collections) Edgar Degas froze the unmistakable gesture of upflung arm and out-thrust hip so characteristic of the Spanish dancer.[3] In Paris Toulouse-Lautrec painted the cultural transferences in Spanish Dance in his *Marcelle Lender Dancing the Bolero in "Chilpéric"* (1895–96, National Gallery, Washington, D.C.).

In an age rife with Hispanism, the vogue for all things Spanish—prevalent in England and on the Continent—crossed the Atlantic and brought Iberian dance to Americans. One of those who best understood its gestural possibilities for the visual arts was a celebrated Austrian ballerina named Fanny Elssler (1810–84), who introduced theatrical folk dance, especially Spanish dance, into ballet. That momentous fertilization would enrich both classical dance and the visual images made from it.

To understand that hybridization we must first understand something of the appeal exerted by nineteenth-century ballerinas on the visual arts. Théophile Gautier, the French poet turned journalist, had focused on the romantic ballet as a kind of living painting or moving sculpture, emphasizing dance's revelation of "physical pleasure and feminine beauty." Gender roles were indeed integral to the European ballet; women's delicate ethereality was augmented as they began rising on their toes as early as 1818, then rising even further as they were lifted by their male partners. The ethereal Marie Taglioni (1804–84) achieved enormous fame as the epitome of this kind of dance. Both in her lifetime and later, her dancing became the stuff of indelible legend and a frequent subject for visual artists. An American who saw her dance in Paris in 1836 reported that "her dancing excels that of any other woman. . . . It is not only in great agility and dexterity, but it is the perfection of grace and beauty, and addresses itself to the imagination, as it is, in fact, half the time something between earth and heaven."[4]

Although Americans clamored for Taglioni to visit these shores, and although she frequented the space "between earth and heaven," she never drifted over to the United States. Disappointed Americans, then and later, had to be content with visual images of the otherworldly dancer. But those were plentiful and persistent: long after her feet came to a final rest, and nearly a century after her heyday, the

American sculptor Joseph Cornell breathed new life into her legend. Indeed, through Cornell the iconolatry accorded to Taglioni and other romantic ballerinas of the nineteenth century was revived and a precedent set for dancer-worship far into the twentieth. This Cornell accomplished through his unrelenting artistic focus on dancers and the object-world they inhabited. Cornell invented new, miniature worlds for them in works such as the box constructions he dedicated to Taglioni, including *Taglioni's Jewel Casket* (1940; fig. 65). The complex dual layers of Cornell's mirrored box contain a glass necklace, jewelry fragments, and more than a dozen cubes of glass, explained in the following inscription which the artist included with the box:

> On a moonlight night in the winter of 1835 the carriage of Marie Taglioni was halted by a Russian highwayman and that enchanting creature commanded to dance for this audience of one upon a panther's skin spread over the snow beneath the stars. From the actuality arose the legend that to keep alive the memory of this adventure so precious to her, Taglioni formed the habit of placing a piece of artificial ice in her jewel casket or dressing table, where, melting among the sparkling stones, there was evoked a hint of the atmosphere of the starlit heavens over the ice-covered landscape.[5]

Lined with deep blue velvet, the box's interior recalls the night sky, while the movable "ice" cubes within—an eerie conflation of the sensory and the cerebral—suggest Cornell's affinity for Duchampian random or chance arrangements. Throughout his career Joseph Cornell was a balletomane, finding in its romantic phase (as well as in later dance) the subjects for a number of his sculptures and montages. He assembled a sizeable collection of dance photographs, prints, and drawings, which he often incorporated into his work. For Cornell, collecting was a pursuit enjoyed for its own sake, since he took great delight, as he said, in the "fascinating and still existing possibilities of fresh finds in forgotten tomes and bins, the least trifle ever absorbing and welcome to the devotee of the Romantic Ballet."[6]

Besides Taglioni, Cornell celebrated several other ballerinas in his work, dedicating miniature and magical worlds to them in his box constructions and the covers he designed for periodicals.[7] Here we can mention only a few more of his richest, most insistent visual expressions. Perhaps Cornell's best-loved ballerina was Fanny Cerrito, praised in her day for her rapid footwork and exuberant energy. Cornell made it his personal mission to retrieve the nearly forgotten memory of Cerrito from old books and dusty prints, particularly from a sentimental 1842 souvenir portrait print of her by the Austrian artist Josef Kriehuber. Rummaging through one of New York's used bookstalls in the summer of 1940, Cornell found the print and was immediately taken with Cerrito's image, which prompted a fantastic series of epiphanies of the dancer over the next twenty-five years. His long series of works relating to Cerrito became a serial meditation on the passage of time, the miracle of the creative act, and the complex puzzles he created to surround his mysterious iconography.

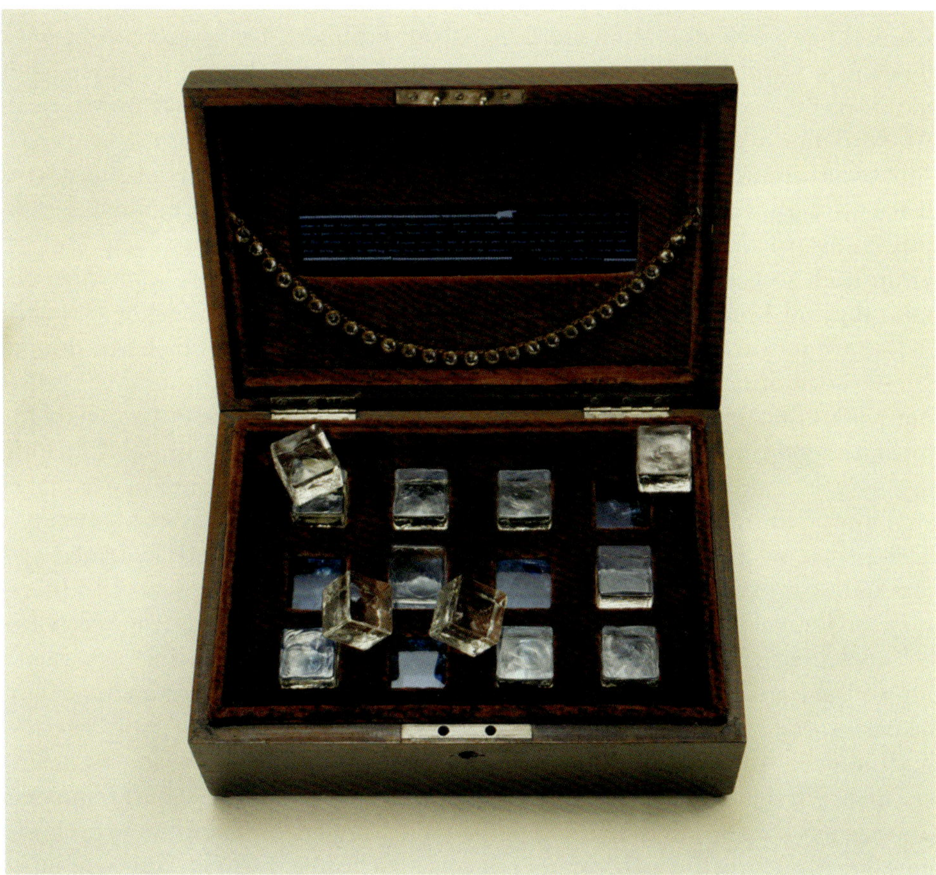

**Figure 65** Joseph Cornell, *Taglioni's Jewel Casket*, 1940, wood box containing glass ice cubes, jewelry, etc. 4 ¾ × 11 ⅞ × 8 ¼ inches. (Museum of Modern Art, New York, Gift of James Thrall Soby, 474.1953; art © The Joseph and Robert Cornell Memorial Foundation/ Licensed by VAGA, New York, New York; image © The Museum of Modern Art/Licensed by SCALA/Art Resource, New York)

Although—or perhaps because—she had never danced in the United States, Cerrito materialized to the highly suggestible Cornell on the streets he frequented in modern New York. As he said, "the figure of the young danseuse stepped forth as completely contemporaneous as the skyscrapers surrounding her. . . . Like the capricious *Ondine* of her favorite ballet she seemed once more to have assumed mortal guise."[8] Cornell proceeded to execute a series of works devoted to Cerrito in *Ondine*, a ballet whose eponymous sea sprite vacillates between her love for a mortal man and her own immortality. Embedded in Cornell's work, Ondine became a metaphor for eternal youth and for nature's sublimity. There were also deep metaphysical components of his Ondine boxes, especially those executed during World War II. A Christian Scientist and ardent pacifist, Cornell contrasted the hideous spectacle of war (discord resulting from erroneous thought) with the creative act in ballet or the visual arts.[9] Transformed and disguised, Cerrito appeared again and again to

Cornell—as a ticket taker on the Long Island Railroad, as a guard closing windows in a Manhattan warehouse, in aquatic ballets at the Hippodrome—but mostly as the undying *Ondine* (*Portrait of Ondine,* 1940, Smithsonian American Art Museum, Washington, D.C.). On a more complex level, Cornell invoked a subtle and ironic nostalgia in Cerrito-inspired *Window Facades* of the 1950s, laden with allusions to Apollinaire's poetry and to Duchamp's punning, fenestrated construction *Fresh Widow* (1920, Museum of Modern Art, New York).[10] From such scenes Cornell continued to create visual responses containing his metaphysical beliefs on the ontological nature of substance, being, and time.[11] Before we return from a Cornell-driven detour into Romantic ballet to resume an extended discussion of Spanish dance, we can summarize his unique contributions to the art of the dance: First, Cornell was responsible in large part for introducing twentieth-century art audiences to the earlier stars of the Romantic ballet, little remembered outside dance circles. Moreover, he Americanized it, as seen above, through his pursuit of souvenir materials from American sources as well as through his encounters with dancers in New York—both imagined and real (as with twentieth-century ballerina Tamara Toumanova). Cornell's incessant time travel links the fragile tradition of Romantic ballet to its modern legacy in American dance. More concretely, Cornell invented a whole new genre for a visual arts interpretation of dance in his box constructions and collages: he used specific references—names, dates, and places to revive memory in ways both allusive and poetic. And he combined symbolic objects—sequins, feathers, photo fragments—as Proustian evocations of the dancer herself, emblems of poignant connection to her and perpetual reminders of his own wistful longings. Finally, Cornell wittily referenced other art forms to enrich his own: nineteenth-century souvenir prints, Seurat's dancers, and early film clips of dancers such as Loïe Fuller.[12]

Returning to the American artists' responses to Spanish Dance, American visual artists abroad had long since discovered it to be an appealing, exotic subject. Its attraction made itself felt on the young American Thomas Eakins (1844–1916) during his trip to Spain in 1869–70. Having spent some months in Paris at the Ecole des Beaux-Arts and then in the atelier of Jean-Léon Gérôme, Eakins, eager to move from drawing into full compositions in oil, headed to Spain. There he studied Velázquez in the Prado before moving on to Seville, where he consciously began a new, post-student phase in his work. Taking on the challenge of Spain's brilliant sunshine and bright color, Eakins soon hired as models a family of itinerant street performers—parents who played instruments while their young daughter Carmelita Requena danced. First he sketched a portrait of Carmelita in oil, perhaps as a preliminary study for the group (1869; fig. 66). Its lively brushwork and brilliant red-green contrasts show Eakins's interest in capturing the immediacy of outdoor light and the brightness of the costume itself. Of posing Carmelita, the painter wrote home, "Some candy given me, I ate a little and then gave the rest to a dear little girl, Carmalita [*sic*], whom I am painting. . . . She is only seven years old and has to dance in the street every day. But she likes better to stand still and be painted. She looks down at a little card on the floor so as to keep her head still and in the right place."[13]

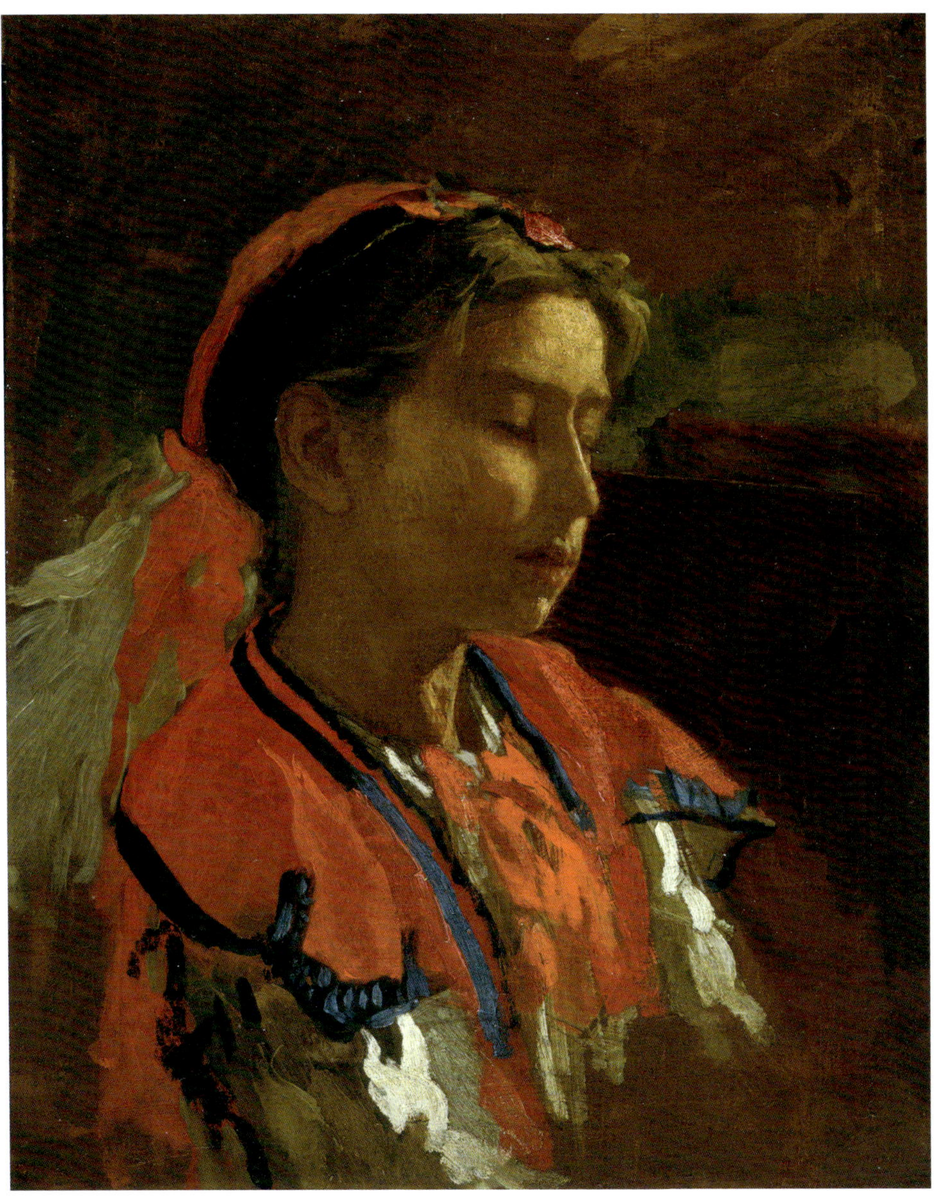

**Figure 66** Thomas Eakins, *Carmelita Requena*, 1869, oil on canvas, 21 × 17 inches. (Metropolitan Museum of Art, New York, Bequest of Mary Cushing Fosburgh, 1978, 1979.135.2; image © The Metropolitan Museum of Art/Art Resource, New York)

For three months Eakins labored on the family group, one of his first finished compositions now known as *Street Scene, Seville* (1870; fig. 67). For that painting he posed the family in sunlight and shadow against a wall on which he recorded the vernacular touch of bullfight graffiti. A woman watches from a nearby window. In their work—and it is work, not spontaneous or celebratory performance—the family members gaze downward, father and mother at their instruments, little Carmelita concentrating dutifully on her steps. In the attempt to capture a transient moment by way of dance, Eakins had perhaps bitten off a bit more than he was then ready to chew. He could not quite realize the liveliness he sought in choosing a dance subject: his figures, even the young dancer, retain a certain posed woodenness. "Picture-making is new to me," he confessed upon the completion of *Street Scene*. "There is the sun and gay colors and a hundred things you never see in a studio light, and ever so many botherations that no one out of the trade could ever guess at."[14] Did Eakins's difficulties lie in representing the dance itself, or were his "botherations" merely technical? Whatever their cause, it would be eight years before Eakins returned to the subject of the dance.

For Eakins, the subject of Spanish dance, especially with a child dancer and a folkloric rather than theatrical setting, provided entrée into the local color of Seville. For his contemporary Mary Cassatt, Spain represented freedom to travel and to combine lessons learned from its masters with more modern

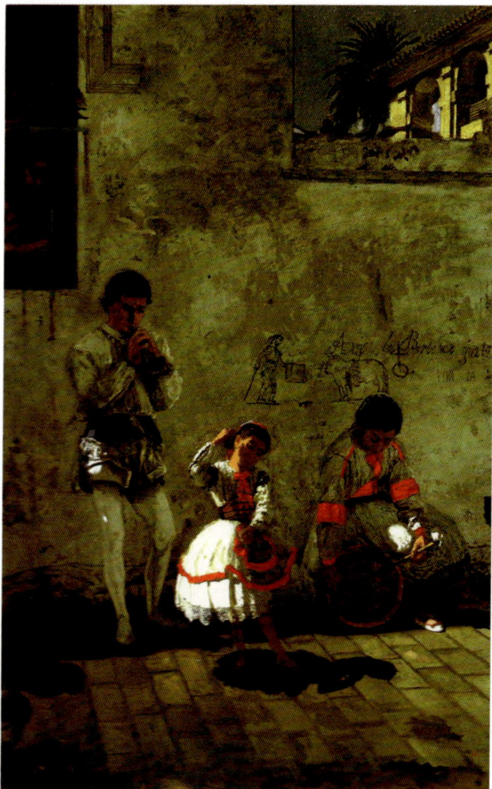

**Figure 67** Thomas Eakins, *Street Scene, Seville*, 1870, oil on canvas, 63 × 37 inches. (private collection)

developments. Long resident in Paris, Cassatt had been pressed to return to the United States during the Franco-Prussian War, but she departed again for Europe in 1872, soon after the war's end. Following a stay in Parma, where she had painted *The Bacchante* (discussed above), she moved on with great anticipation to Spain, where the work of Velázquez aroused her excited admiration. Settling in sunny Seville for the winter of 1872–73, Cassatt wrote to her friend Emily Sartain that Spain "has not been 'exploited' yet as it might be and it is suggestive of pictures on all sides."[15] Soon she fastened on several Andalusian subjects she thought would appeal to American collectors, including a *Spanish Dancer Wearing a Lace Mantilla* (1873; fig. 68). Cassatt's dancer pauses to give the artist opportunity to celebrate her "rich dark coloring" framed by cascades of lace and a delicate fan. In its firm handling of volumes and planes, Cassatt's *Spanish Dancer* perhaps owes a debt to Velázquez or Manet. Like their best portraits, her Spanish dancer is a distinctive, even exotic, portrait, but—unlike many lesser genre painters of her day—Cassatt eschewed the practice of posing sitters in exotic costumes as a means of introducing themes of sexual fantasy. Instead, Cassatt's Spanish dancer, given quiet dignity and reserve, represents a public performer posed in an intimate interior. She anticipates the subtle issues of domesticity and public–private spatial dichotomies Cassatt would explore within the circle of Degas and the Impressionists in the later 1870s, culminating in her shift to avant-garde compositions of women and children in the 1880s.[16]

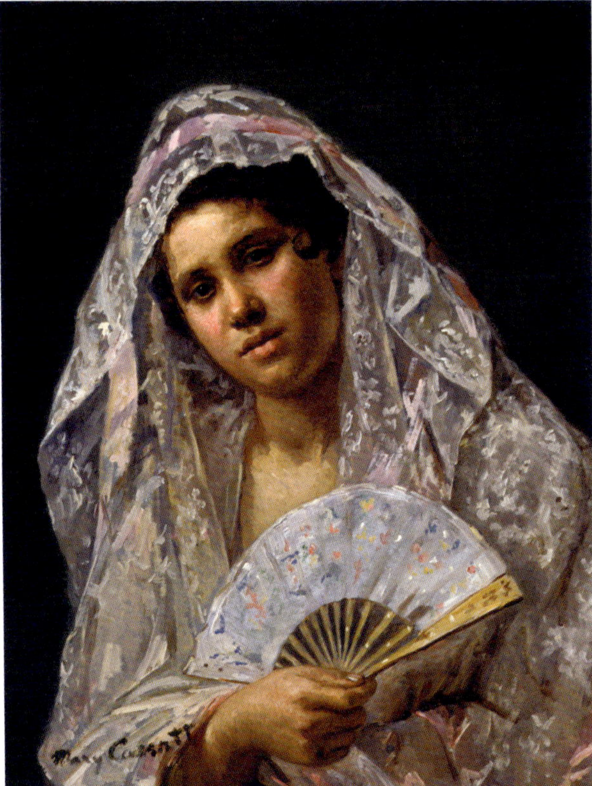

**Figure 68** Mary Cassatt, *Spanish Dancer Wearing a Lace Mantilla*, 1873, oil on canvas, 25 ⅝ × 19 ¾ inches. (Smithsonian American Art Museum, Gift of Victoria Dreyfus, 1967.40)

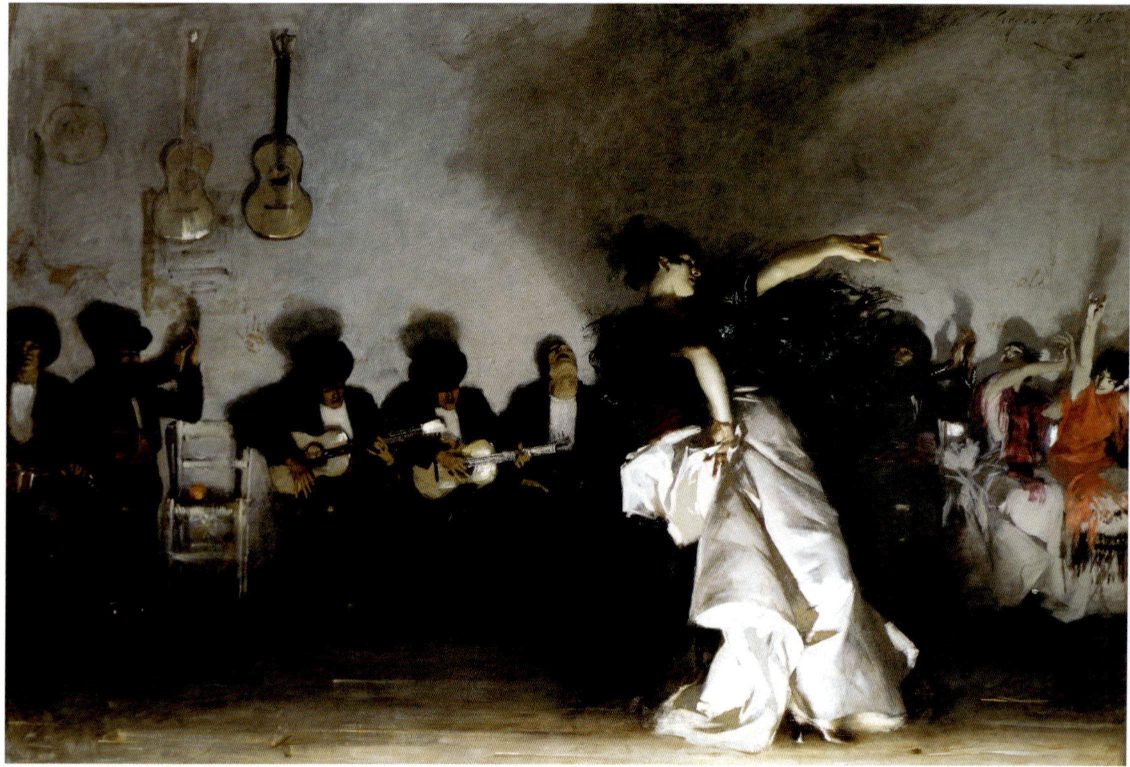

**Figure 69** John Singer Sargent, *El Jaleo*, 1882, oil on canvas, 91 ³/₁₀ × 137 inches. (© Isabella Stewart Gardner Museum, Boston)

Other American artists looked to subjects of Spanish dance for a more deliberate sensuousness they could not find—or express—in American dance subjects. Spanish dance, more than most other kinds, seemed capable of encompassing life's primal acts: of love, loss, tragedy, compensation. No American took up the subject of Spanish dance to greater effect than John Singer Sargent (1856–1925) whose monumental *El Jaleo* (1882; fig. 69) is ignited by an unmistakably erotic charge passing between dancer and spectators. One of the notable features in Spanish dancing, wrote Havelock Ellis, "lies in its accompaniments, and particularly in the fact that under proper conditions all the spectators are themselves performers. In flamenco dancing, among an audience of the people, every one takes a part by rhythmic clapping and stamping, and by the occasional prolonged 'olés' and other cries by which the dancer is encouraged or applauded."[17] Those actions collectively define Sargent's title *El Jaleo,* which names not only the source of the dance (the *jaleo de jerez*) but invokes simultaneously, as Trevor Fairbrother points out, the term's broader meaning of ruckus or hubub.[18] Sargent possessed a definite appetite for such theatrical chaos, his excitement rising with the energy of the performers. In two studies of a Spanish dancer that likely precede and predict the dancer in *El Jaleo*, Sargent's rush of fevered line and dramatic flamenco gesture convey the artist's own participatory response (*Sketch of a Spanish Dancer*, c. 1879–90, Isabella Stewart Gardner Museum, Boston; and

*Study for Spanish Dancer* (1882, Dallas Museum of Art 1974). Other painters followed flamenco, but perhaps Sargent succeeded best in integrating spectator, dancers, and musicians into a unified tableau.

Sargent, like Eakins before him, had gone to Spain to study Velázquez. During nine months there in 1879, he made small sketches of flamenco dancers, weaving them into the *El Jaleo* composition the next year. Musicians and a male singer—eyes closed and head thrown back—form a frieze of figures against the back wall, interrupted by a lone empty chair—the dancer's?—on which a single orange, symbol of Andalusia, reposes. (No matter that Sargent's model was herself a French dancer who posed for him in the studio). Farther right along the eleven-foot horizontal expanse of *El Jaleo* Sargent positions the dancer herself, seen in profile in the strong light and shadow of the tavern. She manages a voluminous skirt, beneath which we catch just a glimpse of stamping foot. Out of an inky darkness, in a dangerously caressing flamenco gesture, emerges her right hand. We can scarcely escape the Dionysiac mood. Sargent's room pulses with ecstasy. Robert Hughes speculates that *El Jaleo* might be the first American painting that "celebrates the Dionysiac urge, a visceral joy in movement and music. . . . For once, Puritan decorum is overcome."[19]

Sargent's *El Jaleo* was the foreign sensation of the Paris Salon of 1882 and is widely regarded now as the first masterpiece of Sargent's early career. But it was not received with universal enthusiasm at its Salon debut. Sargent's friend Henry James remarked that "*El Jaleo* sins, in my opinion, in the direction of ugliness, and, independently of the fact that the heroine is circling round uncommoded by her petticoats, [it] has a want of serenity."[20] If there were sins, one wants to argue to Mr. James, they were sins arising out of Sargent's own appetite for the theatrical—sins deliberately, defiantly committed. Had an artist ever tried harder to undermine serenity in a painting, to foment tension, both psychological and formal? While spectators (and we with them) devour the dancer's flashy display, we glimpse in her shadowy face the inward, trancelike state flamenco can summon. Sargent's virtuosity with the brush is so confident that he can almost forget about it, paying tribute instead to the technical virtuosity of the dancer.

*El Jaleo*, both damned and praised for its sensuality, set up some of Sargent's future portraits, such as the scandalous *Madame X* (*Mme Gautreau* (1883–84, Metropolitan Museum of Art, New York) painted two years later. In appearance and proud demeanor, the two subjects might be dangerous sisters: both black-clad figures seen in profile, they are at once sexually aware and elusive. Sargent aestheticized both women into objects of desire, one disturbing by the intensity of her movement, the other by the tension within her stillness. Both, but especially the initial breakthrough of *El Jaleo*, accomplished for the artist what he sought. Says critic Trevor Fairbrother, Sargent's choice of El Jaleo "gratified his need for a release from the primness of his Anglo-Saxon Protestant cultural heritage through esoterically coded sensualism."[21]

Sargent made several more studies of Spanish dancers in the wake of his travels to Spain and Morocco. And the subject reappeared in his New York work with the arrival of the celebrated Spanish dancer "La Carmencita," whom Sargent propelled to lasting fame in a full-length 1890 portrait (fig. 70).

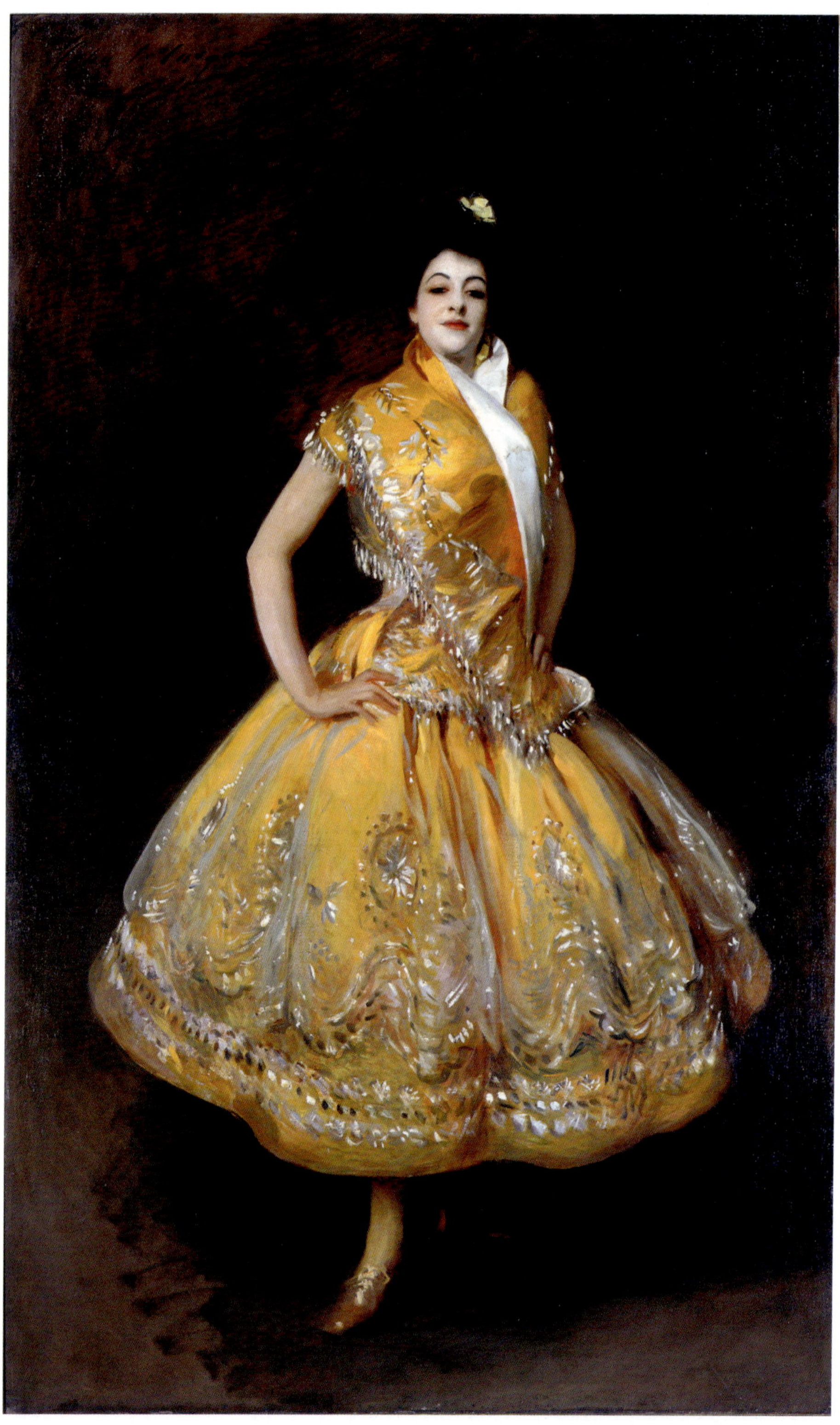

**Figure 70** John Singer Sargent, *La Carmencita*, 1890, oil on canvas, 90 × 54 ½ inches. (Musée d'Orsay, Paris; photo: Réunion des Musées Nationaux/Art Resource, New York)

By contemporary accounts, Sargent's Carmencita was (as a performer) reportedly less brilliant than others of lesser reputation. But she managed to convey a suppressed fire, by way of her "intriguing and exotic personality," which sparked a vital connection to audiences wherever she performed.[22] "Her dancing had set the town on fire in that Age of Innocence of New York," wrote a critic in the *Times*.[23] Sargent's portrait begins to suggest the force of that personality. She agreed to pose for Sargent, but, straight from the cabarets of Spain, Carmencita was a wild, restless beauty, alternately sullen and childish. As a dancer whose being came alive in movement, she found it difficult to pose. To keep her amused and focused, Sargent resorted to games such as painting his nose red or slowly eating his own cigar—the latter of special delight to the dancer. Offered six hundred pounds for the portrait when it was exhibited, Sargent turned down the sum, saying that he had spent much more for the bracelets and gifts necessary to keep Carmencita happy.

In the resulting portrait, Carmencita's bold carriage—arched back, hands on hips, flashing eyes, uplifted chin—conveys something of her fiery, even defiant spirit. But at the same time, the dancer's power is undermined by the excessive decorativeness of her costume and the artist's virtuoso rendering of it. Like his idol Velázquez, Sargent makes its surfaces—orange, black, and silver—shimmer and rustle. Carmencita's is a costume not unlike that worn by Fanny Elssler, but, buoyed by layers of petticoats, the dress threatens to take over the dancer within, suggesting nothing so much as the shape of a saucy, bouffant lampshade. In its theatricality and superficial brilliance, Sargent's *Carmencita* lacks the physical intensity of the dancer in his *El Jaleo*. And the artist knew it: when *Carmencita* was acquired for the Luxembourg, Sargent regretted that it would represent him, calling the work "little more than a sketch."[24]

What Sargent reported of Carmencita's behavior in words, his compatriot William Merritt Chase (1849–1916) captured with his brush. Painted in the same year as Sargent's, Chase's portrait of the Spanish dancer (1890; fig. 71) exudes a confident liveliness achieved in part by the painter's broad, dashing brushstroke. It is a showy tour de force, with roots in Velázquez, Manet, and the Impressionists, from whom Chase learned a directness and spontaneity perfectly congruent with Carmencita's flashy presentation and missing from Sargent's portrait. Chase's *Carmencita* is eminently self-possessed, her power as a performer sharply enhanced by Chase's customary isolation of the figure, conscious placement of props, and dense surfaces.

Spanish dance subjects proved amazingly durable and versatile for later visual artists. During World War I the Ballets Russes's Diaghilev and his circle haunted Madrid's flamenco cafés, resulting in a whole cycle of Spanish-inspired dance works.[25] European painters such as Natalia Gontcharova and Henri Matisse took up Spanish dance themes with enthusiasm.[26] Back in the United States, Man Ray, whose avant-garde associations and technical innovations made him a leader in New York Dada, found inspiration in a troupe of Spanish dancers. A fairly representational drawing called *Spanish Dancer* (1918, location unknown) finds an organizing pattern in the concentric ovals of her skirt. That pencil drawing likely preceded several more abstract Spanish

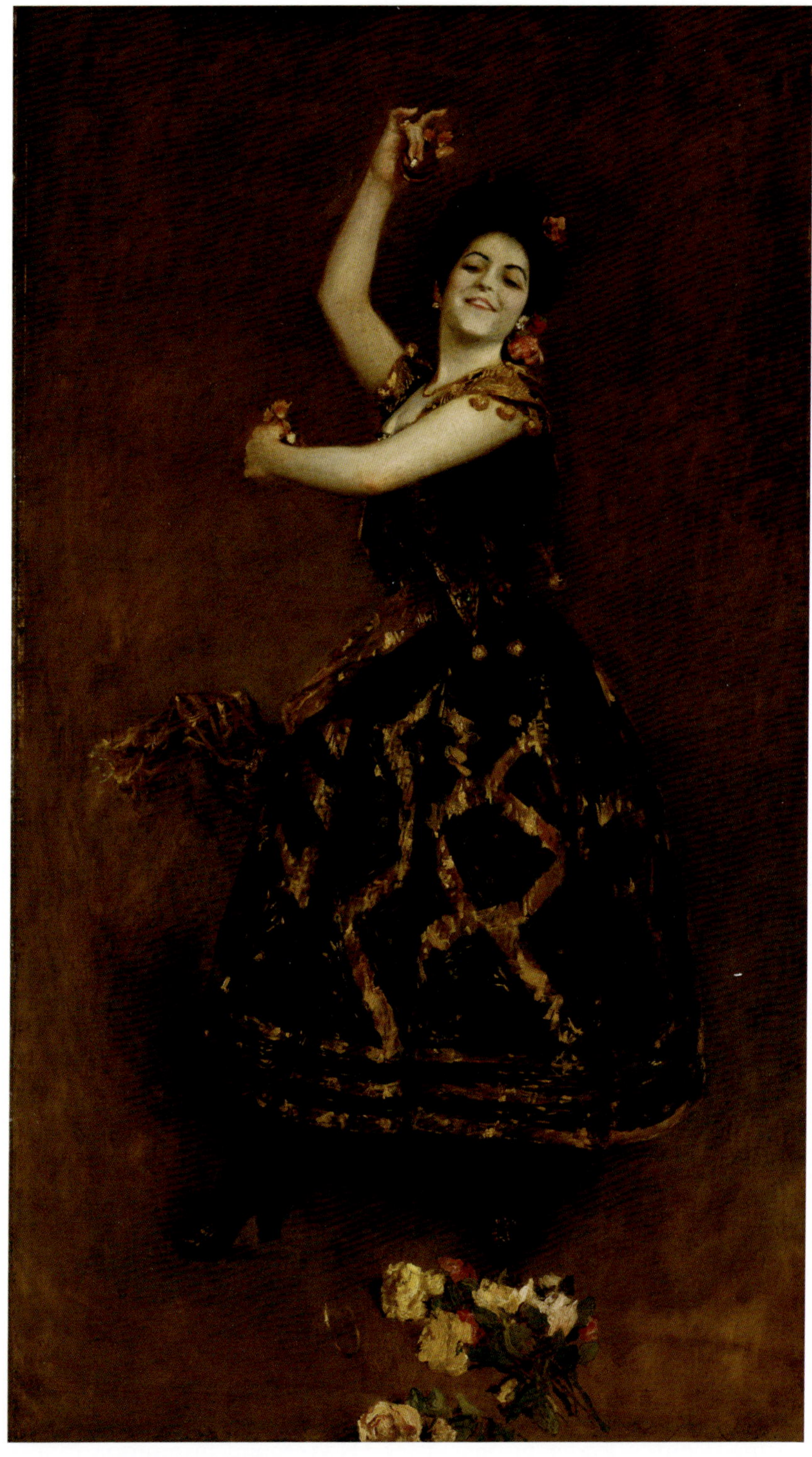

**Figure 71** William Merritt Chase, *Carmencita*, 1890, oil on canvas, 69 ⅞ × 40 ⅞ inches. (Metropolitan Museum of Art, New York, Gift of Sir William Van Horne, 1906, 06.969; image © The Metropolitan Museum of Art/Art Resource, New York)

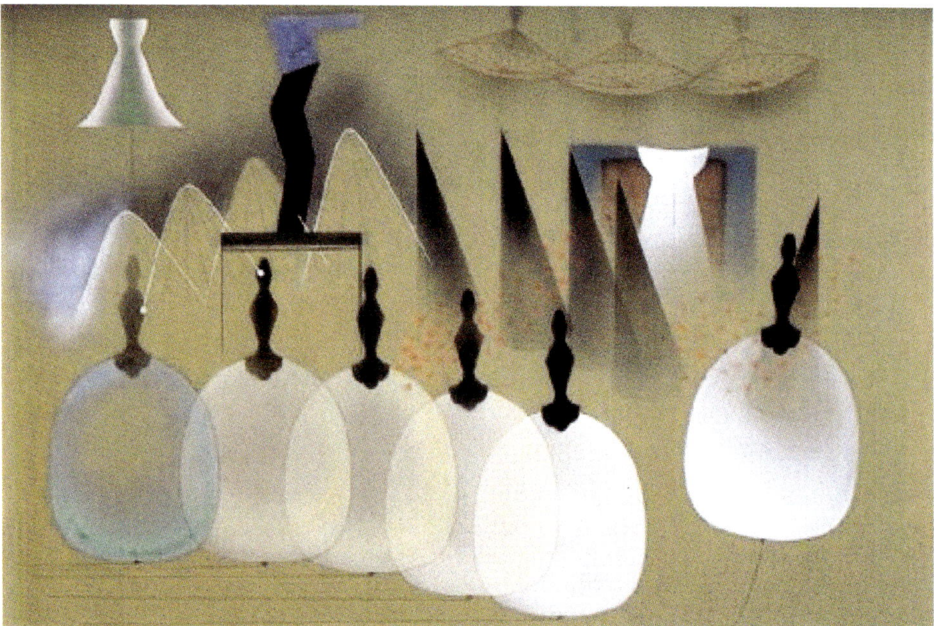

Figure 72 Man Ray, *Seguidilla*, 1919, airbrushed gouache, ink, pencil and colored pencil on paperboard, 22 × 27 ¹³⁄₁₆ inches. (Hirshhorn Museum and Sculpture Garden, Smithsonian Institution, Joseph H. Hirshhorn Purchase Fund and Museum Purchase, 1987)

dance subjects from 1919, including his *Seguidilla* (fig. 72), an abstraction of a Castilian dance with distinctive rhythmic and visual features. Overlapping translucent fans in the foreground, handles upward, suggest the full-skirted figures of female dancers. They are six in number, like the shadows in the artist's earlier *Rope Dancer* (1916; see chapter 8), and they are tethered, again similarly, with ropes or strings. Trailing their strings, the dancers in *Seguidilla* resemble balloons as well, especially as the one on the far right floats up and away from the others. Behind them, the fragmented male torso of a flamenco dancer pauses in midstep on table top amid airy conelike forms suggesting Spanish mantillas. Nearby, a drift of red dots scatters like sequins on a flamenco costume. How creatively has the artist adapted the rhythms of dance to the visual rhythms of his compositions. In *Seguidilla,* the entire effect is evanescent, appropriately so for Man Ray's new medium of airbrush. He called his sprayed paintings *aerographs,* and reveled in his newfound ability to paint "without touching the canvas; this was a pure cerebral activity. It was also like painting in 3-D, to obtain the desired effect you had to move the airbrush nearer or farther from the canvas."[27] Like the dancers whose movements inspired him, Man Ray choreographed his dance-derived paintings, floating the passion of the Spanish dance within a whole range of fluid or staccato pictorial rhythms.

## Spectacular Vernacular: Importing the Cancan

While Americans were still responding at home and abroad to Spanish dance, new excitement was generated with the arrival in America of the "high-kickers," the female dancers of the cancan and the chahut. They had been seen first by foreign visitors to Paris. Students, tourists and thrill-seekers, first from Britain and later the United States, reveled in these dances as forms of protest against authority, the bourgeoisie, and the spirit of order and propriety. Dancers such as La Goulue, Jane Avril, and Nini Patte-en-l'air brought an electrical charge to the stage, their heads thrown back, legs flying above their heads in startling and sudden high kicks, followed by frantic pirouettes and a wild run among the spectators, ending finally in an abrupt stop, sliding horizontally into "splits" on the floor. Toulouse-Lautrec and Seurat captured this frenetic energy.[28] But Americans traveling to Paris, including Winslow Homer, had begun to record the frenzied cancan two decades earlier. Homer, then a young illustrator, had a studio in Montmartre during part of a ten-month Paris visit stretching from late 1866 to the fall of 1867. His wood engraving *A Parisian Ball—Dancing at the Mabille, Paris* (fig. 73) was reproduced in *Harper's Weekly* November 23, 1867. In this lively illustration a large crowd looks on as both women and men kick up their heels, skirts flying high. By their dress we can tell that Homer's cancan dancers are not stage performers, but presumably young social dancers daring and athletic enough to engage in the riotous cabaret sensation of the day. Such scenes were wilder than the usual fare on the pages of American family journals

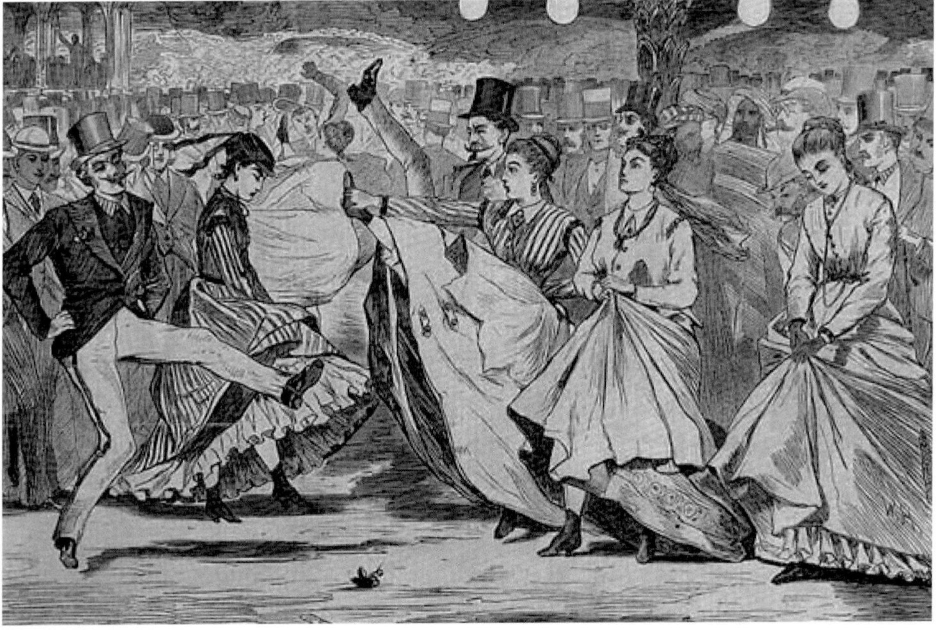

**Figure 73** Winslow Homer, *A Parisian Ball—Dancing at the Mabille, Paris*, 1867, wood engraving, 9 ⅛ × 13 ⅝ inches. (from *Harper's Weekly*, November 23, 1867)

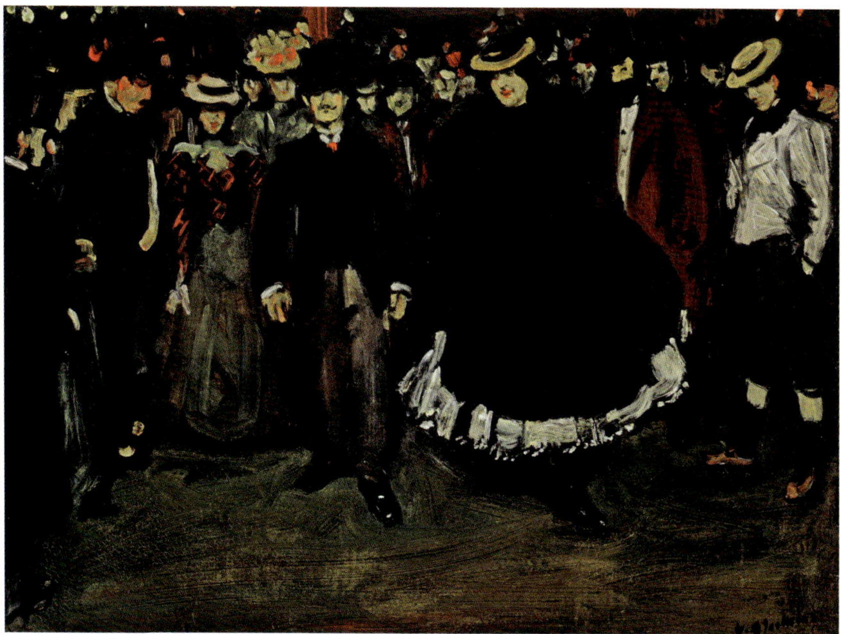

**Figure 74** William Glackens, *Bal Bullier*, 1895, oil on canvas, 23 ¹³⁄₁₆ × 32 inches. (Terra Foundation for American Art, Chicago, Illinois, 1999.59; image: Terra Foundation for American Art, Chicago/Art Resource, New York)

of the day. The editors of *Harper's*, perhaps to forestall predictable criticism, appended a long, censorious article to Homer's dance illustrations. "We shall not venture," intoned the editor, "to look into the abyss on the brink of which these frenzied men and women are dancing, and this too curious crowd of spectators is treading. This is work for the severe and steady eye of the preacher and moralist."[29]

Just two years later the irrepressible Mark Twain (Samuel Clemens), gathering material for *Innocents Abroad* (1869), professed shock at the naughty antics of the Cancan dancers. Twain reported that he dutifully covered his face with his hands, but managed to peek through the fingers. Upon its release, his book became wildly popular, no doubt tempting hordes of other Americans to jettison their *faux* innocence—or perhaps Yankee hypocrisy—in the dance halls of Paris.

An American painter who sampled the broad range of public entertainments offered in Paris dancehalls was William Glackens (1870–1938), who arrived in 1895 with his friend and mentor Robert Henri. Keen to paint real life as encountered in the streets, Glackens, well trained as a magazine illustrator and newspaper artist, applied his reportorial skills to the lively nightlife of Montmartre. "The Paris cafés are a never ending source of inspiration to me," he wrote to an American friend.[30] In tune with the alluring realism of Manet and the caricatured demimonde subjects of Toulouse-Lautrec—combined with a dash of Yankee ambition bent on elevating his career status—Glackens undertook to transform himself that year from illustrator to painter.[31] Still, his early canvases, among them a scene from the *Bal Bullier* (1895; fig. 74), rely heavily on his reporter's ability to grasp and interpret the nuanced interactions among diverse social classes in a distinct setting. In *Bal Bullier* Glackens's broad brush-strokes compress a dense crush of bodies within the dimly lit dancehall interior. Onlookers, pressed mostly to the top of the composition, surround a couple dancing at the center: a man stiffly attired in top hat and formal suit pairs with a more relaxed, flirtatious young woman, likely a working-class *grisette* trying out the cancan as part of her evening's entertainment. Animating the dark-toned composition are bright flashes of petticoat ruffle, shirt fronts, hands, and faces—bravura touches that anticipate Glackens's later affiliation with Henri and the group of progressive New York painters known as the Eight.

Another American visual artist who recorded the wild hilarity of turn-of-the-century Parisian nightlife was Alfred Maurer (1868–1932). His *Le Bal au Moulin Rouge* (1900–1902; fig. 75) and *Le Bal Bullier* (c. 1901–3, Smith College Museum of Art, Northampton, Mass.) capture, even more than Glackens's more timid composition, the high-kicking abandon and color of the dancers in those notorious clubs.[32] Maurer, who began as a commercial artist in New York, sailed for Paris in 1897, making him one of the earliest of a generation of American modernists abroad. In Paris Maurer explored a series of styles, absorbing innovations from late Impressionism and Tonalism before moving into the modernist circles where Cézanne and Matisse held sway. Known later for his still life and landscape paintings, Maurer at the turn of the century chose the subjects of Moulin Rouge and Bal Bullier dancers to convey the infectious energy of a Paris whose raucous welcome extended to all visitors adventurous enough to step into its living spectacle.

The Polish-born American sculptor Elie Nadelman (1882–1946) was a life-long devoté, wherever he lived, of music halls, the circus, and all forms of dance. Resident in Paris from 1903 until 1914, he read Baudelaire, discussed modern art with Leo and Gertrude Stein, and developed a career as a sculptor of contemporary life. His artistic heroes also appreciated dance: Guys, Daumier, and Degas, but especially Lautrec and Seurat. But unlike most of these, Nadelman made no portraits of individualized dancers, concentrating instead on types, and studying proportion, silhouette, and definitive gesture. Although these were the years of the Ballets Russes in Paris, Nadelman preferred the mocking grace of the noisy café-concert, where brief, high-energy dance routines culminated in a smashing finale. There he found the famous dance move that defined an era—the high-kicking cancan. Likely Nadelman knew Seurat's famous *La Chahut*, an image of the cancan in Seurat's neo-Impressionist manner (*Study for Le Chahut*, 1889–90, Albright-Knox Museum, Buffalo).

Based on his own observations of the cancan and likely of Seurat, Nadelman made several versions of his own *High-Kicker*, now known simply as *Dancer* (c. 1920; fig. 76). In New York, where he pursued his career after the outbreak of World War I, Nadelman also discovered American vaudeville, in which he discerned rich veins of folk tradition, a style of American artistic expression whose forms he avidly collected (along with old theatrical photographs and dance programs) and incorporated into his simplified figures. *Dancer* may, in fact, be based on a photograph owned by Nadelman of the vaudeville performer Eva Tanguay. Probably the sources for his high-kicking dance sculpture are multiple, both

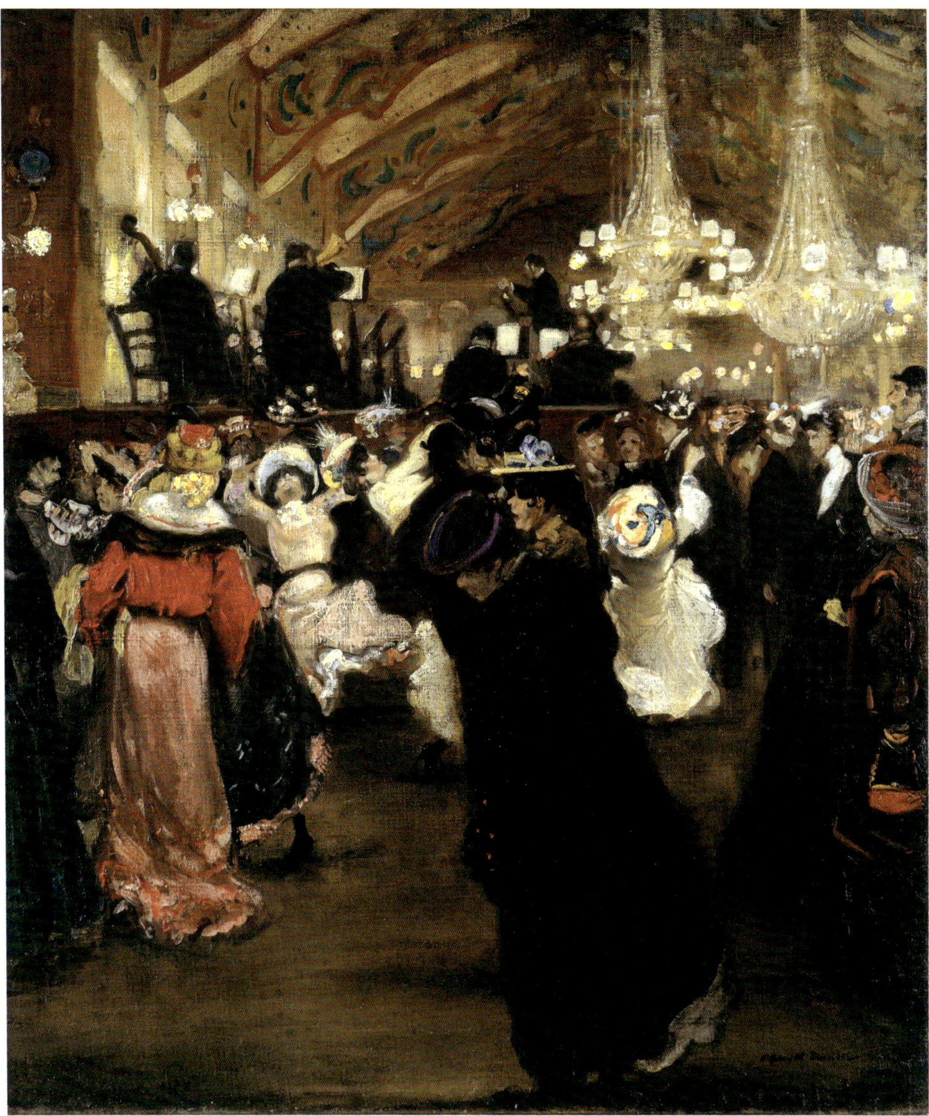

**Figure 75** Alfred Maurer, *Le Bal au Moulin Rouge*, 1900–1902, oil on canvas, 36 ½ × 32 ¼ inches. (Curtis Galleries, Minneapolis, Minnesota)

remembered and revised. She is a hybrid Franco-American dancer, on one hand oddly calm and remote, on the other stylish and *outré*, like the naughty can-can itself. In at least one of these *Dancer* sculptures, Nadelman wittily accentuated the latter qualities when he wiped off a layer of gesso to reveal the red cherrywood cheeks of the dancer beneath. In this, as in many of Nadelman's other dancers, the figure is defined by a single unified movement that dictates a degree of abstraction, here her scissor-like split kick, part of her Vaudeville routine. Future sections of this study will revisit Nadelman's revealing dance gestures, inspired variously by classical subjects and folk art forms, and presented in highly diverse moods.

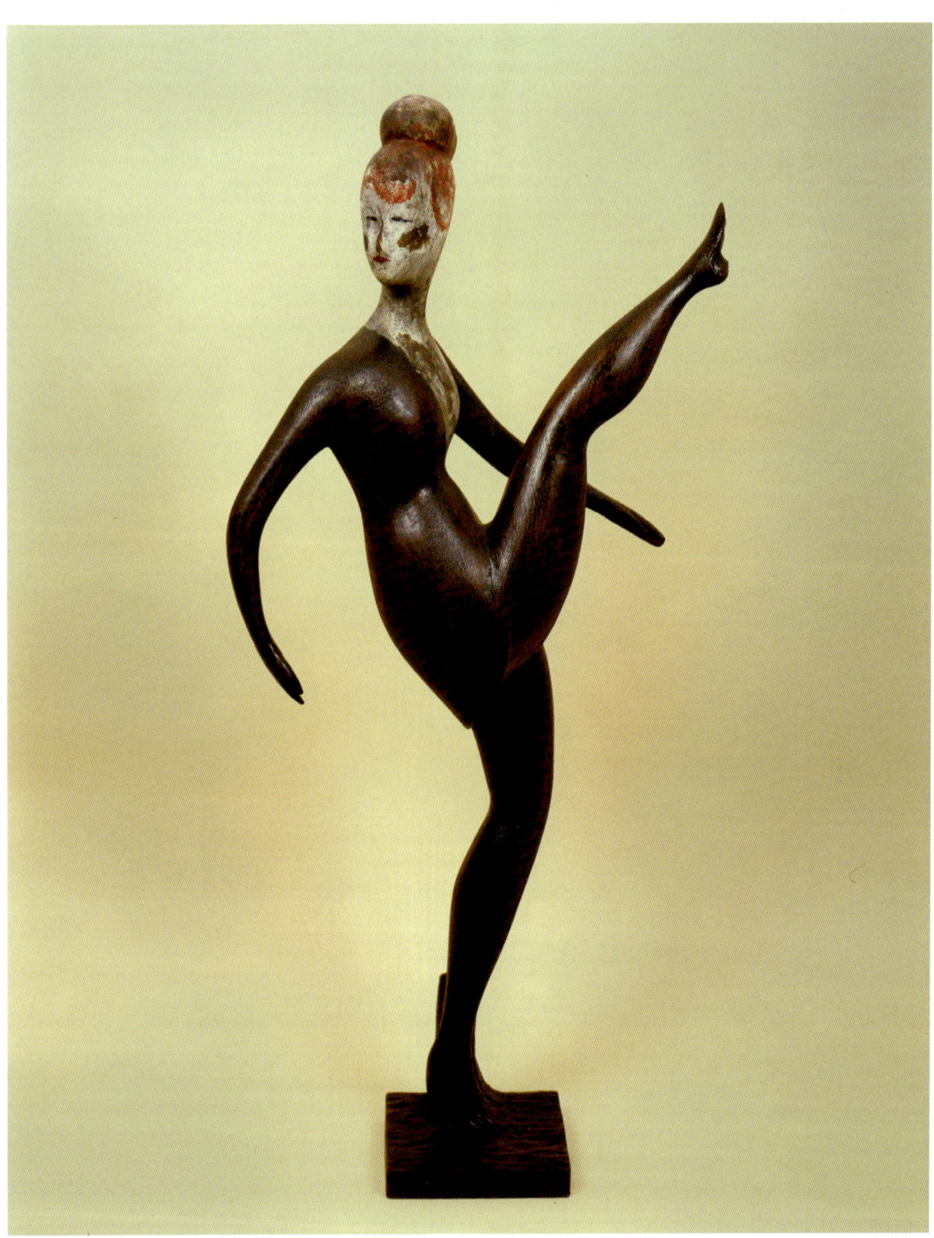

**Figure 76** Elie Nadelman, *Dancer [High-Kicker]*, c. 1920, cherry wood with painted gesso, h. 28 ½ inches. (private collection, photo courtesy Gerald Peters Gallery, New York)

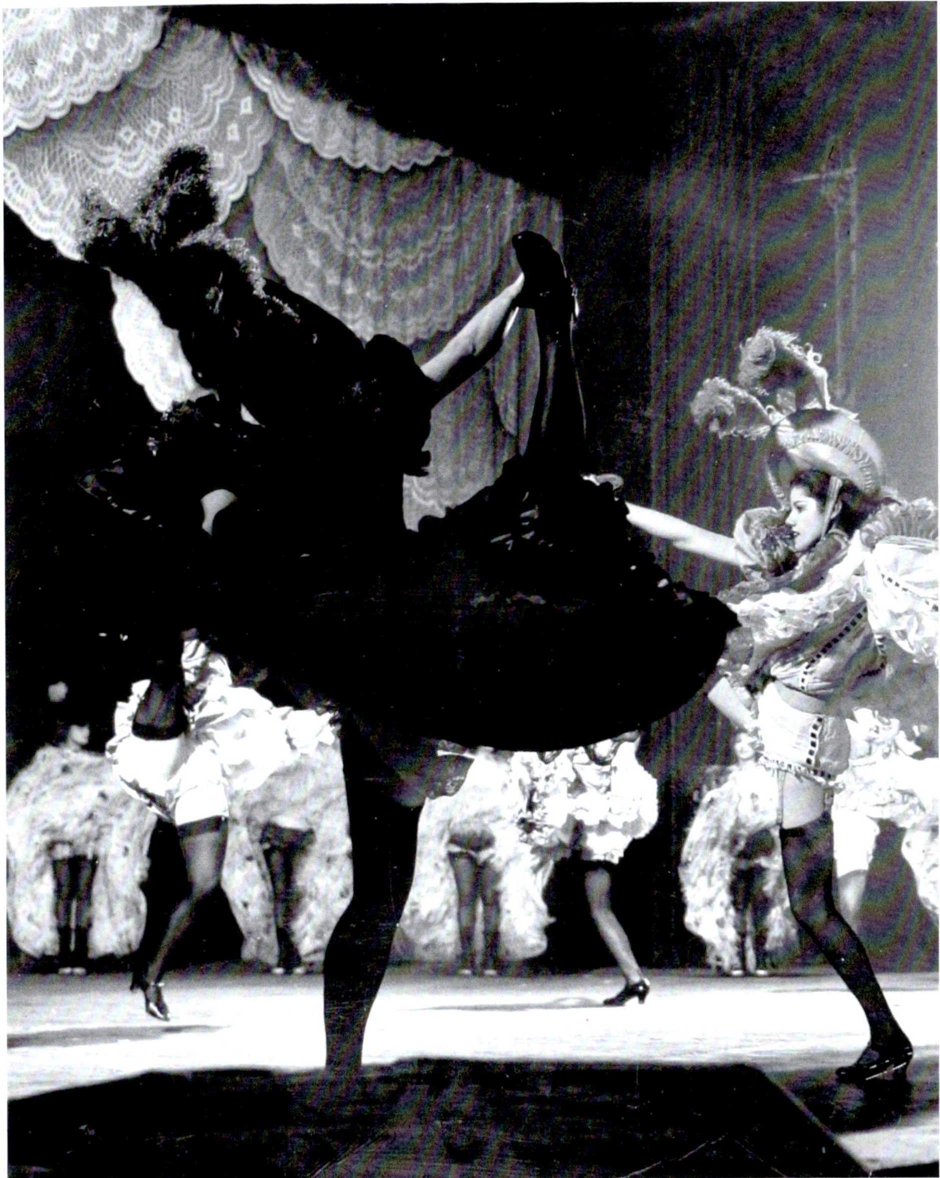

**Figure 77** Harold "Doc" Edgerton, *Can-Can Dance*, 1940, gelatin silver print. (University of New Mexico Art Museum, 96.5.93; © Harold and Esther Edgerton Foundation, 2010, courtesy Palm Press, Inc.)

In contrast to the smooth, unified treatment of Nadelman's high-kicker, American photographer Harold (Doc) Edgerton (1903–90) created a much more complex portrait by means of an electronic lamp of his own invention. Edgerton's high-voltage flash was of such intensity and brevity that it could make even fast-moving objects appear to stand still. It was a perfect foil for the mass of swirling skirts in Edgerton's *Can-Can Dance* of 1940, which sweeps the viewer into the infectious energy of the dance (fig. 77).

Just a few years later, American artist Joseph Cornell, in a departure from his own Romantic-ballet works, discussed above, created a whimsical dance-themed construction based on the *opéras bouffes* of the nineteenth-century composer Jacques Offenbach (1819–80). This mixed-media piece, which Cornell titled *A Pantry Ballet (for Jacques Offenbach)* (1942, Nelson-Atkins Museum of Art, Kansas City, Mo.) is a "crayfish ballet," featuring a bevy of red toy crustaceans sporting ballet skirts and lined up in dance formation. Like Offenbach, Cornell built into his construction elements of political and social satire, obliquely referencing wartime Paris, the occupying German troops, and remarks on the human condition presented in rebus-like form.

Taking what he needed from the world of dance and extending his delight in images that transgress boundaries between high and popular culture, Cornell (like Nadelman) took a cue from Georges Seurat, who had earlier burlesqued both the circus and the dance. Cornell borrowed Seurat's circus image for a collage he said was "dedicated to those persistent dancers, the Clown, the Elephant and the Ballerina (or Equestrienne)" (fig. 78).[33] Framed by illusionistic torn paper, Seurat's circus dancer nearly flies off the cover of *Dance Index*, the journal for which Cornell created it in 1946.

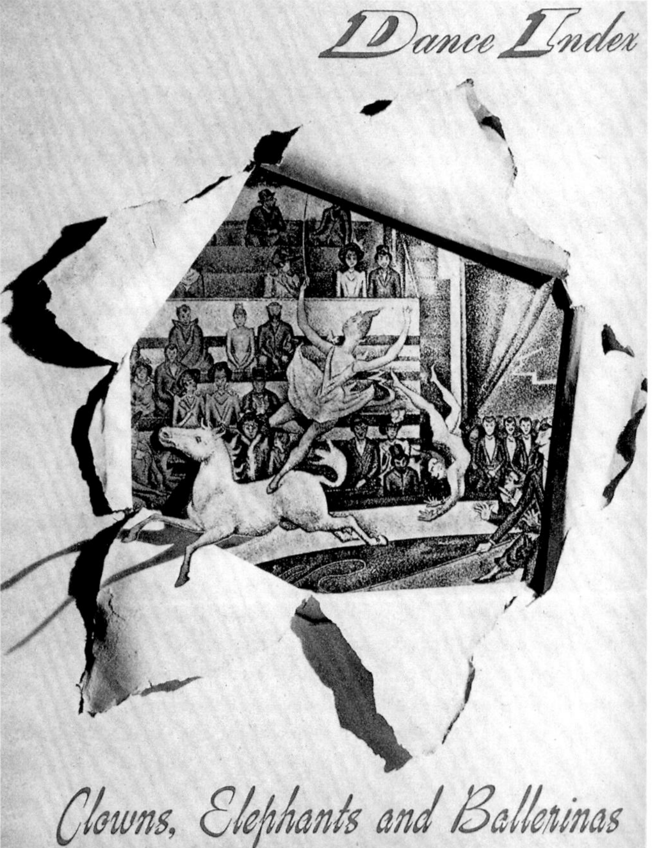


**Figure 78** Joseph Cornell, *Clowns, Elephants and Ballerinas.* (cover of *Dance Index*, June 1946)

## Matisse and the Romantic Sublime: The Surviving Legacy of the Archaic Circle Dance in American Art

Henri Matisse has exerted a profound legacy on both European and American art, not least through his paintings of dance subjects. His monumental *The Joy of Life [Le Bonheur de Vivre]* (1905–6; fig. 79) contained several lessons for American artists, uniting Matisse's iconography of dance with his complementary manner of execution. First owned by Gertrude and Leo Stein, American patrons of the European avant-garde in Paris, the painting hung in the Steins' apartment, where it was seen by a steady stream of visitors, including the many American artists who frequented their informal salon. More Americans saw it in 1912, when it was reproduced in *Camera Work,* and its renown was further enhanced upon its inclusion in the famous Armory Show of 1913.[34]

Recognizing that the artist can freeze and deaden gesture by fixing too closely upon it, Matisse explained, "I never force my hand in drawing. On the contrary, I am like the dancer or the tight-rope performer who begins his day with several hours of loosening-up exercises, so that every muscle in his body responds freely when, before his public, he wishes to translate his emotions into slow or fast dance movements, or by an elegant pirouette."[35]

*The Joy of Life* is a grand fable of innocence and experience, a Romantic fantasy of the free, dancing, and desiring self. Matisse's color is pure sensuality,

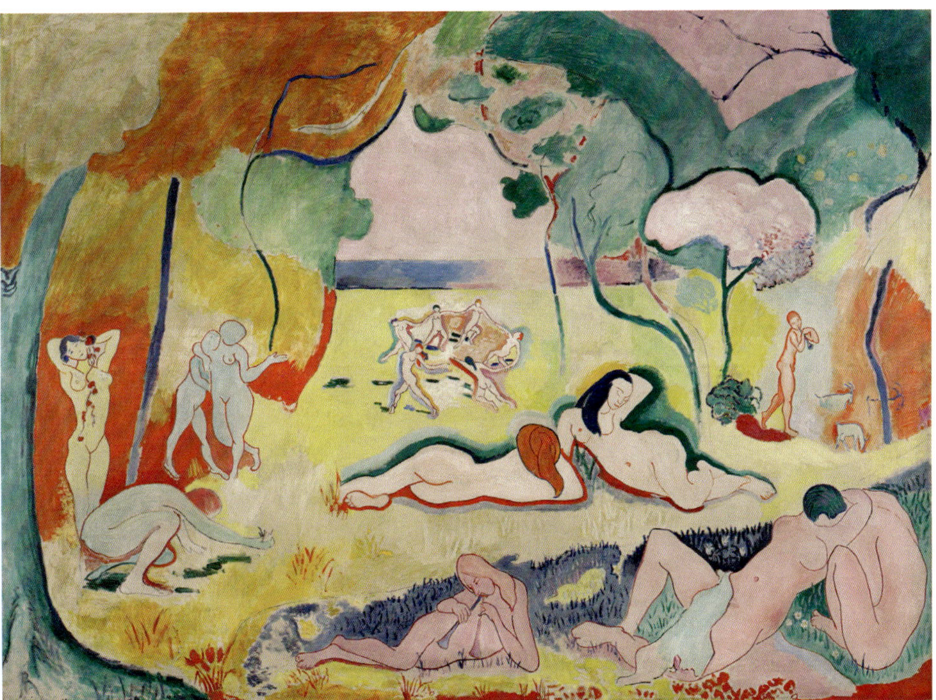

**Figure 79** Henri Matisse, *The Joy of Life [Le Bonheur de vivre]*, 1905–6, oil on canvas, 69 ½ × 94 ¾ inches. (Barnes Foundation, Merion, Pennsylvania, BF719; photo © 2010, reproduced with the permission of the Barnes Foundation)

and the undulating rhythms in the contours of the foreground nudes find echoes within the canopy of trees overhead. If the foreground of the painting is all languorous pleasure, the background figures provide contrasting action. Here Matisse introduced a *ronde*, or *reigen*, a traditional dance of circling figures with its roots in antiquity but with later ritual practice in European folklore. The circle dance performed various functions: inviting pagan gods to join human company, synchronizing human activity with seasonal cycles, or as a dance of love. Such survivals of Dionysian activity were historically opposed by the Church, which saw in them links to malefic practices. But that had not kept European artists from using the round dance as motif throughout the centuries. In Italy, Botticelli's Three Graces from *Primavera* dance in their own small circle, and the traditional dance of Apollo and the Muses was painted as a round dance in works by Mantegna (on prominent display at the Louvre) and Giulio Romano.[36] French artists such as Poussin, Fragonard, Ingres, and Carpeaux all produced variants of the subject, as did Auguste Rodin, whose images of *La Ronde* in drawings, prints, and sculpture were known to Matisse.[37] Finally, Matisse apparently saw the round dances of Catalan fishermen on the French Riviera during the summer of 1905, after which he introduced for the first time the circular dance motif into *The Joy of Life*.

From *The Joy of Life* Matisse had learned that dance can embody, at least in the fevered imagination, the living, pulsing eroticism of the world. In the painting's contrast between calm and excitability he found a visual metaphor for balancing the physically expressive with the poetically expressive. And he had made reference through dance to a continuous narrative of peoples, regions, and rhythmic connections. In such basic configurations as the circle dance, something might be discovered about the ideology of connection, or about the collective beliefs held by a people. Examples of such preclassical dance forms abound from the ancient world, as well as from Matisse's own day: circle dances of Native Americans; Rodin's drypoint etching *La Ronde*; the circle dance in Stravinsky's *Le Sacre du Printemps*; and Henri Rousseau's *Le Centenaire* (seen in the New York Armory Show and discussed in chapter 10).[38]

In his explorations of dance subjects Matisse learned what American visual artists were discovering as well: that rhythmic visual patterns might reveal vestiges of folk culture in closer touch with the unconscious than with the conscious world.[39] But in painting his dancers as nudes Matisse fixed their anonymity, perhaps their interchangeability within the patterns of pagan or folk culture. That his dancers seem to be people of color only connects them more firmly to the universal commonalities of human desire. Matisse's dancers circle—surging, reaching, bending, leaping—and enclose a space of creativity within which dance and painting coexist. Their limbs describe sweeping curvilinear shapes, creating a vocabulary of grand gestures, spirals, and grids. The complexity of Matisse's explorations of dance movements seems to owe something to another very old idea, the Pythagorean notion that nature and music—even mathematics—form part of a single system embracing both the human and the celestial (as in the music of the spheres). But Matisse expressed it in visual rather than philosophical terms. He would summon variants of that vocabulary in his important subsequent paintings of the dance, becoming highly geometric in his remarkable dance mural at the Barnes Foundation (1932?). By that time, Matisse had gleaned many lessons and had teased out, over decades, many nuances of meaning from dance, while influencing countless American artists to look at subjects of the dance with fresh eyes. What must not be forgotten when looking at Matisse's multiple versions of the dance is that the subject served his central and then-problematic concept of *decoration*.[40] Dance, as an expansive activity frequently associated with leisure and pleasure, invited Matisse to create a hybrid of *peinture décoratif* with the *tableau,* that is, to join the scale and planar simplifications of mural painting to the expressive intensity of color inherent in easel painting. In achieving this union of decoration and "high art," Matisse virtually invented a new category.[41] Most subjects would not lend themselves to such cross-categorization, but the Dionysian context of dance in general and Matisse's piping shepherds in particular allowed him both to allegorize and to *decorate*—in other words, to indulge his preoccupation with the harmonious and total organization of the whole.

That preoccupation, legitimized by Matisse's stature and reputation, would expand the range of formal and expressive possibilities for dance subjects among American artists. His use of the dancing group, with its allusions to the primal, folkloric, and collective myths embedded in dance, struck a similar vein in the work of some of America's most inventive artists of the 1930s and 1940s. Aspects of human life writ large—its history, myth, and perennial curiosity for that which lies beyond the immediate—inspired some artists to attempt to recreate a richly resonant past, only partly available to the imagination, attractive precisely because it always remains occluded, ultimately unknowable.

Arshile Gorky, the Armenian refugee painter, wrote to his sisters in 1947 of art's timeless continuum rooted in group experience, a linkage best expressed through the metaphor of dance:

> The tradition of art is the grand group dance of beauty and pathos in which the many individual centuries join in the effort and thereby communicate their particular contributions to the whole event just as in our dances of Van. . . . For this reason I feel that tradition . . . is so important for art. The soloist can emerge only after having participated in the group dance.[42]

Some painters actively incorporated their own mythic consciousness and rhythmic movements into their process. Helen Frankenthaler (1928–2011) famously admired Jackson Pollock's way of moving around and into his canvases, in a kind of idiosyncratic circle dance. Pollock's large-scale *Mural* (1943; fig. 80) contains a tangled frieze of moving forms descended from his totemic figures. In *Mural* we see the remnants of a bacchic dance, a barely controlled, all-enveloping ritual of throbbing gesture.[43] During the later 1940s Pollock turned again and again to the rhythmic inspiration afforded by dance. A critic described a slightly later work as "done in great open black rhythms that dance in disturbing degrees of intensity, ecstatically energizing the powerful image in an almost hypnotic way."[44] Several quasi-figural works from that period were given dance

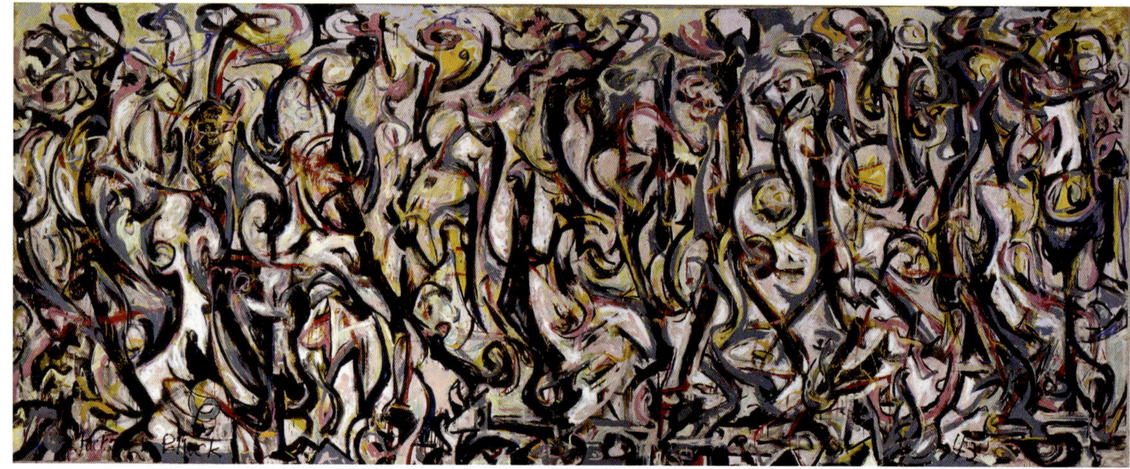

**Figure 80** Jackson Pollock, *Mural*, 1943, oil on canvas, 7 feet 11 ¾ inches × 19 feet 9 ½ inches. (University of Iowa Museum of Art, Iowa City, Gift of Peggy Guggenheim, 1959.6)

titles and feature spindly cut-out dancers pasted onto canvas beneath a blizzard of thrown paint.[45] For Pollock, dance represents (in the tradition of Whitman) the artist's capaciousness, his interchangeability with larger cultural constructs. When Pollock famously declared, "I am nature," he expressed a visual artist's alternative to Isadora Duncan's earlier pronouncement "I am the dance."[46] These three artists—poet, painter, dancer—had learned to absorb and to reinvent— notably, through their *bodies*—an aesthetic of passion, an American response to the liberating synergy of nature, myth, and dance. In Pollock's twenty-foot-wide *Mural,* dance takes its strength from the unity of individuals joining together in collective feeling of joy or significance, an emotion born (as Gorky argued) of moving within a group. For Pollock, as for his many American predecessors dis- cussed above, dance brought alive a fascination with pagan or "folk" cultures, a fascination already introduced to Americans by the cultural lightning bolt known as the Ballets Russes, who revealed to American visual artists ancient paths to passion and ecstasy embedded in rhythmic movement.

# The Ballets Russes and the "Exotic" East

## *Folklore and Modernist Primitivism Invade American Art*

To understand the revolutionary impact of the Ballets Russes, it is necessary to look at its cultural roots in the twin phenomena of modernism and of modernist primitivism, the latter a powerful factor in Russia's modern search for its own cultural sources in folklore, religion, and history. The appeal of modernist primitivism was both broad and deep, beginning with the notion that in some past cultures dance functioned close to the very center of life and death. Seen that way, dance could address some of the fundamental concerns of human existence; it is part of a search for order, certainty, and destiny in life. In India, for example, long tradition holds that the Hindu god Shiva performs the cosmic dance of creation and destruction that keeps the entire universe in motion. Even when life and death were not directly at stake, dance was imagined to have powerful ritual functions in societies. Everywhere, people created rituals to connect themselves with the meaning of human experience (sometimes involving unseen powers) or with the past or the future. In widespread non-Western contexts dancers—like priests, imams, rabbis, shamans, or diviners—can be specialists in ritual, persons who serve as links between the supernatural and human worlds. And dance, like prayer, sacrifice, magic, and divination, can open those lines of communication. In ancient and modern times, recording and preserving those connections often becomes the job of the artist. Art has a major role in dealing with the spirit world, because art can give physical form to what is otherwise intangible; it can make the invisible visible.

Because dance has often been thought to grant privileged access to the primitive, it has intrigued those wishing to resurrect its power and directness. A modern understanding of the "primitive" is part of a constellation of ideas descended from Enlightenment thinkers at the dawn of the early modern era. To them, and to many since, the primitive seemed to resonate with all things "natural," including dance as a universal medium of communication through the "natural" movements of the body, uncorrupted by constructed language.[1] Such cultural longings reveal a nostalgia for an imagined earlier purity, when movement was untainted by artifice. Dance, as we have begun to see, has been called upon repeatedly to figure forth the notion of "natural" movement and "free" bodies. T. S. Eliot wrote, "Anyone who would contribute to our imagination of what ballet may perform in the future should begin by a close study of dancing among primitive peoples."[2] That kind of dancing has been thought to be *powerful* and *authentic*, important aspects of its appeal to both modern dancers and to visual artists. The dancer, working with the body's movements, creates a powerful illusion on a seamless fabric of gesture, while the visual artist conjures an illusion of space from pigments and canvas. Visual artists have wanted to tap into dance's capacity to express meanings and ideas with greater economy, force, and precision than other forms of expression, including most verbal or graphic languages. (Mallarmé observed that dance is writing with the body.)[3]

There are ironies at work here: the imagined undifferentiated unity of the primitive world is itself a myth. And Western (including Russian) attempts to reenact or resurrect a unified primitive, however sincere, are necessarily filtered through dissociated modern sensibilities. Some in the arts recognized the problem, even hoping (however naively) that a return to deep cultural roots might enable the divided modern consciousness to reconcile instinct with intellect. Or that Western culture might be rejuvenated by tapping into the uncorrupted energies of societies in a supposedly earlier stage of development. We might object now to blatant cultural appropriations and mistranslations, but those retrospective criticisms should not discredit the array of creative attempts by artists and choreographers to recover the imagined unities and vanished power of "primitive" dance.

Modernist primitivism and the Russian search for its own past—these were sources that struck a positive chord among Americans in search of their own past. Americans glimpsed a potentially useful model in the recognition by many progressive Russians that the arts—painting, sculpture, architecture, music, and dance—offered a means for staking claim to the new century and, at the same time, for reclaiming a proud past. After generations of rabid consumption of Western cultural forms, Russians in the mid-nineteenth century had rediscovered a yearning for the indigenous sources of a purely Russian art. Still lingering was an ancient peasant culture rooted in mystical religious beliefs. At the turn of the new century a vein of abstraction in Russian icon painting, added to Old Russia's patterned folk art traditions, collided with a whole range of radical new art from Paris and Munich, assembled in Moscow by collectors Shchukin and Morosov. The Russian intelligentsia encountered more modernist ideas on the pages of avant-garde publications such as Sergei Diaghilev's *The World of Art (Mir Iskusstva)*. Soon, intellectual ferment in Russia erupted in new and incendiary ways. Educational reform, sexual emancipation, symbolist aesthetics, religious mysticism, and revolutionary politics—these were ingredients in a radical mix fueling the Russian imagination with visionary, uncompromisingly utopian values. This blending of ancient sources and new abstract idioms was nowhere more visible than in the Ballets Russes.

The Ballets Russes, dream of entrepreneur Diaghilev, was descended from Russia's Imperial Ballet but was born in Paris, where its opening in 1909 ushered in a new era of modern ballet. Even earlier, as American critics were quick to point out, the ubiquitous Isadora Duncan had been a major influence on the new choreography developing in Russia. Duncan had gone to Saint Petersburg in 1904–5, dancing barefoot in a flowing Greek tunic. Following her lead, future Ballets Russes choreographer Michel Fokine began to invent continuous, naturalistic dance passages involving the whole, freely moving body.[4] Rigid torso, classical five positions, and pointe shoes were abandoned. Arts writer Sheldon Cheney declared that the innovation of Diaghilev's Russian ballet "dance-dramas" was due to its expressive effects, seen in stage sets and in movement itself: "Aside from the conjunction with music and dependence on emotional as against imitative use of line and color in the backgrounds, there is here the central emphasis on movement instead of story—and movement is (thanks very largely to our American Isadora Duncan) in the best modern dancing wholly abstract and expressive."[5]

Between 1909 and 1913 Diaghilev's Ballets Russes introduced Parisians to a new, modernist remix of forms, assimilating primitive forms into classical or traditional art in performances of Stravinsky's *The Firebird* (1910) and *Le Sacre du Printemps* (1913), as well as the slightly later Picasso/Satie/ Cocteau *Parade*. Such productions successfully blended the modernity of Fokine's choreography with Vaslav Nijinsky's brilliant dance, Igor Stravinsky's startling original music, and the stage decor of Léon Bakst, Alexandre Benois, and Nicholas Roerich. Diaghilev wrote of his evolving aesthetic of dance: "The more I thought of that problem of the composition of ballet, the more plainly I understood that perfect ballet can only be created by the very closest fusion of three elements—dancing, painting and music."[6] Diaghilev strove mightily to achieve a complete theatrical synthesis, a new gospel of creativity ready for dissemination to vast new audiences.

As early as 1910 the Metropolitan Opera had considered inviting the Russian Ballet to New York, but they moved at a glacial pace, allowing pirated versions of the Paris works to be presented in 1911 by the unscrupulous if enterprising American dancer Gertrude Hoffman.[7] Thus, when the genuine Ballets Russes finally crossed the Atlantic in 1916, New York audiences had already glimpsed something of the brilliance of their European productions. In purely vernacular terms, the Russian company generated new appetites for color, pattern, and style. As critic Carl Van Vechten noted, "The Russian Ballet, on its decorative side, is entirely responsible for the riot of color which has spread over the Western world in clothes and house furnishings."[8] Still, nothing had fully prepared American critics or audiences for the cultural tidal wave that swept ashore. The Russians danced two seasons at New York's Metropolitan Opera House, followed by a cross-country tour (1916–17) that played fifty-two cities over a four-month period. The company, comprising more than a hundred dancers, was imposing in size, positively stunning in influence. Thousands of Americans, including many visual artists, witnessed these performances, and some of them took away unforgettable images. In Philadelphia, just ahead of the Ballets Russes tour in the spring of 1916, locals were treated to an exhibition by the Philadelphia Watercolor Club featuring some of Léon Bakst's original costume and stage designs for the Diaghilev troupe. Included, although Anna Pavlova had by that time left the company, was Bakst's costume for her (1913; fig. 81). Upon seeing the performances, Philadelphia artists were so taken with the integrated music, sets, and costumes of the Ballets Russes that they borrowed its pagan themes and emotive color schemes for a series of Artists' Masques held in 1915 and 1916.

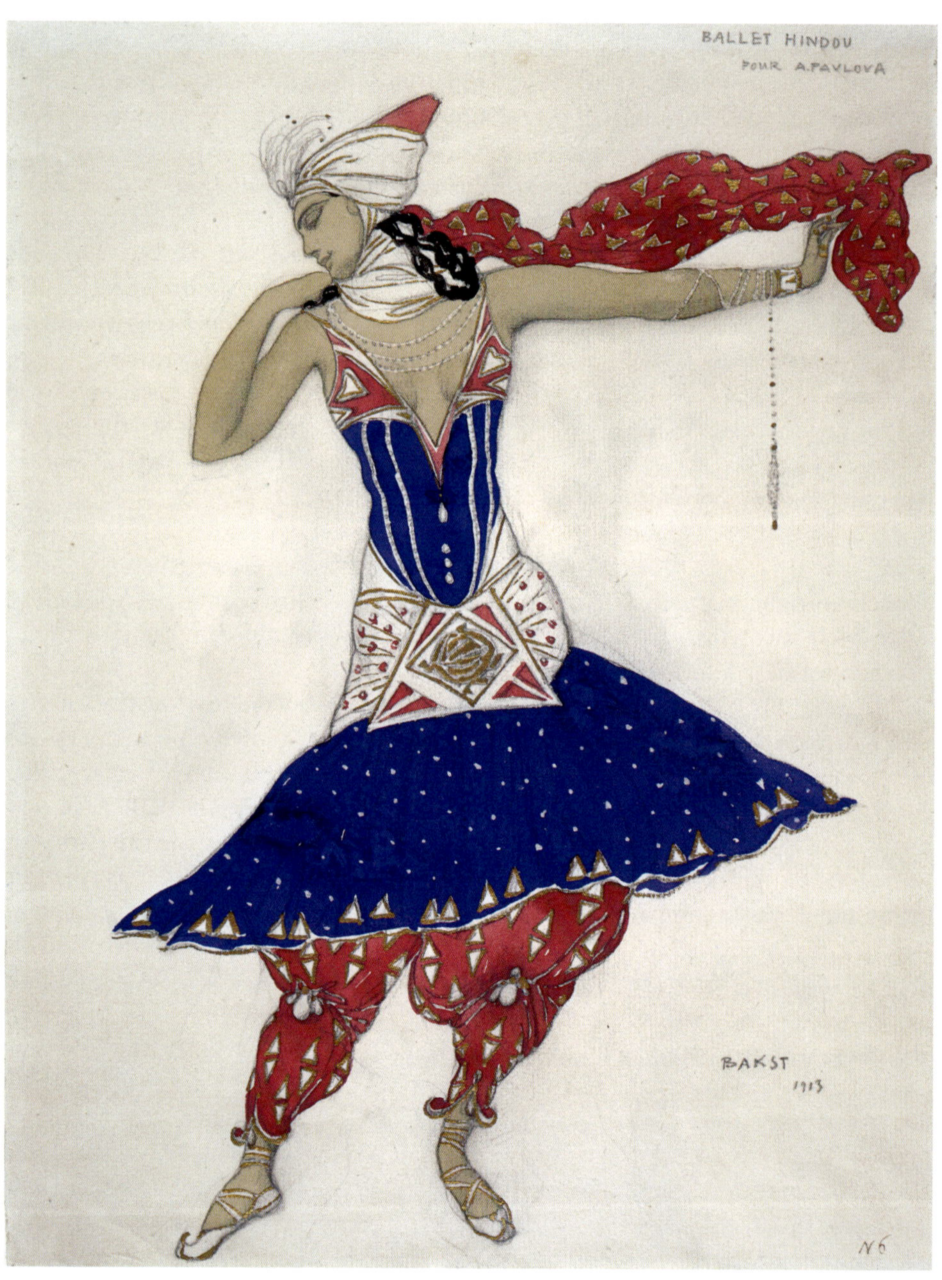



**Figure 81** Leon Bakst, *Costume for Anna Pavlova in the Ballet Oriental Fantasy*, 1913, pencil and watercolor on paper, 12 ⅕ × 9 ½ inches. (© Isabella Stewart Gardner Museum, Boston)

These theatricals—essentially costume pageants featuring some experimental light-ing, music, and dance—awakened many Philadelphians to a conscious connection with avant-garde modernism.[9]

Besides its pure visual appeal, Americans embraced the Ballets Russes for its new sensuality, emanating both from its execution and its roots in earthy pagan folklore. Even as it explored aspects of modernist form, many Ballets Russes pro-ductions, because of their romantic evocation of distant places and times, were no threat either to classical ballet or—at least at first—to representational paint-ing. In fact, the Ballets Russes would help to reinvigorate classical ballet as a flexible, living creative vehicle. The Russian dancers brought new drama to the ballet, injecting bold acting into their performances—certainly an attraction for visual artists. Theirs was a new directness of expression: no wasted movements, bursts of pure feeling. Besides that, Americans reacted strongly to the colorful, folkloric aspects of the Russians. Audiences exhibited, as paraphrased by one dance historian, a "dumfounded gape in the face of the 'optic intoxication' of this modern [Russian] dance, which awakened 'all our latent and barbaric sensi-bilities."[10] Critics saw more: moving patterns that blended artistically with decor and music, stunning modernity, and, not least, "a fund of traditions which these modern Russians had absorbed, questioned, and now transcended."[11] In other words, with its cross-country tour, the Ballets Russes invasion swept American critical opinion before it, becoming the very epitome of artistic dance.

## Acts of the Air: The Influence of Nijinsky and the Russian Ballet in American Art

Among the boundaries annihilated by the Ballets Russes was that between tra-ditional ballet and opera. In their dazzling productions, dance often replaced the customary function of voice. Dancer-choreographer Vaslav Nijinsky, especially, understood that dance could function as a new form of abstracted voice. It was a voice not unlike that of the revolutionary James Joyce, whose startling use of language paralleled the sensation—and sometimes the consternation—created by the unprecedented movements of Nijinsky. Here is Joyce on Nijinsky:

> —Dawncing the kniejinsky choreopiscopally like an easter sun round the colander, the vice! Taranta boontoday. You should pree him prance the polcat, you should sniff him wops around, you should hear his pied-igrotts schraying as his skimpies skirp a . . .

> —Crashedafar Corumbas! A Czardanser indeed! Dervilish glad too.[12]

Within the near impenetrability of Joyce's language we sense the excite-ment but not the specifics of Nijinsky's revolutionary dance. How did he move, what made him modern, and why did he inspire so many visual artists to record and interpret his energies? To begin with, by breaking down the dancer's line into discrete movements of ankle, foot, or hand (as in a clenched fist), Nijinsky orchestrated and inserted them, like the notes of a song, into newly visual operatic forms. At the same time, Nijinsky forsook the three-dimensional shapes of the academic ballet in favor of dancers moving in profile, slicing through the air, or in hunched positions stamping their feet. Having just seen Nijinsky in *L'Après-midi d'un Faune,* Rodin told a favored American student that the performance "was Youth in all its glory, like the days of ancient Greece, when they knew the power and beauty of a human body, and revered it. Such grace, such *souplesse!* An evening to be remembered forever."[13] To help him remember, Rodin made a sculptural study of Nijinsky (c. 1912, private collection, New York) in which he balanced the dancer on one foot, his body curled in upon itself as if to contain and enclose energy in the sharp angles of elbows and knees. It is movement broken into a concentrated gesture, music into a single note, sound into phoneme.

Nijinsky's creation of flat archaic shapes in his *L'Après-midi d'un Faune* and *Till Eulenspiegel,* as well as his angular gestures and leaps, inspired many visual artists. New York artist and illustrator Clara Tice (1888–1973), a onetime student of Robert Henri, bridged the worlds of dance, high fashion, and caricature, all leavened with the nimble irreverence of Dada. When she saw Nijinsky perform in New York (likely in the fall of 1916), Tice drew him nude, stylizing his angular, two-dimensional movement in an ink drawing of taut energy, in which the dancer's hands mime the horns of the faun (c. 1916; fig. 82). Nijinsky's faun turned up everywhere. For the grounds of her California estate, famed Italian opera soprano Amelita Galli-Curci (1882–1963) commissioned sculptor Allan Clark (1896–1950) to model two sculptures, a *Satyr* and a *Nymph,* inspired by Nijinsky's performance in *Faune.*

Another American painter forcibly struck by the Ballets Russes was Charles Burchfield (1893–1967), who caught a performance in Cleveland during the company's celebrated fifty-two-city American tour in 1916–17. Still an art student, Burchfield—eager for new inspirations in design—noted, "I was enthralled by them and loved the costume designs of Bakst."[14] His Cleveland School of Art teacher Henry G. Keller reinforced the Russian Ballet experience in class discussions, and soon Burchfield, who shied away from painting the human figure, was inspired to undertake a series of rhythmic personifications of tall, gesticulating sunflowers—surrogates, perhaps, for Nijinsky and his fellow dancers. To one of his 1916 orchestrations of sunflowers, the young watercolorist bestowed the apt title *Dancing Sunlight* (private collection).

Nijinsky's stylized gestures were so radical that they presented an almost metaphysical conundrum: observers didn't know what they were looking at. Intrigued, many visual artists and writers bent their most creative efforts to finding out. James Joyce had to invent a new word to describe Nijinsky's leap, which the writer saw as a troubled fury transmitted by blood from Taglioni to the hyperkinetic Russian. Nijinsky carried, according to Joyce, a "pantaglionic affection through his blood like a bad influenza in a leap at bounding point."[15] The unprecedented look of Nijinsky's movements also struck cultural historian Frederick Karl, who pronounced them a lever of modernism: "The image there, the memorable one," writes Karl, "is of the leap, that leap which Nijinsky made

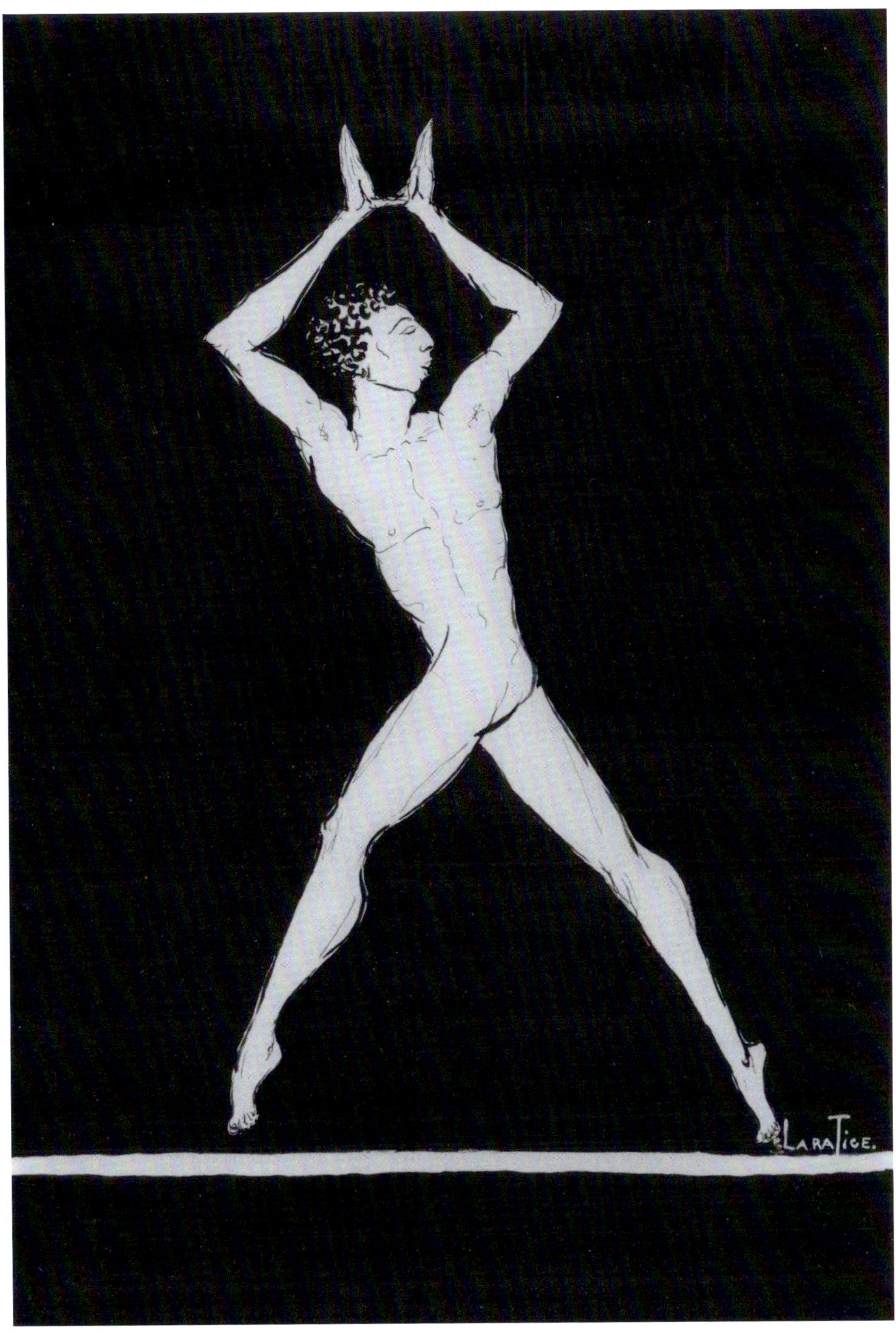


**Figure 82** Clara Tice, *Nijinsky Dancing [L'Après-midi d'un Faune]*, c. 1916, Indian ink on paper, 21 ¾ × 14 ⅞ inches. (Francis M. Naumann Fine Art, New York)

his own. That spatial arc characterizes not only dance, but the entrance into Modernism itself."[16]

Such shapes and geometries within dance were still new and, to many Americans, shocking, like all those loudly deplored modern paintings. Why would an art form such as dance, capable of sublime grace and beauty, turn to such crooked, preposterous shapes? One critic summed up a common view of the use of abstraction, whether in dance or the visual arts: "[P]art of our objection to futurism and cubism in painting is not that we can't understand them but that we don't want to understand them." Not until long after his death did Nijinsky receive widespread recognition for ushering ballet into modernism.[17]

Nijinsky's contributions emerged both in formal/technical terms and in thematic ones. His choreography was one of the major aesthetic threads on the loom of modernist primitivism, a weaving together of ideas from folklore, myth, and a romanticized pagan past. Especially in *L'Après-midi d'un Faune* and *Le Sacre du Printemps,* the effects were determinedly "primitive," the space deconstructed in analytic fashion. *L'Après-midi,* set to Debussy's music of the same title (1912), was a precisely organized series of flattened, archaic, frieze-like images of a faun disturbing the serenity of nymphs in a glade. In *Le Sacre du Printemps,* an ancient Slavic tribe calls on their gods for springtime renewal of the earth, accomplished in the end only by human sacrifice. The hunched, stamping choreography, incorporating ancient circle dances and combined with Stravinsky's pounding music—written, as he said "with an ax"—seemed to onlookers nearly bestial.[18] Aghast at its power and unsure what to make of this new "primitive sublime," the Parisian audience rioted at the premiere—famously—and a new creative model staggered forth.

Contrasts were stark and deliberate: temporal rhythms associated with industry were contrasted with those of nonindustrial cultures, whose rhythms range from those of seasonal change to the stamping foot rhythms of dance. Nijinsky touched a nerve in an emerging modern consciousness, and his early ballets caused an uproar and brought him notoriety. *Le Sacre du Printemps* was said by Riviere to have "alter[ed] the very source of all our aesthetic judgments."[19]

Beyond the Paris of Nijinsky, Diaghilev, and Picasso, modernist primitivism was rising in many places, and encompassed a range of ideas that would embrace such far-flung sources as the revival of paganism and Russian neo-Slavism. Diaghilev's five seasons in Paris had stirred appetites there for the exotic, pagan, and revolutionary in dance and music.

American painter Florine Stettheimer saw Nijinsky dance in Paris in 1912. She recorded in her diary for June 7 that

> Nijinsky the faun was marvelous. He seemed to be truly half beast if not
> two-thirds. He was not a Greek faun for he had not the insouciant smile
> of a follower of Dionyson. He knew not civilization—he was archaic—
> so were the nymphs. He danced the Dieu Bleu and the Rose in which he
> was a graceful as a woman and Scheherazade. He is the most wonderful
> male dancer I have seen.[20]

When Stettheimer returned to the United States at the onset of World War I, she translated these vivid visual memories into paint. Over the next few years the male dancer became a major source of romantic symbolism for her. She painted Nijinsky crouching near her as a pagan faun in *Sunday Afternoon in the Country* (1917, Cleveland Museum of Art) and included him as the central figure in her *Music* (c. 1920; fig. 83). In the latter work Nijinsky stands, arms upraised, in a characteristic pose similar to the way he was photographed for his role in *Le Spectre de la Rose* (1911; fig. 84). Stettheimer's *Music*, a dream fantasy of the Ballets Russes, mingles Freudian theory with a certain comedic aspect, teasing the conventions of masculinity and emphasizing Nijinsky's androgyny. Stettheimer shows his feet *en pointe* (no male dancers, including Nijinsky, ever danced thus) and he wears, instead of a leafy tunic, a one-piece body stocking covering decidedly female breasts, above which rise the dancer's own muscular arms and chest.[21] Stettheimer here extends Nijinsky's subversion of the old travesty paradigm, in which a woman (*la danseuse en travesti*) filled male roles in romantic ballet, a complex persona playing to the many nuances of desire represented in nineteenth-century ballet audiences. The travesty dancer exhibited to advantage a splendid female figure while aping the motions and steps of the erstwhile male performer in such roles. But she never pretended to be a man, despite portraying such characters as hussars, toreadors, and sailors. A curious

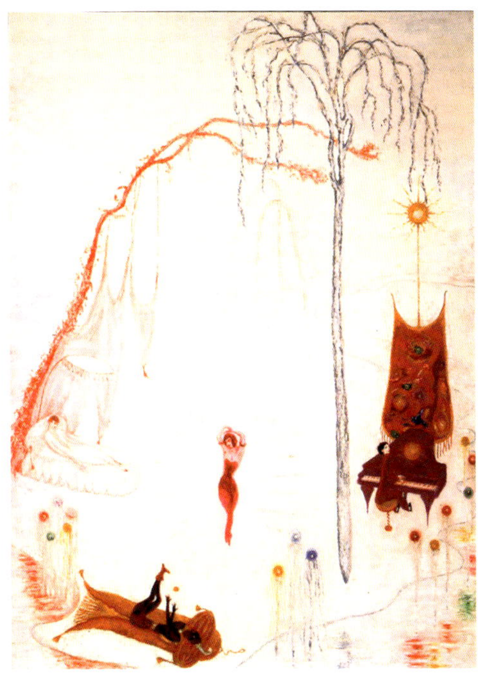

Figure 83 Florine Stettheimer, *Music*, c. 1920, oil on canvas, 69 × 50 ½ inches. (Rose Art Museum, Brandeis University, Waltham, Massachusetts, Gift of Joseph Solomon, 1956)

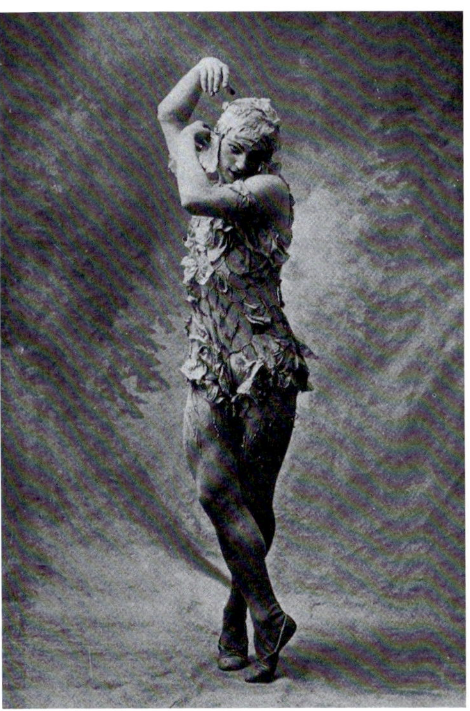

Figure 84 E. O. Hoppe, *Vaslav Nijinsky in Le Spectre de la Rose*, photograph, 1911.

breed of masqueraded transvestite, she provided the antiheroic, demuscular-ized presence critics called for and audiences favored. As dance historian Lynn Garafola explains, "What audiences wanted was a masculine image deprived of maleness, an idealized adolescent, a beardless she-man."[22] Only with the revolu-tionary aesthetic introduced by Diaghilev's Ballets Russes was the travesty par-adigm shattered. Particularly in the roles created for Nijinsky, a new, androgy-nous iconography emerged, obviating former gender categories and allowing the return of strength and athleticism in male dancers. This is the new, hybridized sexuality Stettheimer painted for Nijinsky in *Music*.

But the rich, dance-saturated iconography of the painting does not end with Nijinsky. At the left, and in the direction of Nijinsky's coy glance, a sleeping Stettheimer reclines on an elaborate canopy bed. Her dream fantasy in *Music* includes yet another Russian dancer, Adolph Bolm, whom she depicted in body paint and costume as the Moor in *Petrushka*. Near the bottom of the canvas Bolm reclines on a divan, arms and legs extended upward, juggling a coconut. When Bolm agreed to pose for Stettheimer, the two became good friends. She often visited him backstage, where she dispensed advice on stage makeup, and the Bolms joined lavish house parties given by the Stettheimer sisters.

Dance, and performance in general, played an increasingly important role in Florine Stettheimer's subsequent work. Perhaps inspired by the Russian dancers she admired, she moved from the relatively static poses of Nijinsky and Bolm in *Music* to compositions such as *Natatorium Undine* (1927; fig. 85), in which dancers and divers, moving like Bacchantes, disport themselves freely near the water's edge. Stettheimer taught herself, through watching dancers, how to paint movement, an accomplishment Parker Tyler called "the trait of one who con-sciously studies motion; it is a dancer's as well as, in Florine's case, a painter's art."[23] Its apex would appear in Stettheimer's set and costume designs for various avant-garde ballets and operas, especially her collaboration with Virgil Thomson and Gertrude Stein in *Four Saints in Three Acts* (1934).

Many other American visual artists fell under the spell of the Ballets Russes, whether in Paris or in the United States. American modernist H. Lyman Sayen, for example, painted an abstract interpretation of *Schéhérazade*, which had pre-miered in Paris in 1910 and was repeated in New York in 1916, with music by Rimsky-Korsakov, choreography by Michel Fokine, and costumes by Léon Bakst. Adapted from the prologue to *The Thousand and One Nights*, *Schéhérazade* as choreographic drama evoked romantic visions of the ancient East, propelled forward by the modernist innovations of Sayen's colorful abstraction (1915, Smithsonian American Art Museum, Washington, D.C.).

Inspired by Ballets Russes star Ida Rubinstein (1885–1960), American sculp-tor Jo Davidson (1883–1952) witnessed the company's performances during his residence in Paris, creating a bronze portrait of the celebrated dancer in 1909 (fig. 86). Although a graceful dancer, Rubinstein was not a great one. But she had other talents: trained in mime and recitation, she possessed a flair for the dra-matic, an inclination that would later lure her away from dance into a period of serious dramatic performance. Rubinstein was also exceptionally beautiful, which attracted many visual artists to her. And, not least, she was an heiress who used

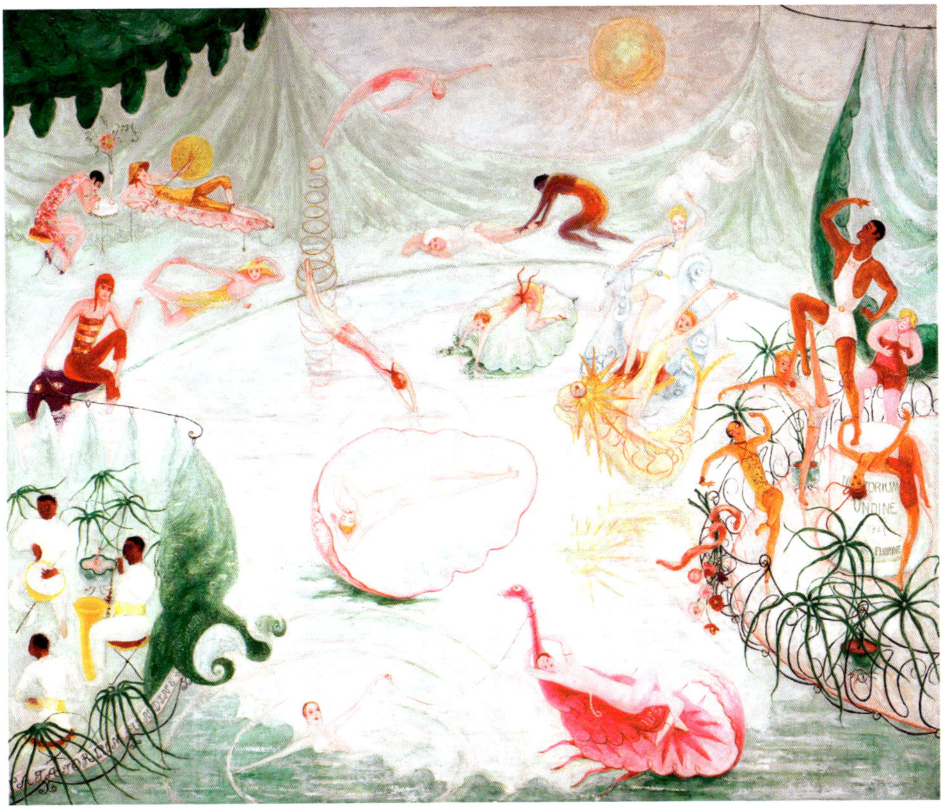

**Figure 85** Florine Stettheimer, *Natatorium Undine*, 1927, oil on canvas, 50 ½ × 60 inches. (Frances Lehman Loeb Art Center, Vassar College, Poughkeepsie, New York, Gift of Ettie Stettheimer, 1949.5)

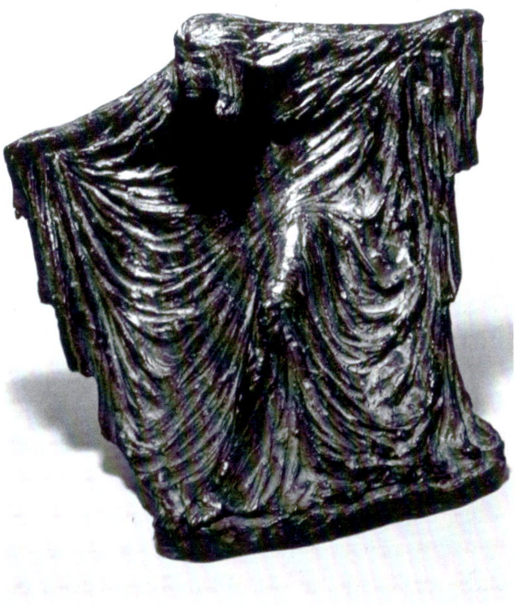

**Figure 86** Jo Davidson, *Ida Rubinstein*, 1909, bronze, 11 ¼ × 11 ½ × 6 ½ inches. (Vanderbilt University Fine Arts Gallery, Nashville, Tennessee)

her considerable fortune to commission dance works and to form her own dance troupe, which toured Europe until the 1930s. Davidson's early bronze depicts Rubinstein dancing the title role in the 1909 ballet *Cleopatra*, choreographed by Michel Fokine for the Ballets Russes's first Paris season with a cast that included both Pavlova and Nijinsky. In Davidson's swirl of bronze, only Rubinstein's head and knee project from heavy draperies which surround her like a tent, nearly obscuring the dancer's body but revealing her penchant for the dramatic.

These dancers and choreographers—Ida Rubinstein, Nijinsky, Fokine, Adolph Bolm, Tamara Karsavina, and especially Anna Pavlova, came to symbolize the golden age of Russian ballet, and—aided by the inimitable Sergei Diaghilev—led its diaspora to the West. By 1910 former imperial ballerina Pavlova had already left the Ballets Russes, departing soon after its Paris debut for extended tours in the United States. She appeared at the Metropolitan Opera in 1910, and for the next fourteen years her passionate leaps and graceful poses thrilled American audiences from coast to coast. Artists clamored to capture her seemingly weightless flight across the stage. The versatile realist George Luks, whose *Spielers* (fig. 10) and *Cake Walk* (fig. 37) we have already encountered, demonstrated his abiding interest in all kinds of dance when he painted the ballerina in her New York debut (1910; fig. 87). Photographer Herbert Mishkin captured her at the Met in *The Dragonfly*, in fluttering draperies reminiscent of Art Nouveau subjects. *The Dragonfly* became a staple in the Pavlova repertoire and inspired other images of pale ethereality and lifted grace.[24]

Most famous of all Pavlova images in American art are those by Malvina Hoffman (1887–1966). A student of Rodin, Hoffman found, like her teacher, much sculptural potential in the forms of the dance. Between 1910 and 1914 she received regular critiques from him and took his advice to focus closely on the study of anatomy. Moving in the circles of Parisian artists and literati, Hoffman became acquainted with Matisse, Gertrude Stein, and Romaine Brooks. At the time, Rodin was making many studies of dancers—visiting Cambodian troupes, the Japanese dancer Hanako, and drawings of Loïe Fuller, whose voluminous draperies Rodin turned into rhythmic line.

In Paris, Hoffman's first important sculptural group was based on Pavlova and Mordkin dancing the *Bacchanale*, a London performance that electrified the sculptor. "Fireworks were set off in my mind," recalled Hoffman. "Here were impressions of motion of a new kind, of dazzling vivacity and spontaneity and yet with a control that could come only from long discipline and dedication. . . . I went to further performances, standing up when necessary, and made sketches. These precious sketches I took back to Paris."[25] There, under the guidance of her mentor Rodin, Hoffman worked up a maquette for a bronze piece. Looking at her first study Rodin advised her, "When you carry joy to its full intensity like this, you are already on the borderline of exquisite pain. Don't forget that these dancers could be drunk with joy or mad with despair. It is all so closely interwoven in human life!"[26] Hoffmann won a first prize at the 1911 Paris Salon for this piece. Another version, over life-size, of *Bacchanale Russe* (aka *Bacchanale*) 1917, was cast as an outdoor sculpture and installed at the Luxembourg Gardens in Paris as well as at the Cleveland Museum of Art (fig. 88).

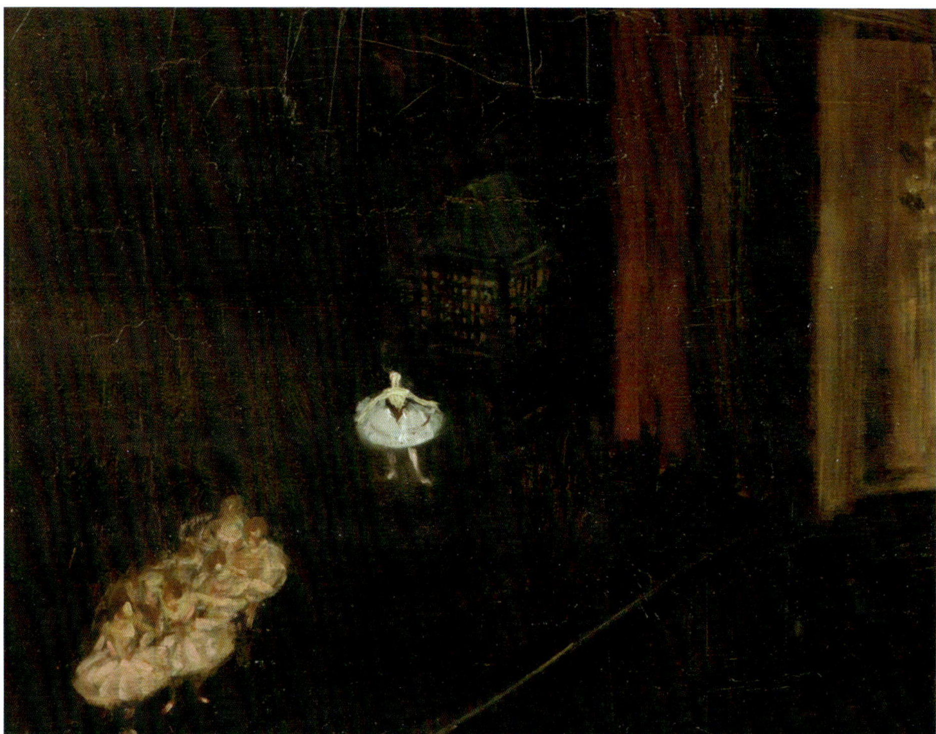

**Figure 87** George B. Luks, *Pavlova's First Appearance in New York*, 1910, oil on canvas, 16 ½ × 20 inches. (Munson-Williams-Proctor Arts Institute, Museum of Art, Utica, New York, 58.296)

To experience for herself the dance-derived intensity Rodin saw in her work, Hoffman later took up the study of ballet. Once, while performing *Autumn Bacchanale* for Pavlova, the frenzied sculptor danced with such fervor that she "saw the lights go red and fade out into oblivion" just as she fainted in mid-dance.[27] By that time, Hoffman and Pavlova had become friends, having been introduced in New York when Pavlova was performing at the Metropolitan Opera. Seeing Hoffman's several previous efforts, observed from afar, to capture her in dance, Pavlova responded warmly to the young American and arranged a permanent observation spot for her in the theater wings. From that post Hoffman made many studies of the Russian and soon began a new study of Pavlova dancing the *Gavotte,* a work for which the dancer also posed in the sculptor's studio. Pavlova wore a diaphanous yellow dress, high-heeled golden slippers, and a yellow bonnet with long streamers (1915; fig. 89). Cast in bronze, the *Gavotte* was much appreciated for its airy, seemingly effortless grace, a pose the sculptor achieved in reality only after many preliminary drawings and test armatures of hands, arms, and feet.

Pavlova especially liked one of the unused sketches for the *Gavotte*, a pose with head thrown back, and suggested that it become a poster (1918; fig. 90). Hoffman drew it in black and white with touches of red, the first in a series of posters she made for the Russian Ballet. For seven years dancer and artist

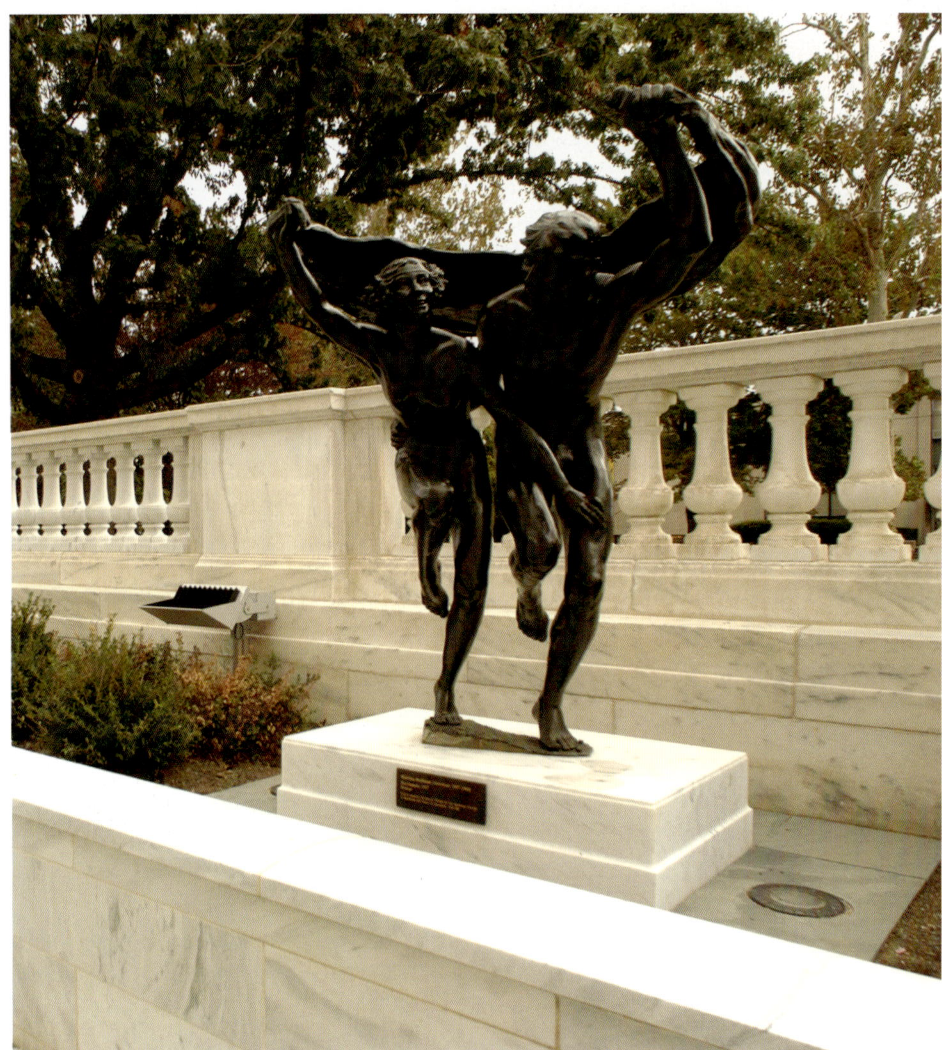

**Figure 88** Malvina Hoffman, *Bacchanale Russe* (aka *Bacchanale* or *Pavlova and Mordkin Dancing the Autumn Bacchanale from Glazunov's Seasons*), 1917, bronze with green-black patina on stone base, approx., 62 × 58 × 48 inches. (Fine Arts Garden, Cleveland Museum of Art, Cleveland, 43.384)

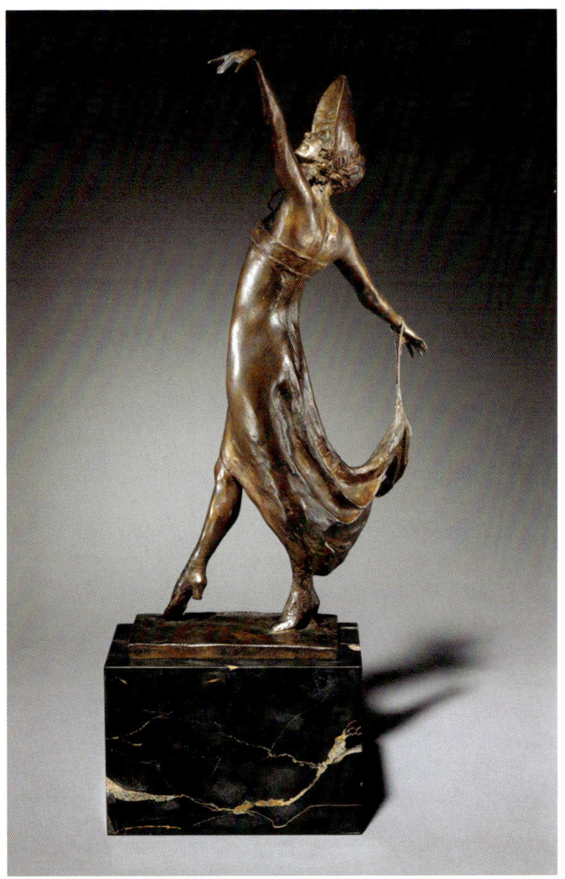

Figure 89 Malvina Hoffman, *Pavlova Dancing the Gavotte*, 1915, bronze, gilt patination, h. 14 inches. (Cleveland Museum of Art, 23.725)

Figure 90 Malvina Hoffman, poster of Anna Pavlova dancing the *Gavotte*, 1918.

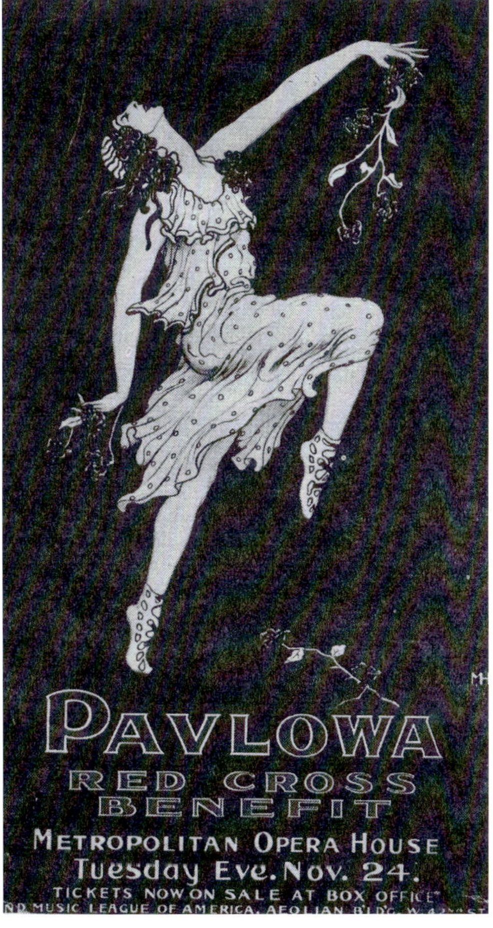

collaborated in what became a joint project to preserve the dynamics of dance in sculptural form.

The most ambitious of Hoffman's Pavlova subjects was an imposing sculptural frieze of twenty-six panels created in 1924. Its fifty-two dancers were modeled by Pavlova and her various Russian dance partners. In preparation for this work, Hoffman recalled, "I made innumerable studies of [Pavlova] in action on the stage. Sometimes I wold be in the wings and sometimes in the audience. We would examine them together after the performance and decide which ones seemed to catch a movement accurately and which ones suggested the action just previous and just after the movement we wished to capture. By this method we collected about one hundred and fifty poses, from which we selected the twenty-five for the bas-relief frieze of *La Bacchanale*" (fig. 91).[28] Of these impressive poses photographer Arnold Genthe wrote, "No good dance motion picture was ever taken of Pavlowa. One might say that the only thing approaching it is the splendid frieze that Malvina Hoffman did of her with Mordkin in the Bacchanal in about thirty different poses."[29] What Hoffman's paired dancers capture is a mutuality of energy, of bodies intoxicated with the sheer pleasure of movement released in Dionysian abandon.

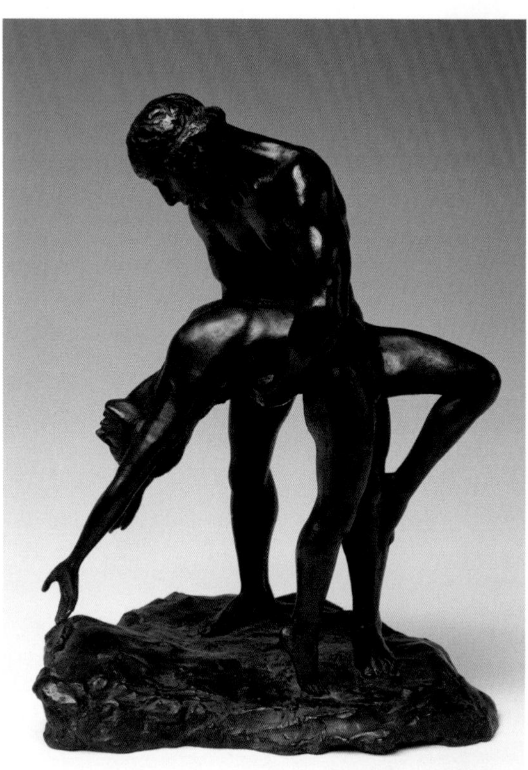

Figure 91 Malvina Hoffman, *Bacchanalia (Pavlova and Mordkin)*, 1914, bronze, h. 12 inches. (Santa Barbara Museum of Art)

Seeking respite from the intensity of the frieze, Hoffman turned to individual sculptures of Pavlova, using plaster, wax, marble or bronze. Her life-size marble portrait *Anna Pavlova* (1924–25; fig. 92) is a half-length version of the dancer with hands folded over her breast, pensive in mood. "[Pavlova] and I had enjoyed the contrast of quietude after all the poses of vigorous action in the dance that we had interpreted together," remarked Hoffman of this piece.[30] The sculptor carved Pavlova in a serenely detached manner reminiscent of the Italian Renaissance sculptor Francesco Laurana (c. 1425–c. 1502), noted for his marble portrait busts of aristocratic women. Like Laurana, Hoffman achieved elegance by reducing detail and concentrating on an essential geometry of forms, severely rendered in harmonious balance.

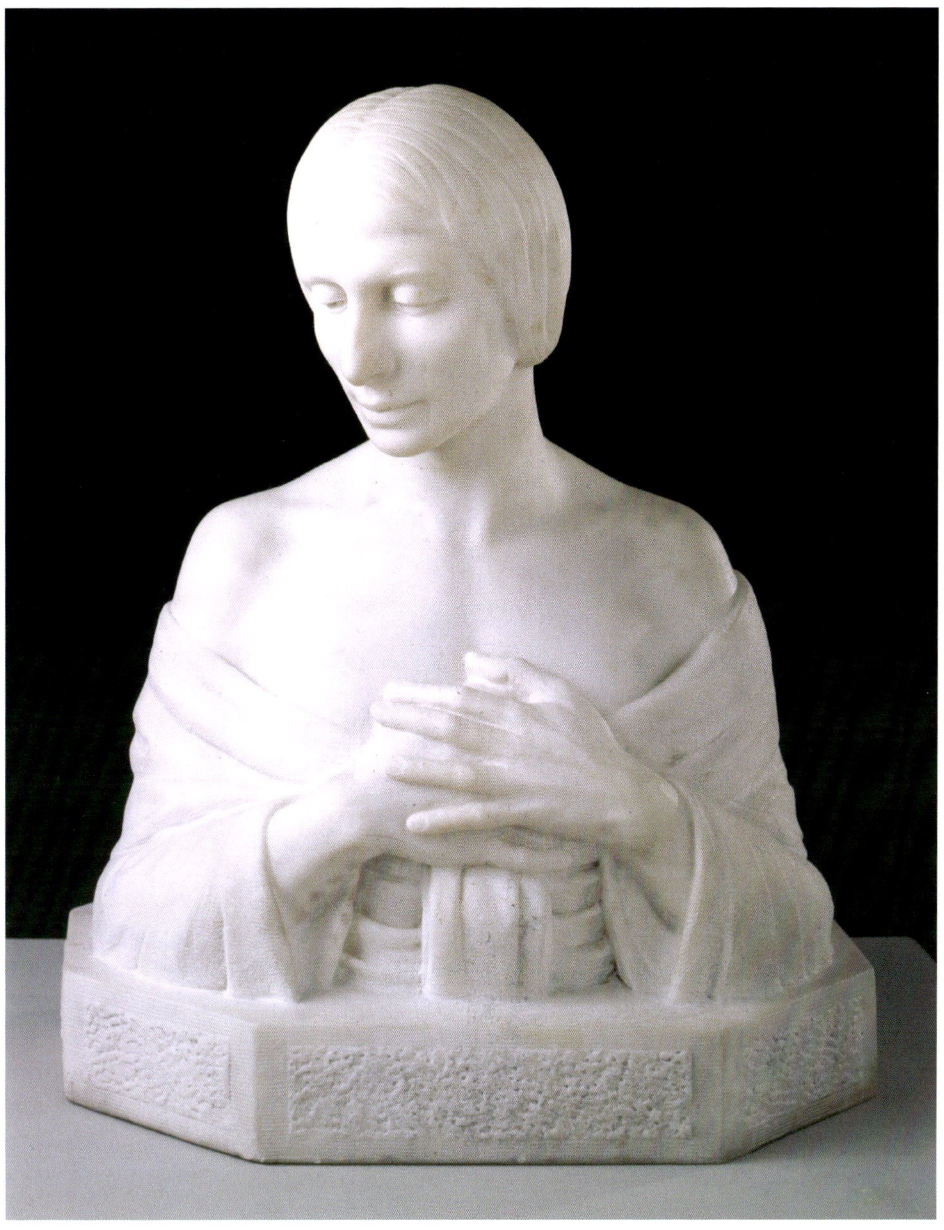

**Figure 92** Malvina Hoffman, *Anna Pavlova*, 1924–25, marble bust, 26 × 20 × 12 inches. (El Paso Museum of Art, Robert and Pauline Huthsteiner Trust Fund Purchase, 1981.26.1)

Still, despite her elegance, Hoffman's marble Pavlova is not idealized; she is a real, recognizable portrait down to her uneven nose.

Fired by her early training under Rodin in Paris, her extended sojourns there over many years, her own passion for the dance, and her worldwide travels documenting the peoples of the world, Hoffman came to envision dance as a bridge between cultures, a language with the power of universal expression. She was that rarest of creatures, an artist of sustained vision who used her technical skill and her resources to document in her own art the energy and exquisite refinements of another.

In Paris, European artists such as Bakst, Braque, de Chirico, Derain, Ernst, Gris, Matisse, Miro, Picasso, Rouault, and Utrillo designed sets or costumes for the Ballets Russes. That history of collaboration, between progressive visual artists and new dance forms, helped to challenge the artistic conservatism still prevalent in the United States. Here, visual artists responded in diverse ways to its unprecedented forms and to the modernist stylizations they saw in performances.

American painter Max Weber (1881–1961) was uniquely equipped by heritage, training, and temperament to interpret Russian dance for Americans. Born in Russia and brought to America at age ten, Weber studied art in New York with the innovative composition teacher Arthur Wesley Dow. By 1905 Weber had saved enough money to travel to Paris, arriving at the precise moment when he could best assimilate the innovations of Cézanne, Rousseau, and especially of Matisse, with whom he studied. Equally interested in Cubism and in the relevance of "primitive" cultures to modern sensibility, Weber grew increasingly fascinated with the concept of the Fourth Dimension, which he described in an article as "a great and overwhelming sense of space-magnitude in all directions at the same time."[31] Weber experimented with visually representing the space–time continuum in a number of subjects, finding in dance the potential for expressing a new complexity of time. What Weber learned was that a dancing figure embodies a near-simultaneity of events in memory—color, rhythm, and pattern experienced all at once.

Once back in the United States, he worked repeatedly with images of dancers in both paintings and sculpture, assimilating Parisian aesthetics into a search for a native vocabulary of forms. Weber's bronze *Spiral Rhythm* (1915, Hirshhorn Museum, Washington, D.C.) translates that revolving aspect of time into firm, solid form. As he wrote, "Art is the very fluid of energy made concrete—the rhythmic spiritual energy revealing more and more, opening infinity."[32] Transferring that energy into two dimensions, Weber painted a highly kinetic and complex work, his *Russian Ballet* (1916; fig. 93). Not coincidentally, it was painted the same year Diaghilev's troupe made its New York debut. Placing his foreground figures against the kaleidoscopic color of Russian stage decor, Weber pairs rich textures with the aggressive shapes of Cubo-Futurism to convey the splintered movements and fractured time of modern ballet.

While Weber responded generally to the Russian Ballet's unprecedented visual impact, other artists looked specifically at individual dancers, especially Nijinsky. Jo Nivison Hopper, who had already sketched Isadora Duncan in her 1915 New York performances, watched Nijinsky from the wings, trying to fix

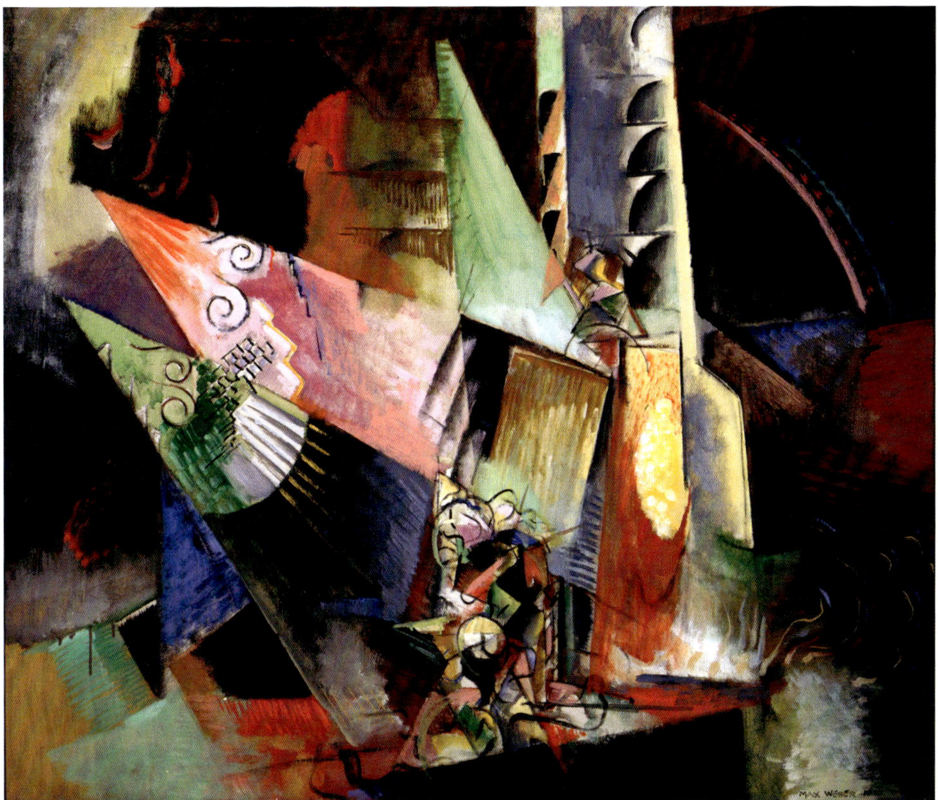

**Figure 93** Max Weber, *Russian Ballet*, 1916, oil on canvas, 30 × 36 inches. (Brooklyn Museum, Bequest of Edith and Milton Lowenthal, 1992.11.29)

something of his incomparable energy. She was there obsessively when Nijinsky danced in *Cleopatra* at the Met in 1916. Nivison recalled how she had "strutted in [posing] as one of the musicians in Cleopatra—& how Nijinski had offered to pose for me—& all the enchantment of those nights in the wings snatching at so quick sketches."[33] In a letter to her former teacher Robert Henri, Nivison described those drawings as "just breaths, gasped from the wings where I was allowed to hover while the Nijinsky ballet was here—oh such a heavenly experience—to draw to music—grab what one could."[34] She took some of these drawings of the Ballets Russes and Nijinsky to *The Dial,* but they seem not to have appeared on its pages.

As the Ballets Russes crisscrossed the country on its first American tour, many future artists came under its thrall. In San Francisco young Louise Dahl, a future photographer but then a twenty-year-old design student, witnessed several performances, recalling,

It was the first time that I had ever seen a perfect synthesis of three arts: painting, music, and dance. Nijinsky's modern abstract movements of the dance in *L'après-midi d'une Faune,* for which he did the choreography, was exciting beyond belief. The modern music of Debussy and the modern background set of Leon Bakst were as important as the dance movements, which made the spectacle into one breathtaking whole.[35]

For others in the United States, the Ballets Russes would generate consonances between Russian-style modernist primitivism and Native American ritual. Dancer-choreographer Adolph Bolm may have been the first to see connections between Russian and Native American dance. During Diaghilev's second American tour, Bolm decided to stay on to pursue choreography and teaching in the United States, forming his own Ballet Intime company. While performing in France, many Russian dancers had noted what they viewed as excessive individualism in that artistic world. Instead, the Russians—probably by training—had learned to subordinate personal glory for the collective benefits of the whole company. That collaborative spirit, as well as the ritual framework surrounding much Russian folk dance, undoubtedly prepared Bolm for his encounter with the communal spirit of Native American dance. On at least one occasion Bolm chose to demonstrate publicly the ritualistic aspects of Russian folk dance for a mixed audience of whites and Native Americans at an outdoor performance in Santa Fe, New Mexico. In that small city an annual fiesta celebrating the town's seventeenth-century founding and its multicultural history has been held for nearly a century. In 1921, locals were treated to a firsthand comparison between ceremonials of their region and Russian folk dance. Adolph Bolm, erstwhile star of the Imperial Ballet and the Ballets Russes, more recently at New York's Metropolitan Opera, came to town with a small, well-connected Russian contingent interested in cross-cultural ideas. Before a rapt fiesta crowd in the town's central plaza, Bolm launched into a fully costumed, highly acrobatic performance of a Slavic war dance (fig. 94). Bolm, in contrast to Nijinsky, was a hypermasculine presence who "ranged the stage like a force of nature . . . the barbarian untamed by civilization."[36] Enacting this persona within a tiny anthropological elite (prominent ethnomusicologist Natalie Curtis was also on hand),[37] Bolm struck a

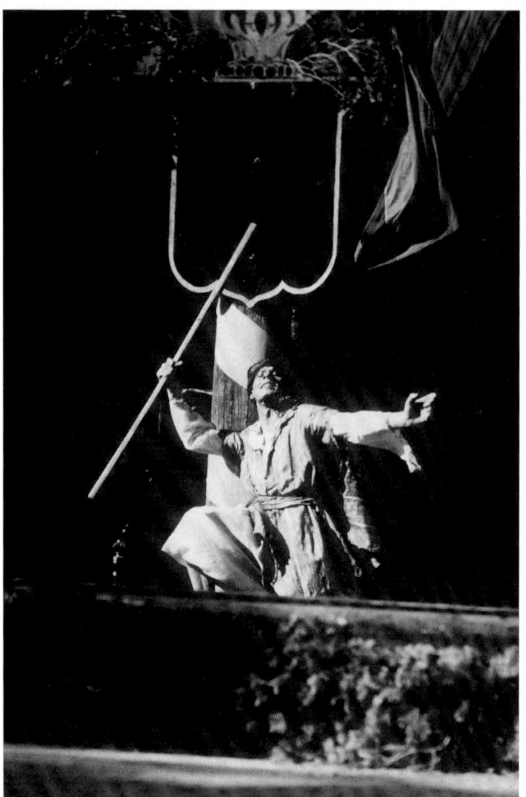

**Figure 94** Adolph Bolm performing Slavic war dance at Santa Fe Fiesta, 1921. (Museum of New Mexico, photo 52850)

powerful chord of cultural relativism. His performance was followed by that of a group of Zuni pueblo dancers who reciprocated with a Yeibichei medicine dance in honor of the Russian visitors.[38] What might Bolm have learned from his exchange of dances with the Zuni? Perhaps he perceived in Native American dance its inherent power as ritual drama, bolstering his own inclination to move classical ballet beyond rigid traditional forms to become an integrated, multisensory spectacle, newly attentive to dance's intimate relationship with the earth.[39]

## Nijinsky Redux: American Abstract Expressionism

Nijinsky's experiments with abstract movement far outlived the dancer himself, provoking artistic responses on both sides of the Atlantic. Nearly four decades after Rodin's study, the American Abstract Expressionist Franz Kline (1910–62) was profoundly inspired by the great dancer. And there was another uncanny connection: in private life Kline was married to Elizabeth Parsons, a ballet dancer who, like Nijinsky, suffered from schizophrenia. When he worked as a commercial illustrator Kline had made several portraits of Nijinsky. To begin with he studied photographs such as that of Nijinsky as the roguish Harlequin Petrouchka (1911; fig. 95). From that image Kline adapted a figurative rep-

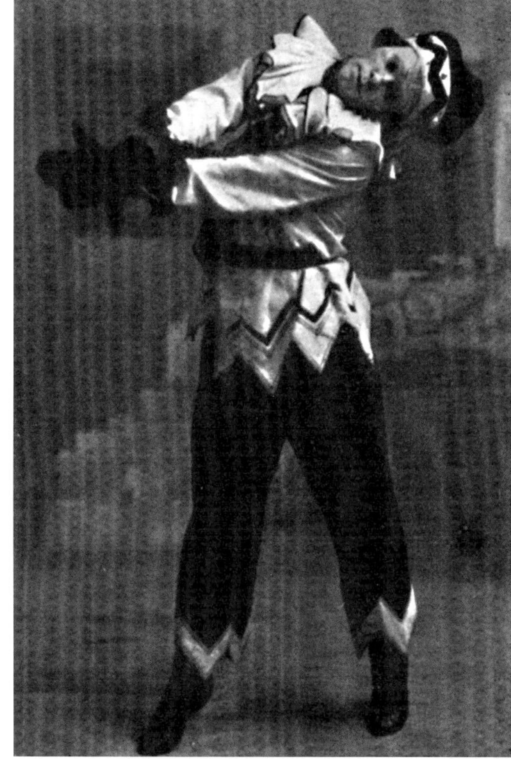

resentation in oil, *Large Clown [Nijinsky as Petrouchka]* (c. 1948; fig. 96), a work that, according to one interpretation, may have been a surrogate self-portrait of Kline himself.[40] Later, Kline mused on Nijinksy's dual roles as athlete and shaman, capable of moving matter and energy beyond conventional bounds. In other photographs of the dancer, Kline studied the Russian's centripetal concentrations of force, as well as his knowledge of physical culture, acrobatics, eurhythmics and sports—forms of movement codified eventually into the study of biomechanics. Kline's abstraction *Nijinsky* (1950; fig. 97), may recognize those diverse sources: it is an assertive black-and-white composition integrating sharp geometric angularities with muscular, enclosing curves and a zigzagging line at bottom left, perhaps a reminder of the neck ruff on Nijinsky's famous Petrouchka costume.[41] Regardless

**Figure 95** Elliott and Fry, *Nijinsky as the Harlequin Petrouchka*, Paris, 1911. (from *Dance Index* 2 [1943])

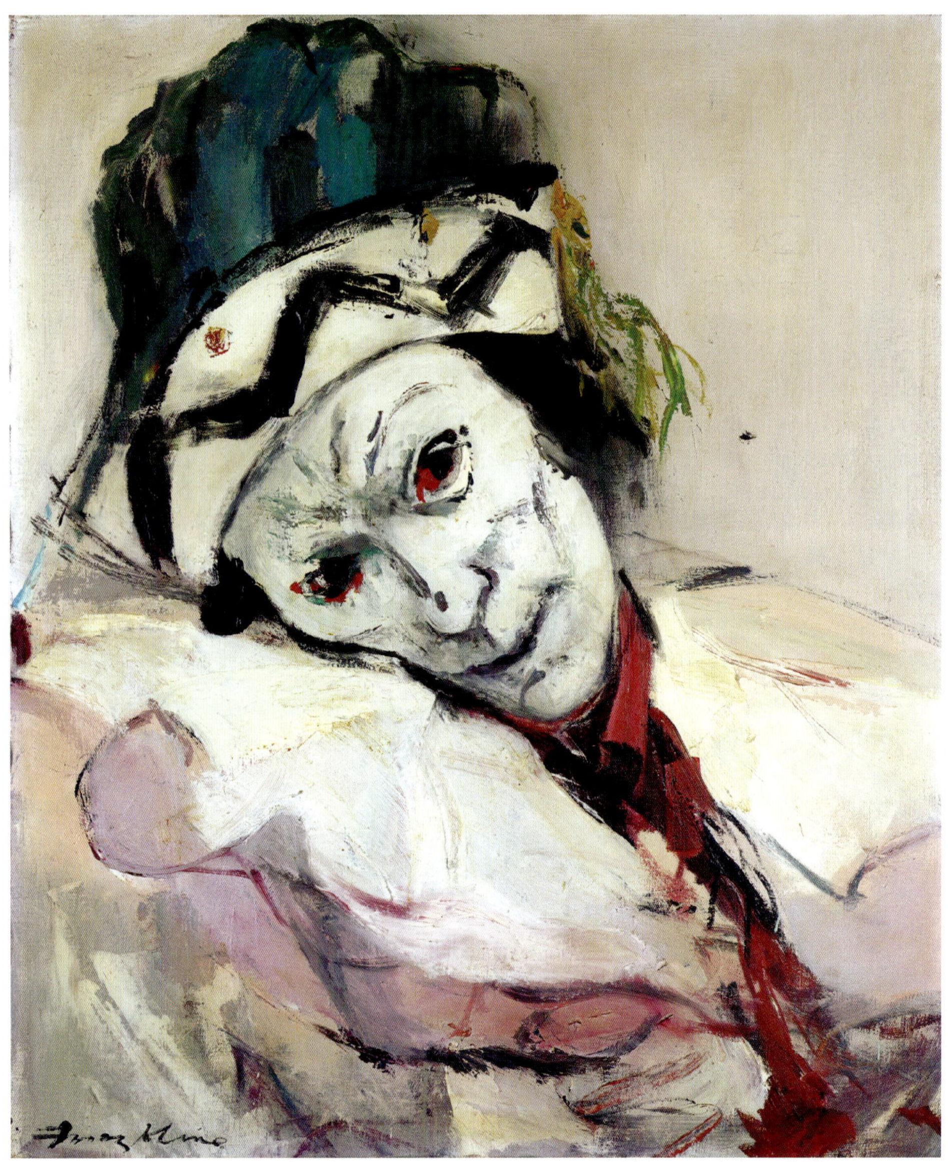

**Figure 96** Franz Kline, *Large Clown [Nijinsky as Petrouchka]*, c. 1948, oil on canvas, 33 ⅛ × 28 ⅛ inches. (Wadsworth Atheneum Museum of Art, Hartford, Connecticut, Gift of Miriam Orr in memory of her late husband, Israel David Orr, and through the courtesy of her daughter, Sulamith L. Orr, 2001.24; image © Wadsworth Atheneum Museum of Art/Art Resource, New York)

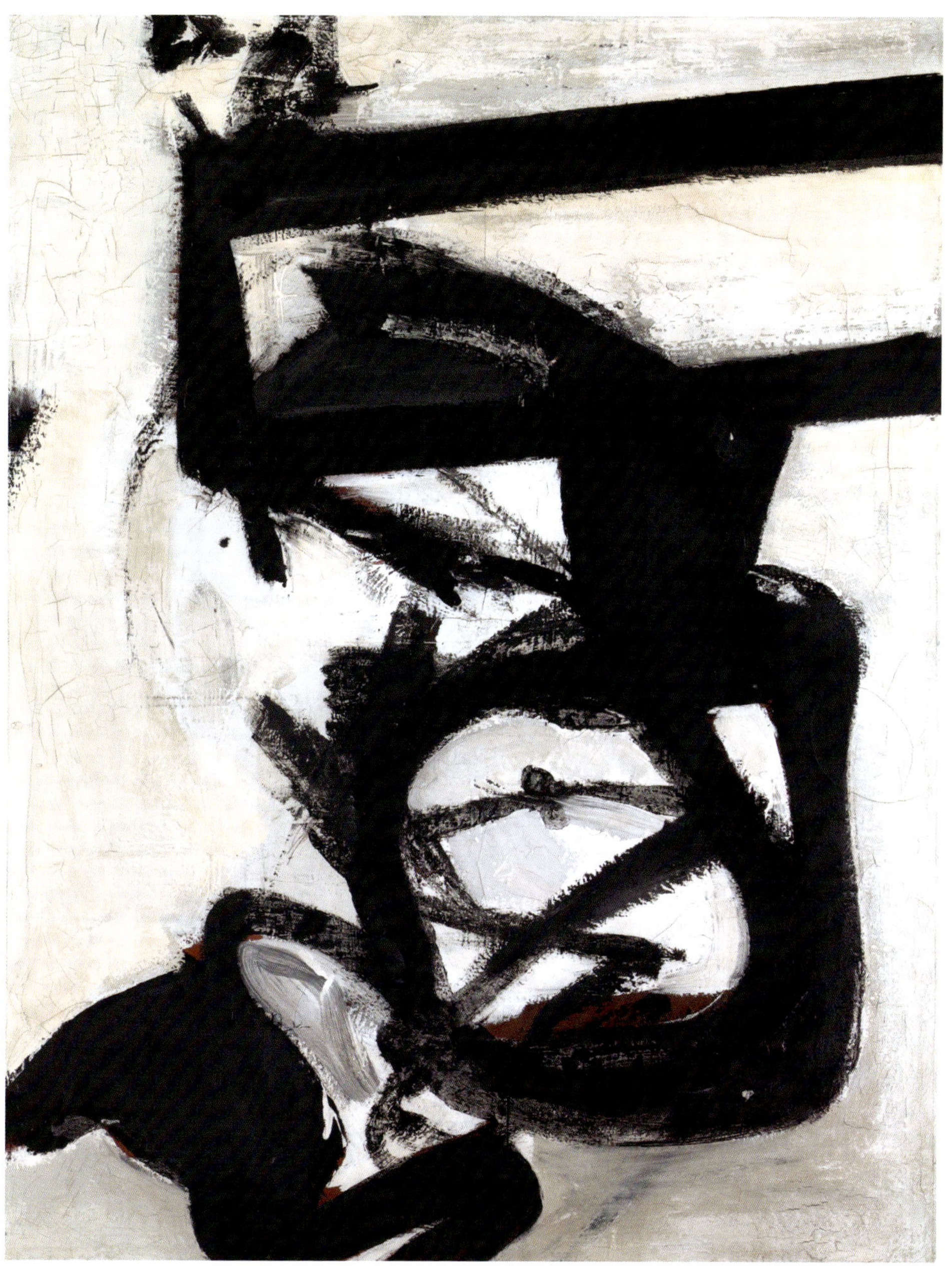

**Figure 97** Franz Kline, *Nijinsky*, 1950, enamel on canvas, 46 × 35 ¼ inches. (Metropolitan Museum of Art, New York, The Muriel Kallis Steinberg Newman Collection, Gift of Muriel Kallis Newman, 2006.32.28)

of the painting's direct connection to the Russian dancer, the breakthrough Kline achieved in 1949–50 saw his compositions reach unprecedented boldness in design and in dimensions. Kline's Abstract Expressionist colleague Willem de Kooning (1904–97) assisted in this process by projecting some of Kline's small calligraphic studies on studio walls with an overhead projector, enabling Kline to envision them as large paintings.

While each was developing new experiments with abstraction, de Kooning and Kline pursued their mutual fascination with Nijinsky's unprecedented movements. Early in the 1940s, before he took up the gestural "action painting" for which he is best remembered, de Kooning studied photographs of the dancer carefully, remarking in 1943 to the dance critic Edwin Denby that "Nijinsky does just the opposite of what the body would naturally do. The plastic sense is similar to that of Michelangelo and Raphael."[42] De Kooning recognized in Nijinsky's movements the countermovement inherent in ballet, raised to a new level of expressive grace. The human figure, while not always present in de Kooning's work, proved a longstanding obsession to him. After painting biomorphic abstractions in the late 1940s, de Kooning shocked the art world by reintroducing figuration in his work. Conscious, as he remarked to Denby, of the master painters of the European tradition, de Kooning's powerful figures of the 1950s are constructed of built up planes of color and interwoven brushstrokes, a technique that adds life to the body, in a manner not unlike the tensions and countermovements he had marveled at in Nijinsky's dancing.

Even as the Ballets Russes made deep impressions on American dancers and visual artists, other European-derived models set up paradigmatic conflicts between the old narrative forms and new ways of representing modernist primitivism. These competing models would preoccupy many artists searching for new expressive possibilities.

## Beyond Russian Dance: American Art Looks East

America's appetite for passion and sensuousness in dance was operating at a high pitch early in the twentieth century. Even as the Russian Ballet was stirring up unprecedented responses in American visual arts, it had to share the spotlight with imported traditions from other parts of the globe. One was the exoticism of Asia, which had long fired the imagination through visual art and was often conveyed through images of the dance. Implicit in the remarkable frequency of dance subjects based on Eastern sources was the belief, common around the turn of the century, that the enlightened art of the future would reflect a West that was conscious of the East. That consciousness was raised when American artists saw Eastern dancers at home and abroad, often in settings such as the large international expositions that purported to present the world's sweeping varieties of cultural experiences.

In the Paris Exposition Universelle of 1889, which marked the centenary of the French Revolution, one of the pavilions pointed up the Dutch colonial presence in Indochina. A Javanese village, or *kampong,* featured performances by a richly costumed delegation of dancers from the royal court. Debussy, Toulouse-Lautrec, Gauguin, and Rodin all responded to the Javanese dance and music at the *kampong*, as did the American John Singer Sargent, whose cosmopolitan existence took him to most such grand expositions. Sargent was instantly drawn to their rich costuming and curiously angular gestures. He immediately put off a visit to Monet at Giverny in order to sketch four of the dancers, apparently gaining access behind the scenes of the Javanese village.

Sargent went on to make many other sketches and three surviving life-sized studies of individual dancers (*Javanese Dancer*, National Gallery, London). Writing of Sargent's dancers the poet Alice Meynell (1847–1922) noted, "The flat-footed, flat-handed action of the extreme East—a grace that has nothing to do with Raphael—is rendered with a delightful, amused and sympathetic appreciation."[43] Sargent's drawings and paintings capture those novel flathanded gestures, which correspond well to the dancer's flowing sash and skirt. In lingering pentimenti of hands, Sargent alludes to a kind of stop-action in their gestures, a detail that prompted scholar D. Dodge Thompson to suggest that the artist also may have been acknowledging contemporary stroboscopic experiments undertaken by photographers Etienne Jules Marey in Paris and Eadweard Muybridge in the United States.[44]

Whatever his intention, Sargent took careful note of the dancers' unique movements, affirming a difference (oversimplified, to be sure) often pointed out by later observers of international dance: that Eastern dance tends to be mostly about the body; while Western dance concerns itself more with the feet.[45] Testing that contrast may have been part of Sargent's interest in Javanese dancers, and his ultimate plan—to combine three of them in a large tableau comparable to his *El Jaleo*—would constitute an aesthetic arena in which to fully study such differences. Or were Spanish and Javanese dance actually more alike than different? A close friend later linked them together as expressive of the artist's personal tastes: "As a young man [Sargent] was, and perhaps remained, especially attracted by the bizarre and outlandish: Spanish dancers (the Jaleo) posed and lit up in enigmatic fashion; Spanish Madonnas like idols, and Javanese dancers scarcely more barbarically improbable. . . . Such were his individual predilections."[46] Unfortunately, personal or professional pressures prevented Sargent's execution of the final work, three dancers in the architectural setting of the Javanese village. He returned instead to the rapid and profitable production of society portraits, a far cry from the exoticism and dynamic movement Sargent craved—and found—in dance subjects. Of Sargent's Javanese dancers, what remains are an entire sketchbook and the large studies, one of which he apparently valued enough to copy for his London colleague Lawrence Alma-Tadema. And, again contrasting different versions of the exotic, Sargent exhibited one of his Javanese dancers in London in 1891 paired with his *Egyptian Dancing Girl*.[47]

Dancers from the "extreme East" endeared themselves to Western audiences and to artists, not all of whom distinguished carefully among their countries of origin. Rodin, who had drawn the Javanese dancers in 1889, brought to his studio in Meudon a troupe of royal Cambodian dancers who performed in Marseilles and Paris in 1906 (*Cambodian Dancer*, 1906, Saint Louis Art Museum). Rodin's pencil and watercolor drawings of them required the artist to work with a haste made possible only by his utter confidence in rendering human movement. He worked out a method for capturing their fugitive grace: without moving his gaze from the subject, Rodin would let the completed sketch drop to the floor, to be succeeded immediately by another. A tinted wash, applied later, fleshed out the contour lines, correcting proportions and enhancing wholeness of the forms. This drawing and others of the Cambodian dancers capture the sharp angularity of their movements, which is not unlike those of the Javanese dancers painted by Sargent. Cambodian dancers underwent methodical training to enable them to exceed the usual range of motion for various joints. Dance historian Curt Sachs described their practice, in which the dancers manipulate each other's joints, bending fingers backward until all the joints crack and forcing their arms backward "until they can move them as much as forty degrees backward at the elbow. . . . And every joint of the body must undergo a training in distortion like that of the elbow."[48] Eventually the sockets and ligaments move with highly elastic resilience and with an angularity recalling the movement of marionettes. All this was new to Rodin, who was captivated by the range and flexibility of their gestures, and whose drawings of them were exhibited in New York as early as 1908.[49]

On the Midway of the 1893 World's Columbian Exposition in Chicago, photographer Eadweard Muybridge (1830–1904) built his "Zoopraxographical Hall." Muybridge, peripatetic pioneer of motion photography, had included photographic sequences of dancers in his 1887 book *Animal Locomotion* (fig. 98), enabling readers to analyze movement more accurately than was possible from a single image. At Chicago, Muybridge's hall was intended to exhibit his work and to hold the crowds he expected would attend his scientific lectures on the analysis of motion. Unfortunately, Muybridge had to compete with the fair's most sensational attraction, the louche Street of Cairo, located right next door. There, Little Egypt performed her sensational gyrations for the crowds conspicuously absent from Muybridge's more edifying environs. When last heard from at the fair, Muybridge was trying to assemble audiences by lecturing outdoors in Jackson Park, charging no admission.

So popular were the Egyptian and "oriental" exhibits in Chicago that they created a blaze of interest in all things from the East. By the next great World's Fair in 1904, the strains of "Meet me in St. Louis, Louis. . . . We will dance the Hootchy Kootchy" echoed from coast to coast. And beyond: in Paris, Diaghilev's Ballets Russes introduced *Cléopâtre* or *Une Nuit d'Egypte* in its first (1909) season, the success of which prompted inclusion of exotic ballets in each subsequent season.[50]

Wildly jumbled exotica was becoming the hottest ticket on the American dance-spectacle circuit. In 1892, the year before Little Egypt vanquished Zoopraxography, the Palisades Amusement Park in New Jersey premiered *Egypt through the Centuries*, a lush visual extravaganza unrolling eleven thousand years of Egyptian history. State-of-the-art equipment—calcium spotlights, incandescent, arc and gas lights—illuminated the park's vast new stage on which hundreds of dancers, jugglers, serpent-swallowers, soldiers, camels, and floats paraded forth. The scale of *Egypt through the Centuries* was unprecedented; it

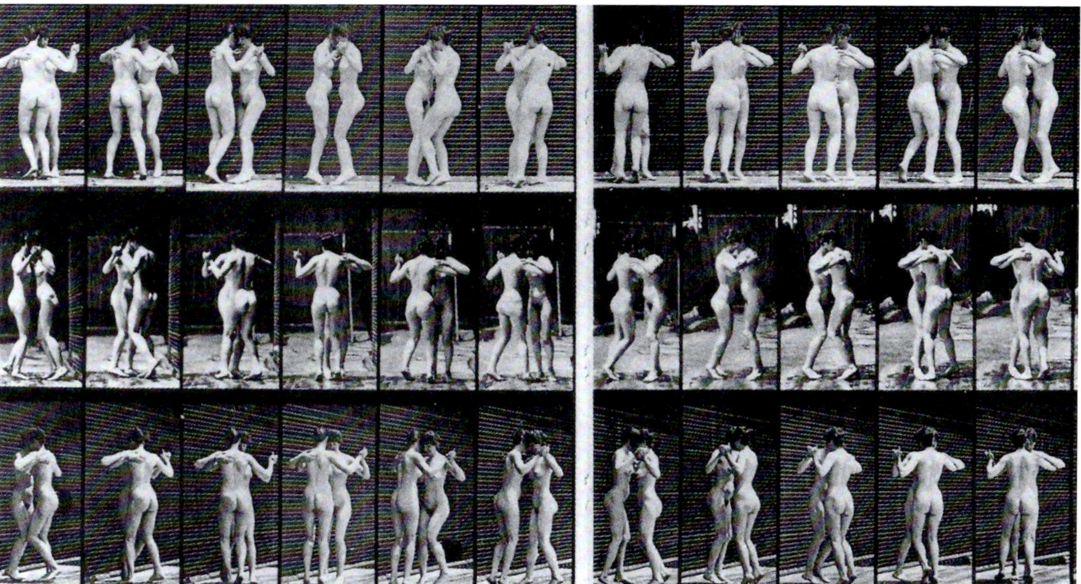

**Figure 98** Eadweard Muybridge, *Nude Women Dancing*, from his 1887 book *Animal Locomotion*.

was Gilded Age American show business at its apogee of excess, and audiences couldn't get enough of it.

## Salomé in American Art: Dance, Seduction, and Death

Dance, through its sense of free-floating, liberated movement and frequently gorgeous costuming, was seen as the perfect conveyance for voluptuous decadence. Often, as discussed earlier, such subjects were of pagan derivation, but others—most notably the biblical femme fatale Salomé—obsessed many fin-de-siècle artists. In Europe, painters such as the academic Henri Regnault (1843–71), Symbolist precursor Gustave Moreau (1826–98), Aubrey Beardsley (1872–98), and the German realist Lovis Corinth (1858–1925) explored aspects of the decorative and the decadent through Salomé.[51] Writers Flaubert and Huysmans seemed haunted by the erotic dance of Salomé, tense with the twin powers of seduction and moral uprightness. Soon (1895) Richard Strauss enshrined her seductions in opera.

The story is familiar: King Herod, mesmerized by his stepdaughter Salomé's dancing, promised her anything. Goaded by her mother Herodiade, Salomé demanded the severed head of John the Baptist. Salomé, as archetypal male destroyer, played directly into fin-de-siècle male anxieties about rising feminism. Her fatal charms proved irresistible to artists on both sides of the Atlantic. In America, the orientalist fantasy of Salomé attracted so many new spectators to theaters that it opened the possibility for dance in America to become a virtuoso, if not virtuous, art.

In 1893, the same year as Chicago's Exposition, Oscar Wilde published his play *Salomé,* for which he envisioned Sarah Bernhardt in the title role.[52] As scripted by Wilde, the play was first banned on the London stage, but in sanitized form it soon became a runaway hit on European stages, and eventually on American ones as well. The American dancer Loïe Fuller was among the first dancers to bring Salomé to life.[53] Fuller's career would take shape largely in France where, starting in 1892, she pursued an uphill battle for respectability as a dancer. She hoped initially to perform at Charles Garnier's celebrated Paris Opéra house, but an engagement there failed to materialize. Instead, her theatrical base became the famed Folies-Bergère, a café-concert of the type painted by the Impressionists, by Degas, and especially by Edouard Manet, whose *Bar aux Folies-Bergère* (1882, Courtauld Institute Galleries, London) was a sensation at the 1882 Paris Salon. These café-concerts were really large, bustling cafés, not theaters, and without theatrical pretensions. Tables with beer-drinking customers filled much of the area, and the larger spectacle, as in Manet's painting, was reflected in a large mirror. As T. J. Clark has written, "the cafés-concerts were meant to be loud, vulgar, and above all modern" and "were characterized by a mingling of the classes, or at least an agreement to listen to the same songs."[54] Or watch the same dances.

Meanwhile, as Loïe Fuller continued to draw crowds at the Folies-Bergère, the decade following Manet's celebrated painting saw unprecedented artistic and social change. In such venues were played out what Norman Bryson has identified as the nineteenth century's "key social processes [such] as urbanization, the proliferation of spectacle, and the development of commodified leisure."[55] From a place where performances consisted of little more than a singer or stand-up comic on stage, the Folies-Bergère evolved into a type of circus, whose acts included animal trainers or acrobats of the type glimpsed in the upper left corner of Manet's painting. With the addition of more elaborate costumes and scenery, it was becoming in the 1890s a kind of grand vaudeville theater where slightly bawdy acts took place in an interior described as "ugly and . . . splendid . . . of an outrageous and exquisite taste."[56]

Determined to refine this garish environment, Loïe Fuller and her "artistic" dances began to broaden the clientele of the Folies-Bergère. Along with the merely curious and the sensation-seeking, her performances attracted some of the most respected artists and scientists of her day, including Sarah Bernhardt, Stéphane Mallarmé, Toulouse-Lautrec, and Marie Curie. Women and children flocked to see Fuller, and Parisian critics started to take her seriously.[57] With mild surprise, one wrote, "there is no pornography, no unwholesome nudity, no coarseness, nothing but the most poetically artistic. This Loïe Fuller is a great, a very great artist."[58] That reputation for wholesomeness, while mostly desirable, imposed its own restraints. Fuller's Serpentine dance, performed with veils and colored lights, was popularly successful, but she still longed for a vehicle to raise her from the music hall to a higher level of artistry. Fuller began to look about for new, artistically representable images in dance. In the Bibliothèque Nationale she found picture books on Oriental dancing and on the painted murals of dancers from Pompeii and Herculaneum; she also read about dancing in the Bible.

She concluded that her methods were not much different from those early dancers, who also relied on silken draperies to enhance their movement. Her legitimization was at hand: "I have only revived a forgotten art," concluded Fuller, "for I have been able to trace some of my dances back to four thousand years ago: to the time when Miriam and the women of Israel—filled with religious fervour and rapture—celebrated their release from Egyptian captivity with 'timbrels and with dances.'"[59] She was convinced that Eastern ("Oriental") dance involved mostly the body's sway and the arms' movement rather than footwork.

Loïe Fuller determined that she would next personify Salomé, bringing her to life through dance and pantomime. In March 1895, she premiered *Salomé*, billed as "a lyric pantomime in one act and five tableaux," at the Comédie-Parisienne. Reaction was mixed: her veils and lights were applauded, her miming dismissed as wooden, with, as one critic said, "the gestures of an English boxer and the physique of Mr. Oscar Wilde."[60] Still, its five dances appealed to public, to press, and, not least, to visual artists. The second act, a Sun Dance, featured Fuller as Salomé dancing before Herod in the rays of the setting sun. With smoke swirling about her, Fuller appeared to be consumed by flames as she manipulated her veils to the swelling strains of Wagner's *Ride of the Valkyries*. The Paris audience ignored the intended allusion to the glories of the setting sun and loudly pronounced it a Fire Dance. It became a sensation wherever Fuller performed it, especially back at the Folies-Bergère (Fuller had not been able to move permanently to her higher artistic station).[61] Fuller's Fire Dance was interpreted in various mediums by a number of visual artists. Most famous is Jules Chéret's (1836–1932) chromolithographic poster of her (1893), of a type so popular that critic Joris-Karl Huysmans advised his readers to ignore that year's Salon paintings and prints in favor of the "astonishing fantasies of Chéret" plastered along Paris streets. Later poster versions of Fuller were made by Chéret's student Georges Meunier and by the Romanian artist Jean de Paléologu (known as Pal). Pierre Roche (1855–1922) cast his Fire Dance image of Fuller in bronze (c. 1894, Maryhill Museum of Art, Goldendale, Wash.), and her Fire Dance was also recorded on film by Pathé in 1906. And, still later, American artist Joseph Cornell used a filmstrip of her *Fire Dance* to make a photomontage, one of his multiple dance designs for Lincoln Kirstein's 1940s journal *Dance Index* (fig. 99).

Fuller's Salomé did not remain her exclusive property. Indeed, multiple Salomés soon graced the stages of theaters in the United States. The premiere of Richard Strauss's operatic version of *Salomé* at the Metropolitan Opera in 1907 spawned dozens of Fuller's dancing clones in the legitimate theater as well as in vaudeville. A Mademoiselle Dazie proved such a draw that she opened a school for Salomés on the roof garden of a New York theater. Eva Tanguay, "The Girl Who Made Vaudeville Famous," also took a lucrative turn as a scantily attired Salomé during this era when vaudeville shifted its focus from sentiment to sex.[62] Two other notable Salomés were Gertrude Hoffman, later the entrepreneur of an ersatz Russian ballet company, and Maud Allan. Allan (1883–1956), a Canadian-born Californian, began her career in Vienna in 1903. Along with Duncan and Ruth St. Denis, Allan became an extremely popular "barefoot dancer" in first decade of the twentieth century. Her representation of the seductive oriental

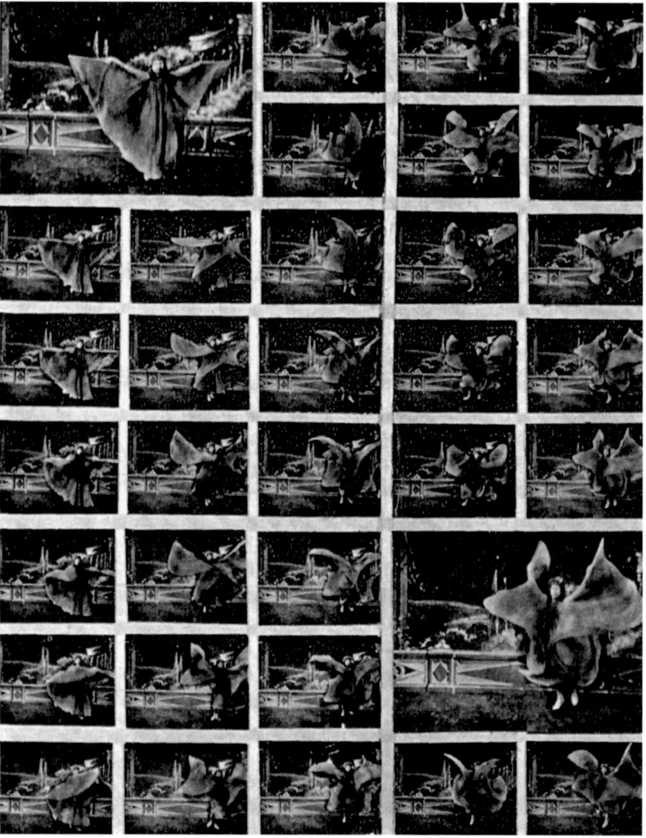

**Figure 99** Joseph Cornell, detail of early twentieth-century photomontage of Loïe Fuller in *Fire Dance*, made from an early
filmstrip, for *Dance Index*, 1942.

princess in "The Vision of Salomé" at the Palace Theatre, London's famous
music hall, extended to more than 250 performances in 1908–9.[63]

American painters who took up the subject of Salomé often placed her
within exotic architectural settings, employing the jewel-like color of Gustave
Moreau's work. Sometimes she danced; sometimes she merely posed; either way,
she reigned as the epitome of Symbolist luxe, eroticism, and decadence. But the
allure of Salomé reached well beyond Symbolism. Robert Henri, a determined
realist, painted two versions of the quintessential femme fatale. Having seen a
performance of Strauss's opera in February 1909 at Hammerstein's Manhattan
Opera House, Henri determined to paint its high point, the notorious "Dance
of the Seven Veils." In most such productions, a professional dancer stepped in
for the lead singer to perform this highly sensual dance, but at Hammerstein's
the celebrated soprano Mary Garden had done her own dancing, dressed in
a pink body stocking. Garden was unavailable to pose for Henri, so when he
set about to paint his Salome in May of that year he hired a model known as
Mlle. Voclezca. In rapid succession Henri turned out two versions of Salome.
The first *Salome* (1909; fig. 100) was rejected when Henri submitted it to the

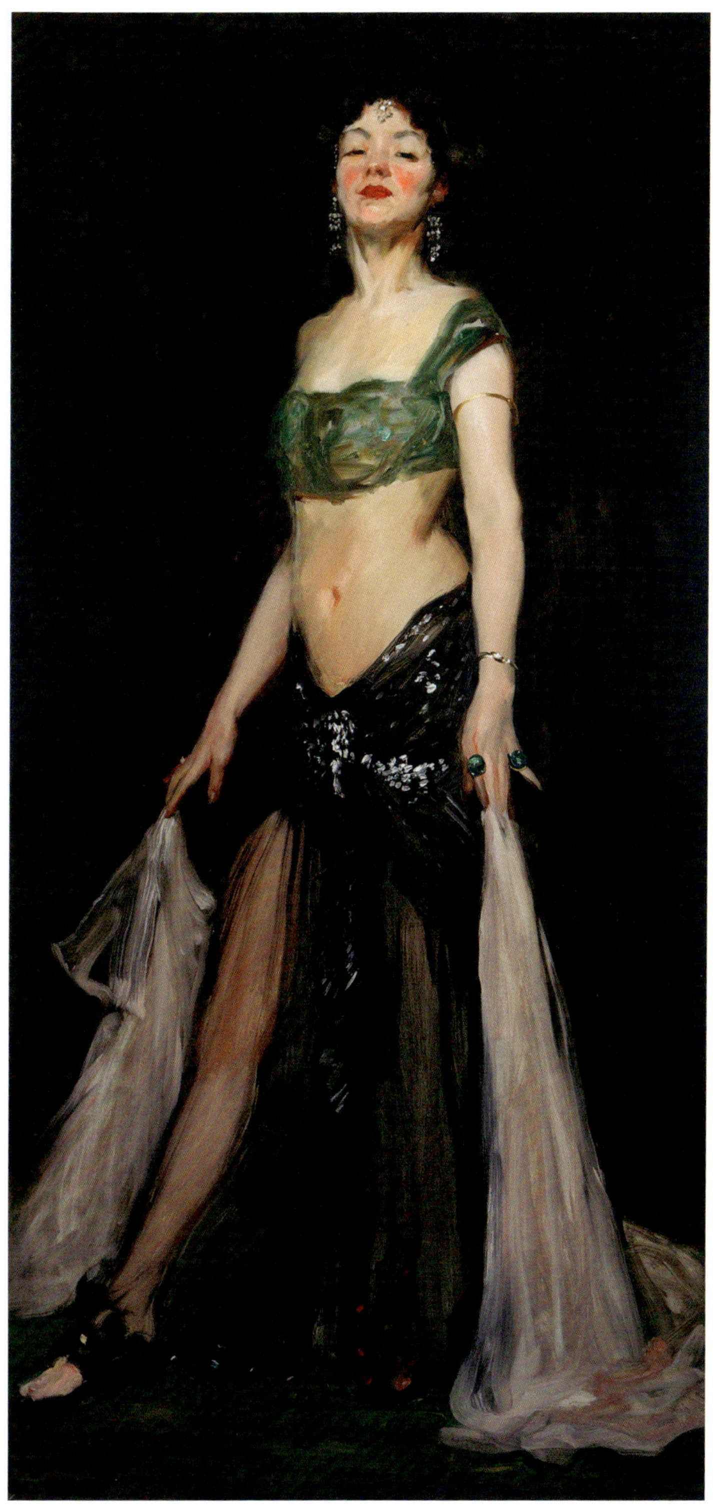

**Figure** 100 Robert Henri, *Salome*, 1909, oil on canvas 77 ¼ × 36 ¹⁵⁄₁₆ inches. (Mead Art Museum, Amherst College, Amherst, Massachusetts, AC1973.68)

1910 National Academy annual, but was shown instead at that year's Exhibition of Independent Artists. The second version, now in the Ringling Museum, Sarasota, was never exhibited during Henri's lifetime. Henri used strong tonal contrasts, liquid blacks, and slashing brushstrokes to bring out the defiant, sensual quality of the Oriental dancer. That sense of vitality, well conveyed on stage by the passionate Mary Garden, was indispensable to Henri, who had absorbed the immediacy of paint application from the work of Velázquez and Frans Hals in particular. Henri's Salome gathers power in the confident spiral of her pose, a kind of organic form likely related to the ubiquitous Delsarte system of body movement and gesture so popular then among actors and dancers.

Painter Edward Hopper, a constant theatergoer, found humor in the craze for Salomé. Instead of painting her, Hopper lampooned both the character and the larger enterprise of modern dance. Hopper's wife, Jo, recalled that Hopper reveled in pantomime, once as a slouching Salomé bearing a grapefruit on a plate in lieu of the Baptist's head, and sometimes posing as Isadora Duncan, swathed in flowing draperies.[64]

If Salome's regular recurrences on American stages demonstrate anything about public taste, it must be that her character answers some kind of perennial desire to witness the body's potential to enact wonderment, to watch as the slow dance of seduction—by turns searching, erotic, ecstatic—works its magic. Power, in the person of Herod, is humbled by eros; in the high-stakes game of sexual favors at the royal level, the world can change, and does, as Salomé entrances her stepfather. As in all biblical stories charged with lustful energy, the outcome is both terrible and fascinating to watch. Although reaching an apex in Symbolist art, Salomé survived into modernism, both in the visual arts and in dance.

American sculptors of every artistic stripe bodied forth their Salomés. As early as 1871 William Wetmore Story (1819–95) carved her lifesize in marble, seated and clothed from the waist down (Metropolitan Museum of Art, New York), while Gutzon Borglum's (1867–1941) *Salome* rises in marmorean dance (n.d., Borglum Historical Center, Keystone, S.D.). Paul Manship (1885–1966) envisioned her as a small bronze (1915, Smithsonian American Art Museum, Washington, D.C.). As abstraction engaged more sculptors, they often chose familiar subjects such as Salomé as starting points for their modernist innovations. Russian American sculptor Alexander Archipenko (1887–1964) exhibited a *Salome* (1910, unlocated) in the 1913 Armory Show.[65] This is a piece in stylistic transition: elongated, slightly angularized, the nude body bends in a great C-shaped curve. Archipenko's *Salomé,* compared to many of her previous artistic incarnations, has been de-eroticized. The sculptor was clearly focused on formal elements, edging toward the Cubist innovations for which he would soon be recognized. Another modernist sculptor, Robert Laurent (1890–1970) carved his *Salomé* in alabaster, a curiously pristine material for a lurid bit of iconography. Like Story's and Borglum's marble versions, Laurent's pale stone sets up strong internal contradictions—themselves inherent in modern consciousness. How do surface textures, color (or its absence) and abstraction affect a sculpture's emotional temperature?

Salomé returned to concert dance in modernist form with the premiere of Martha Graham's 1944 ballet *Herodiade,* staged in a biomorphically themed set

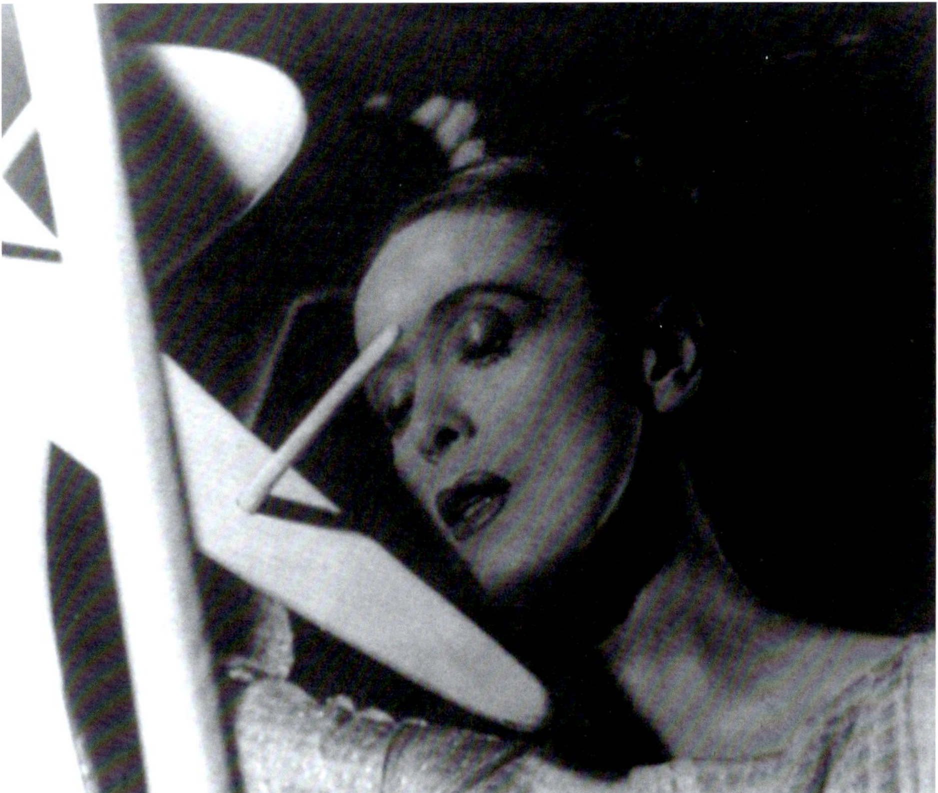

**Figure 101** Martha Graham with detail from Isamu Noguchi set in *Herodiade*, 1944.

by sculptor Isamu Noguchi, who called it "the most baroque and specifically sculptural of my sets." Painted plywood shapes in a chair and clothes rack— curving, interpenetrating, bonelike—anticipate the decisive appearance of Salomé before her mirror, where she sees, in Noguchi's words, "her bones, the potential skeleton of her body. The chair is like an extension of her vertebrae; the clothes rack, the circumscribed bones on which is hung her skin. This is the desecration of beauty, the consciousness of time" (fig. 101).[66]

Robert Henri's interest in dance subjects continued for decades. Beyond his Spanish dancers and Salomé subjects, he continued to seek out and paint dancers both famous and obscure, becoming something of an advocate for them and for the elevation of dance among the arts of the United States. In 1902 Henri discovered a lively Ziegfeld Follies dancer named Jesseca Penn, who announced her intention to become "the greatest dancer in the world." En route to that goal, she slowed her pace long enough to pose for Henri, soon becoming his favorite model. Penn was a stunning redhead with green eyes and a pair of long legs discernible even in his clothed portraits of her. As *Young Woman in Black Jesseca Penn* (1902; fig. 102) Henri painted her life-size, in street clothes, grasping the folds of her full black skirt in her gloved hand, as if about to waltz briskly across the room. Absent the era's usual studio props, she is dramatically self-contained, exuding a frank physical confidence in her superb dancer's bearing. Without

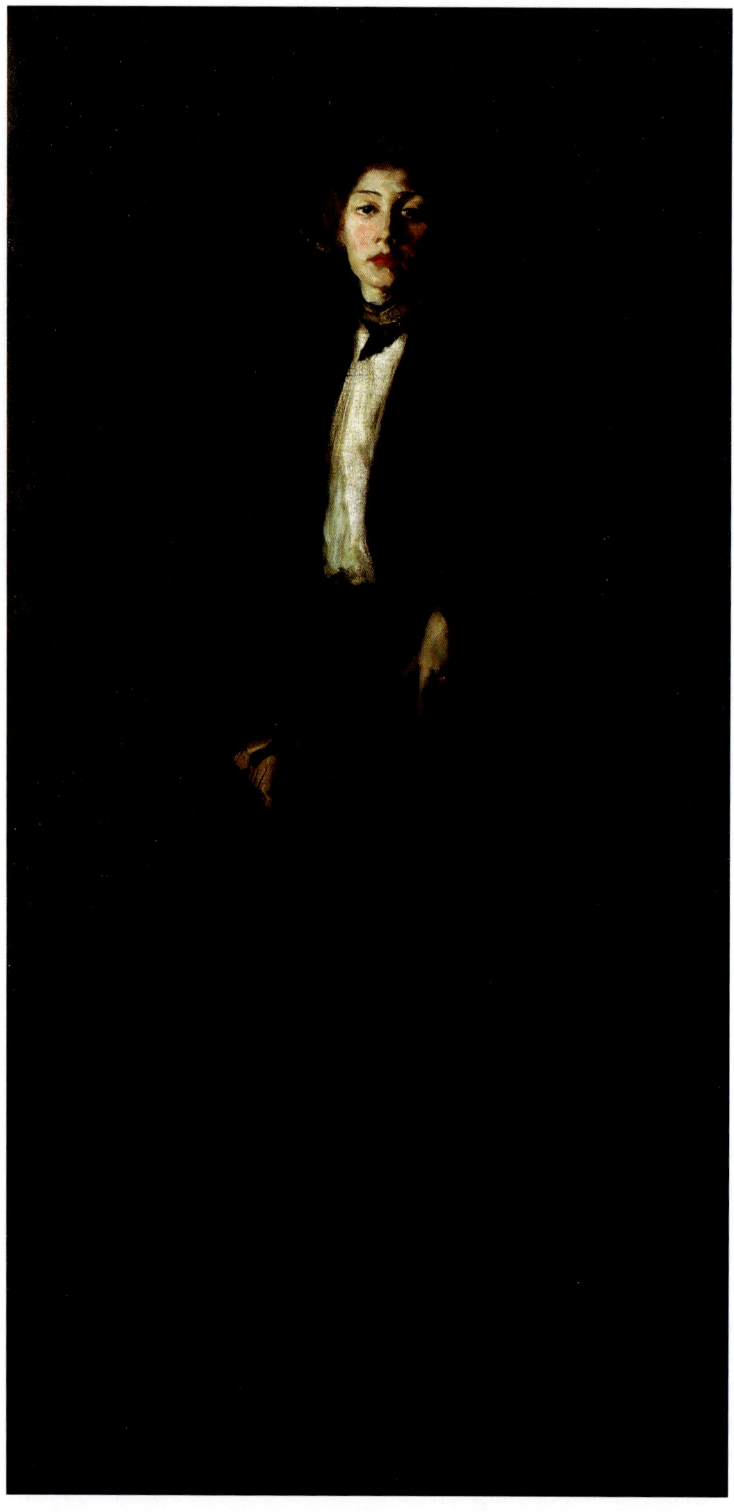

Figure 102 Robert Henri, *Young Woman in Black, Jesseca Penn*, 1902, oil on canvas, 77 × 38 ½ inches. (Art Institute of Chicago, Friends of American Art Collection, 1910.317)

clothes, she must have been even more ravishing. To his diary Henri remarked only that she was "one of the finest nudes I have ever seen."[67] The painter's choice of words is telling: detaching his notice from the specifics of her movements or her anatomy, he sees her (or so he claims) with a purely professional eye, as a studio nude.[68]

From his early twenties on, Henri saw important parallels between his own art and that of dance and theater. Believing as he did that immediate experience should inspire the American painter, few subjects could be more compelling to Henri (and thus to his students) than the urgent temporality of the dance. Its intrinsic vitality especially corresponded to his insistence on expressive energy and immediacy in subjects in general.

In the coming years, especially as a metaphor for ideal motion, dance permeated Henri's thinking. So saturated was he with dance metaphors that they often spilled forth in his lively classes. He exhorted his students to "pretend you are dancing or singing a picture."[69] Henri's vaunted interest in gesture led him to study some of the great dancers of his time, especially Isadora Duncan. Not all dance was of equal interest to Henri, but he found himself deeply in sympathy with Duncan's efforts, calling her "perhaps one of the greatest masters of gesture the world has ever seen; [she] carries us through a universe in a single movement of her body."[70] He saw her dance at the Metropolitan Opera House in 1908, and met her the next year at a party given in her honor by Mary Fanton Roberts, who had arranged Duncan's first public performance in New York. Next, Henri saw her dance to Bach at Carnegie Hall, and when she swept into one of Henri's studio parties swathed in royal purple robes, she became an object of worship for the whole Henri circle.

Henri urged his students to see her performances, sometimes passing along free tickets. To capture the fugitive effects onstage, he invited them, in effect, to think like choreographers, in moving masses and defined moments: "Work with great speed," advised Henri. "Have your energies alert, up and active. . . . Get the greatest possibility of expression in the larger masses first . . . Do it all in one setting if you can. In one minute if you can."[71] Henri and his students (as well as other artists) could often be seen making quick sketches of Duncan from their seats in the audience. Back in class, Henri critiqued a batch of student drawings at one of his usual Friday sessions, remarking, "The Isadora Duncans are very good today. I find this collection very, *very* very interesting. Unusually so. It means that the march on toward individual vision is increasing."[72] As a means of isolating and intensifying that individual vision, Henri urged his students to "concentrate on just the movement of the model," an idea at work in his *Figure in Motion* exhibited in the Armory Show (catalog 835). Although not labeled as such, it is perhaps one of Henri's many studies of Duncan herself.[73]

Ultimately, Henri extended his appreciation of Duncan into a broader, almost universal vein: "Back of her gesture," he concluded, "I see a deep philosophy of freedom and of dignity, of simplicity and of order."[74] For Henri, as for many other artists, Duncan's bearing, gesture, and costume made her performances an intensely visual form of theater. Dance became, in a sense, another of the visual arts.

Other dancers would capture Henri's attention in new ways. Back in New York, he continued his rapid-fire talk, sharing his many enthusiasms with his students. No ivory-tower aesthete, Henri talked often of art's responsibility to society, which to him meant that art students should immerse themselves into the life of their time, absorbing "the great ideas native to the country."[75] Besides dance, classroom conversations bubbled with talk of literature, poetry, and music, mingling Whitman and Emerson with Dostoevsky, Tolstoy, Wagner, Zola, and the omnipresent Duncan. Maintaining his devotion to her largeness of gesture and the vibrancy of her "Duncan Girls," Henri began to extend his appreciation of dance to many other styles and performers—from Kimura, a graceful Japanese dancer performing at the Neighborhood Playhouse, to Ruth St. Denis, Betalo Rubino, and Roshanara, the last three of whom Henri persuaded to pose for monumental canvases recording their great roles.[76]

These portraits were undertaken at Henri's initiative, unabashedly in celebration of their talent. In his dance subjects Henri always tried to capture the unique expressive genius of the sitter, and he turned for a time to Ruth St. Denis, one of America's most famous interpretive dancers. A veteran of many European tours, St. Denis was back in New York in 1919. Henri posed her in the regalia for her celebrated dance enacting the legend of a Kashmir princess imprisoned in the body of a peacock. *Ruth St. Denis in the Peacock Dance* (1919; fig. 103) captures the elegant spirit of the bird in the long, curving shapes of the dancer's body, seemingly paused between avian gestures. Although he had long appreciated the popular forms of dance, Henri now tried to preserve its more artistic forms as distinct from the quotidian variety. The year he painted St. Denis, he wrote to his fellow dance enthusiast Frank Crowninshield at *Vanity Fair* to urge that "such great artists as Ruth St. Denis and the beautiful girl we saw the other afternoon—Roshanara" be given a true Theatre of the Dance in New York "instead of being hampered by vaudevillians and sandwiched between imitations of George Cohan . . . The Dance must come," thundered Henri. "It is too great an art for us through our inertia to miss."[77]

St. Denis inspired artists working in popular mediums as well. Illustrator Marius de Zayas caricatured her famous Cobra dance in 1910 for *Camera Work* (fig. 104). Dance historian J. E. Crawford Flitch described St. Denis's Cobra as

> Strictly speaking, not a dance at all, for it was performed in sitting, crouching or kneeling postures. The dancer appeared in the role of a snake-charmer, and throwing off her mantle revealed her arms clasped over either shoulder, like two coiling snakes. On the first and fourth fingers of each hand two enormous emeralds gleamed like serpents' eyes. The arms slowly unwound and with a curiously sinuous motion began to writhe about her body. They twined, coiled, fought and darted with lightning flashes in all directions, simulating the movements of the reptile with astonishing fidelity. It was a marvellous exercise in the flexibility of the arms.[78]

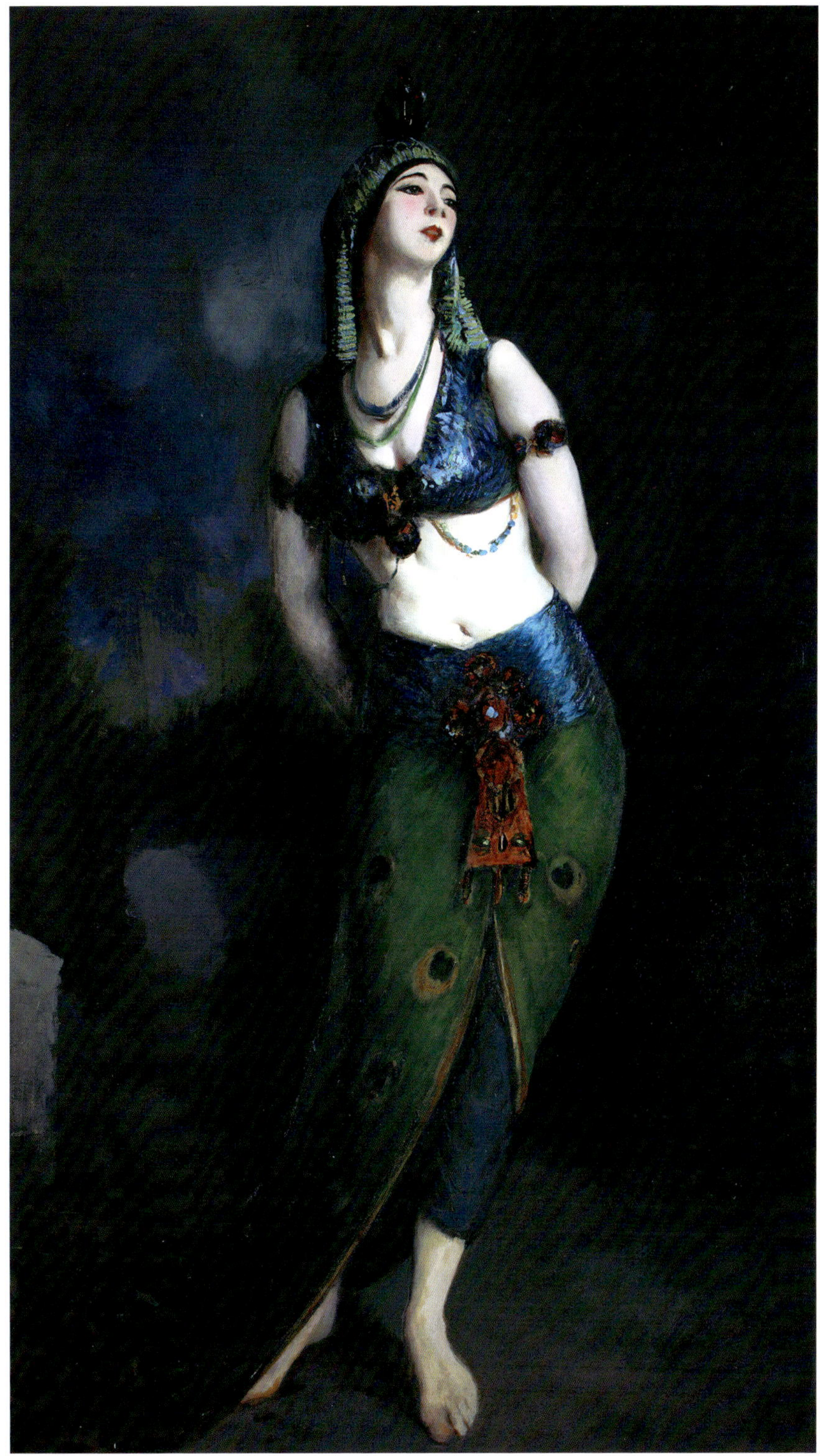

Figure 103 Robert Henri, *Ruth St. Denis in the Peacock Dance*, 1919, oil on canvas, 85 × 49 inches. (courtesy Pennsylvania Academy of the Fine Arts, Philadelphia, Gift of the Sameric Corporation in memory of Eric Shapiro, 1976.1)

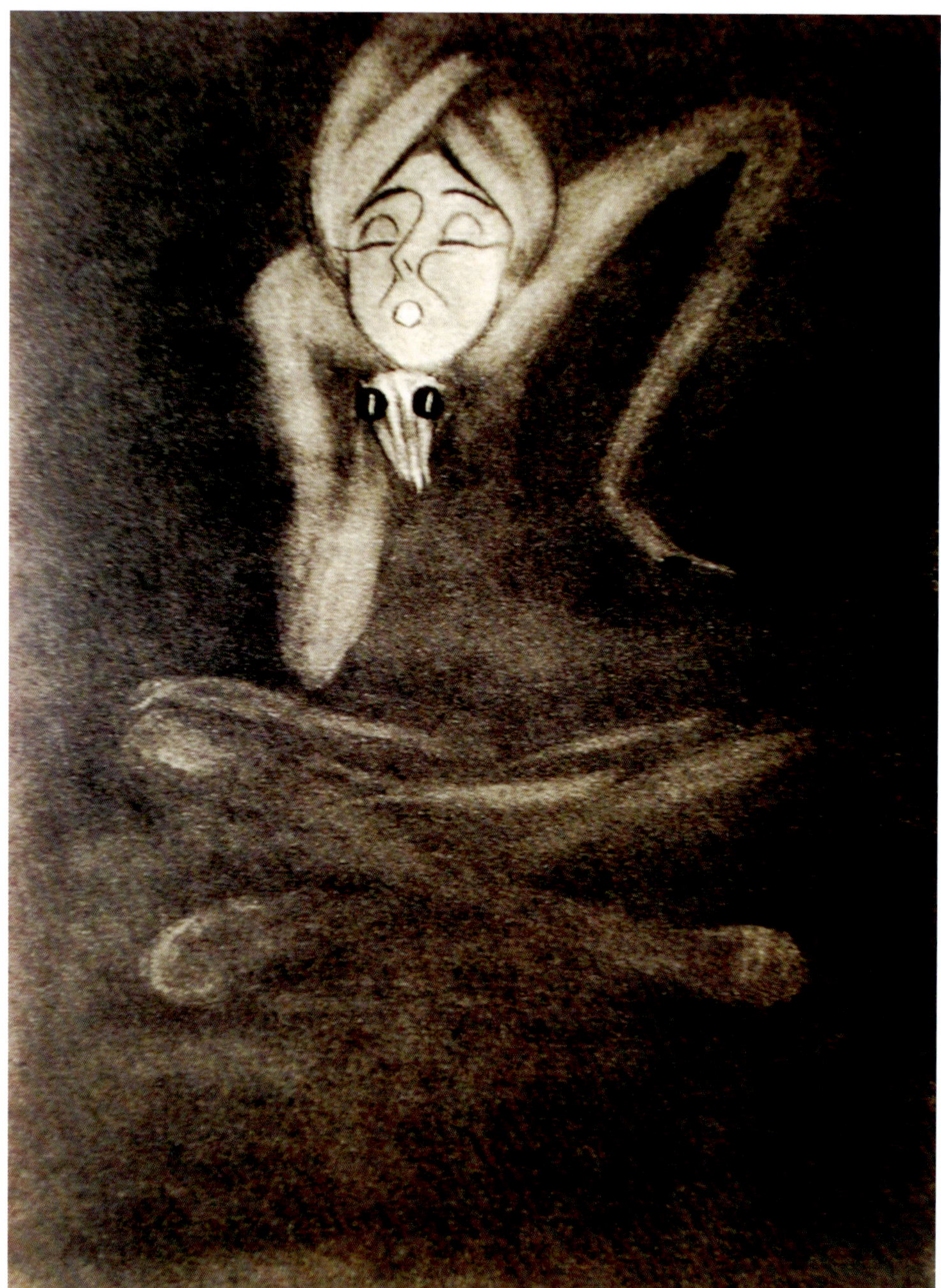

**Figure 104** Marius de Zayas, *Ruth St. Denis in the Cobra Dance*, 1910, photogravure, 8 ⅗ × 6 ⅖ inches. (from *Camera Work* 29 [1910])

St. Denis performed the Cobra wherever she traveled in those years. Especially in Europe she attracted writers and artists to her performances. In Germany in 1906 she discussed poetry and plays with the likes of Hugo von Hofmannsthal and Gerhart Hauptmann and was sketched and painted by various artists. In a 1906 photograph by the German Aura Hartwig, St. Denis poses in her Cobra

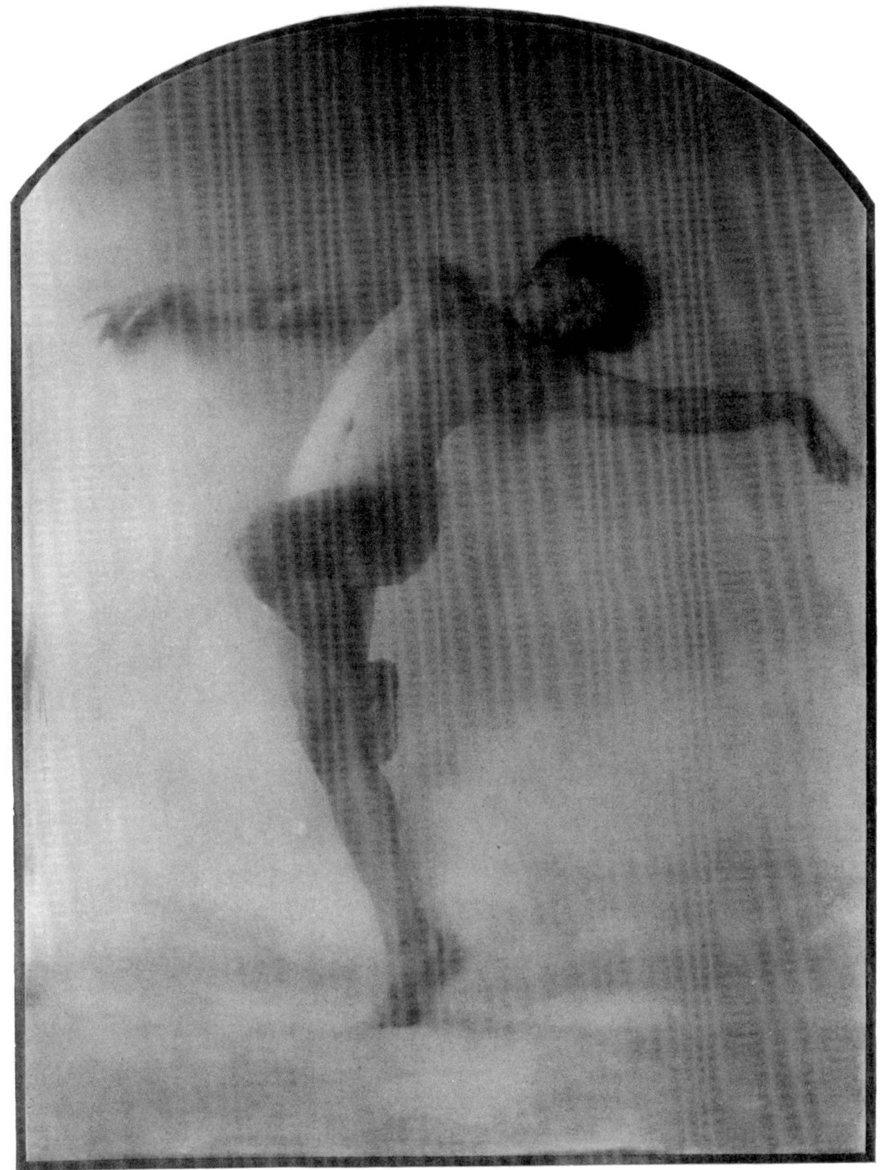

Figure 105 Edward Weston, *Ted Shawn: Dancing Nude*, 1916. (from *Photograms of the Year: 1916*; photo courtesy George Eastman House, 50590)

headgear and facepaint for an artist, probably Count Harry Kessler, who works at his easel, watched over his shoulder by St. Denis's European agent.[79]

The yeasty mix of exoticism, modernism, and new photographic techniques produced some startling, unprecedented innovations. In 1916 photographer Edward Weston photographed St. Denis's partner Ted Shawn, with whom she had recently opened a new dance school, Denishawn. Weston tried a daring new dance photograph of Shawn, a subject of Dionysian revelry. *Ted Shawn: Dancing Nude* (fig. 105) embodies a lively, highly unstable pose in which the dancer rises on one foot, opposite knee raised and arms fully extended.[80] To Denishawn fans, this type of movement was known as a "sculpture plastique," taken from Shawn's eponymous performance of the same year. (St. Denis and Shawn often referred to a dancer's "plastique" in describing movement). Weston apparently achieved the exposure by supporting Shawn, unseen, against the wall behind him, a technical sleight of hand for which some critics faulted him. But Cyrus Dallin, an artist to whom Weston sent the print, responded, "I think the 'dancing nude' almost the most beautiful photo of a dancing figure I ever saw and it has appealed to me so much from its plastic beauty that I have been tempted to make it in sculpture. It is truly quite a wonder from a sculptor's standpoint."[81] Both photographer and sculptor were intrigued by the expanding expressive and mechanical possibilities of dance movement.

Clearly, dance images—often based on the exotic, the "primitive" and the pagan—had captured the imaginations of many American artists during the early part of the century. The waves of Salomés and Scheherazades, as well as Egyptian- and Asian-derived dance flooding American stages, had much to do with that proliferation of visual images. The dancers and visual artists discussed in this chapter awakened Americans to the expression of pleasure in both the physicality of dance and in the physicality of mediums chosen by visual artists. Nowhere is this better evident than in Robert Henri's use of flowing, juicy paint as a tactile presence, available and gratifying to multiple senses. If Isadora Duncan condensed the universality of dance into *exultation*, Henri and the many other visual artists considered here responded with painting and sculpture that gave visual form to the unfathomable, the exotic, and the euphoric. Together, dance and visual art opened new pathways for those perceptions and explored ways of preserving the elusive, evanescent forms and pleasures of the dance.

# Part Three

# "The Complete Actual Present"
## Dancers and Visual Artists Explore the Immediate Cultural Moment (Expressions of Modernity)

Gertrude Stein declared prophetically that "the business of art is to live in the actual present, that is the complete actual present, and to express the complete actual present."[1] Stein, keen observer of modern art and pioneer of the avant-garde in literature, understood the braiding of historical processes with cultural ambitions. Like much of modern visual art, her writing embraced episodic structure, employed movement inspired by life, and took inspiration from popular culture. Picasso said, agreeing with Stein, "To me there is no past or future in art. If a work of art cannot live always in the present, it must not be considered at all."[2] Both Stein and Picasso, each in her or his own way, engaged with the idea of time. Stein explored the possibilities of the stream of consciousness, a term invented by William James. The concept soon fired Stein's imagination, forcing her realization that external things, instead of changing or succeeding one another, in fact did not. Rather, they coexisted, requiring a sentient being to keep them all in mind at once. Before 1910 Picasso and the other Cubist painters were already engaging with time, simultaneity, and the analysis of forms, processes described by Albert Gleizes and Jean Metzinger in their book *Cubism* (1912) as "moving around an object to seize it from several successive appearances, which, fused into a single image, reconstitute it in time." In the visual arts, literature, dance, drama, and music, the overlapping concepts of simultaneity, achronological uses of time, the montage effect, and the fourth dimension all became part of the modernist discourse.

Not all visual artists have agreed with Stein and Picasso, but for many it has indeed been vital to engage with the complexities of time, or at least to express something of the essence of their own time. To the powerful sensual, emotional, and aesthetic responses considered in the previous chapter, we now add another shared by both dance and visual art: a response drenched in time and revelatory of the consciousness of its era. The modern (or what is considered to be so at any given moment) might be expressed in many ways—by addressing new technologies or incorporating new materials, for example—but dance, ever changing, engaging the energies of its era in distinctly physical translations, is a more poetic way to do it.

Dance has been seen as the perfect modernist idiom because it is an art performed in time. Like Cubism and Futurism (and other successor styles) dance necessarily exists in the realm of the temporal, a recognition that has encouraged visual artists to test dance subjects against the most advanced temporal-spatial concepts. Dance feeds into such experiments because it situates the figure in a particular time and place, unlike, say, the timeless, universal quality of the static nude in art. In their evolving arsenal of pictorial means, artists worked on strategies to capture the elusive essences of dance, essences that escaped many writers because they exceeded the power of written language. At the same time dance, typically a more accessible art form than painting, could be engaged to cultivate a broader public taste for modernism. And, not least, it could even serve as an embodied, living link between music and the visual arts.

Like visual art, dance responds to the rhythm of individual emotional life, but also to any era's larger social rhythm. Charles Baudelaire's definition of modernism as the ephemeral and fugitive, as opposed to the immutable, makes dance peculiarly suitable to modernism. In his oft-quoted article "The Painter of Modern Life," Baudelaire summoned before his reader an artist of contemporary manners, "the painter of the passing moment and all the suggestions of eternity that it contains." Manet's *Le Dejeuner sur l'Herbe* seems a response to Baudelaire's call in its open revelations of sexuality taken out of the bedroom or brothel into the outdoors. If Manet's *Le Dejeuner sur l'Herbe* places his viewer in frank confrontation with modernity and contemporary mores, other painters took up Baudelaire's challenge to explore the eternal in the ephemeral. Dance, whose antiquity was unquestioned, seemed so basic and ubiquitous in human activity as to approach the status of the eternal. Dance continues while the world changes around it, and dance, whose only constant is movement, reconciles the paradox imagined by Baudelaire. Both dance and visual art can carry meaningful signs of the contemporary cultural phenomena of any era.

The immediacy, the implicit movement suggested by the dance subject is an aspect of Stein's and Picasso's continuous present. Some dancers, painters, and writers saw it in expansive, philosophical terms: images can become fixed, frozen, and iconic, but if they are images of the dance they contain the capacity, the immanence of change. Dance challenges stasis by investing it with temporality and nowness. Ruth St. Denis talked of "the Eternal Now of the Dance" as equivalent to the experience of life itself. She felt, while dancing, a state of equilibrium, a kind of still point of perfection. In this philosophical position she approached both the thinking of Ralph Waldo Emerson, who reasoned that the highest form of communication was silence, and of T. S. Eliot, who ruminated poetically on the absence and presence, the stillness and movement of the dance:

At the still point of the turning world, neither flesh nor fleshless;
Neither from nor towards; at the still point, there the dance is,
But neither arrest nor movement. And do not call it fixity,
Where the past and future are gathered. Neither movement from nor
     towards,
Neither ascent nor decline. Except for the point, the still point,
There would be no dance, and there is only the dance.[3]

Eliot's words are both allusive and elusive. Dance is a kernel of energy, the latent temporality at the heart of quietude. It is the necessary and inevitable antithesis, without which stillness would lose its meaning. W. B. Yeats, whom Eliot admired for his dramatic innovations, said something similar in slightly different words: "The end of art is the ecstasy awakened by the presence before an ever-changing mind of what is permanent in the world."[4]

# Loïe Fuller, Art Nouveau, and the Technological Present

American-born Loïe Fuller (1862–1928) became, for a few decades, the world's most famous dancer. Her relationship to the exotic dances of the "Orient" has been introduced in a previous chapter, but it was Fuller's parallel promulgation of technology that made her a unique cultural presence early in the twentieth century. In her practical adaptation of science to art, she was regarded as quintessentially American. Largely self-taught as dancer and choreographer, Fuller's colorful background included appearances with American rodeos and the touring Wild West extravaganzas of Buffalo Bill.[1] She dreamed of becoming an opera star as she began her career acting and doing a bit of dancing. Not until 1891, when she conceived a dance routine involving the waving of a filmy robe upon which varicolored lights were projected, did she attract real attention as a dancer. Fuller's act was billed as the "Serpentine Dance," and it would be the centerpiece of her early career because—and this is crucially important—it was seen as "artistic." An early critic in New York declared that the "dancing garments of Miss Fuller, thrown into all sorts of lines and graceful rotatory movements, with ever-changing illumination are infinitely more artistic than the toe-dancing of the greatest *prima ballerina*."[2] And no less a poet than Yeats recalled,

> When Loie Fuller's Chinese dancers enwound
> A shining web, a floating ribbon of cloth
> It seemed that a dragon of air
> Had fallen among dancers, had whirled them round
> Or hurried them off on its own furious path.[3]

In reality, Fuller began in the tradition of "skirt dancers," her yards of billowing costumes controlled by hidden sticks and carefully orchestrated swoops and sways. But her antiformalist approach soon moved her beyond New York's dance halls. The critical praise she received was Fuller's ticket abroad, where greater glory awaited her on the continent. Her timing was remarkably fortunate, for her dance seemed eminently compatible with the ephemeral aspects of Symbolism and its visual expressions in Art Nouveau. Both were vital components of her art, although her use of ephemeral light effects was hardly unique. In late nineteenth-century painting the Impressionists and Post-Impressionists

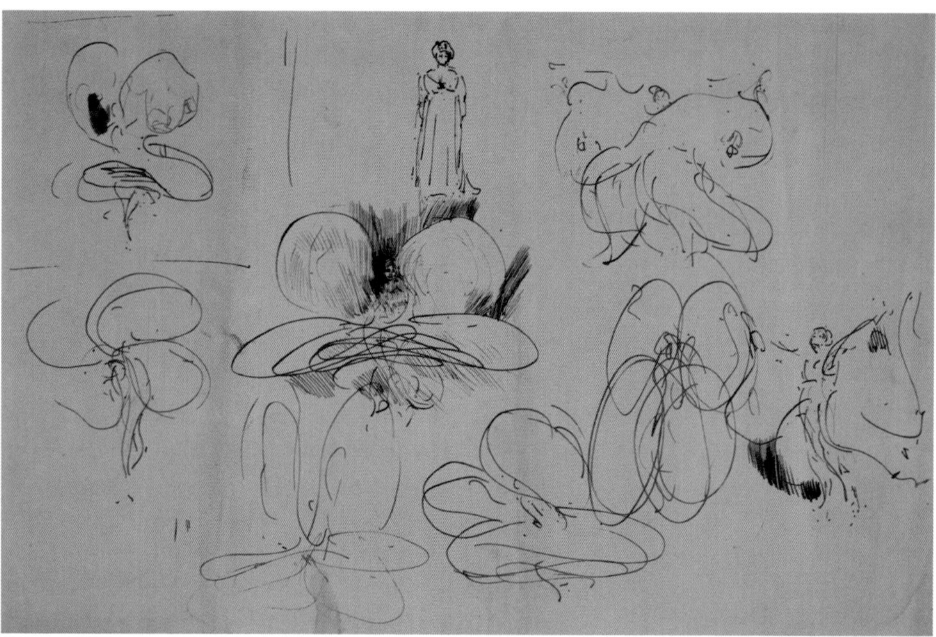

Figure 106 James A. McNeill Whistler, *Loïe Fuller*, c. 1892, pen and black ink on off-white wove paper, 8 ¼ × 12 ⁹⁄₁₆ inches. (Hunterian Museum and Art Gallery, University of Glasgow)

had already shown that changing light effects themselves could create a provocative new visual dance. One thinks of the tremulous light skipping across Monet's sequential cathedral facades, of the glimmer of light on Renoir's dancers, or the shimmering surfaces of Seurat's studies for *Le Chahut*. In Fuller's nonnarrative dances the body nearly disappeared under the abstract play of light on moving drapery. And, like Seurat specifically, she attempted to remove all trace of the artist's personality from the work. What all those visual artists learned, and what Fuller demonstrated onstage, was that light could perform the dance of time. Like light flickering over painted water, dance ennobles ordinary human movement. The convergence of painting's obsession with changing light, combined with the evolving technology changing gaslight to electrical illumination—these things accompanied and influenced Loïe Fuller's innovations in dance.

Among the first visual artists to witness Fuller's performances in Paris was James McNeill Whistler, who, as we have seen, had already drawn and painted many dancers. Not long after Fuller's debut at the Folies Bergère on November 5, 1892, Whistler made a whole sheet of drawings of her (fig. 106).[4] The dancer at rest stands in the central upper portion of the sheet, while in the surrounding images Whistler attempts to capture the swirling, evanescent draperies that describe complex curvilinear shapes around her as she moves. These are patterns comprising airy linear arabesques, which all but obscure the dancer's body in several of the images—exactly the effect Fuller desired.

In this sheet of drawings of Fuller, Whistler went far beyond his earlier dance subjects, which mostly caught dancers at rest.[5] Now, watching Fuller, the artist had something a bit more challenging to draw: ephemeral but readable patterns

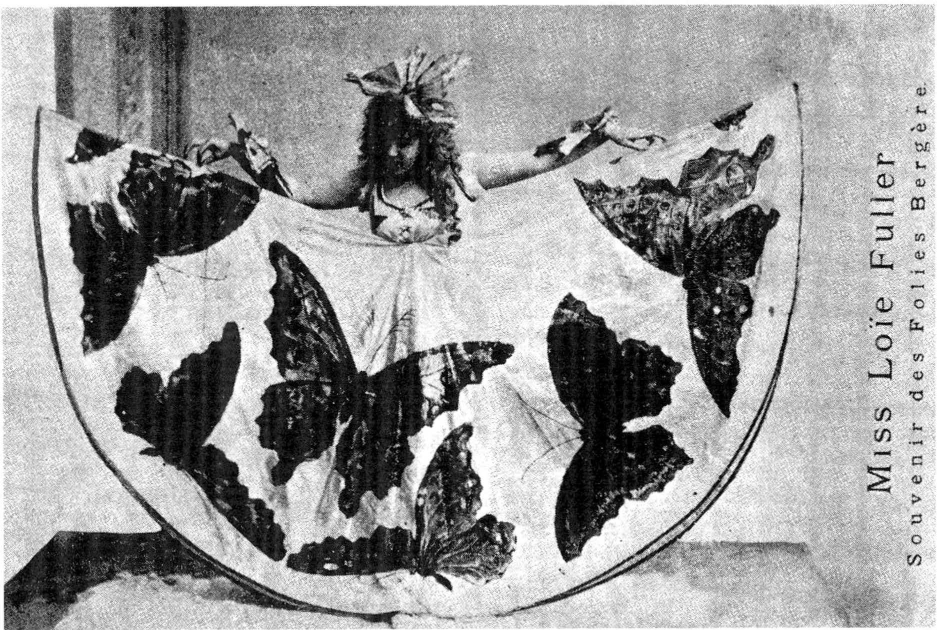


**Figure 107** Anonymous, photograph of Loïe Fuller in moth costume, Paris, 1892.

traced by brilliantly lighted veils. It is as if Fuller's performances sharpened Whistler's ability to catch and record patterns in a dancer's fleeting movements. In later years it was reported by Joseph Pennell that Whistler asked his models to move freely about the studio, pausing when he saw a pose he liked.[6] At work here is Whistler's growing confidence in representing dance movements, grounded in a fundamental knowledge of the human body. Better than his highly finished paintings, Whistler's drawings of dancers show us an eye and mind working in close concert to meet challenges, both technical and aesthetic, first posed to him by drawing the remarkable Loïe Fuller.

Ever the dancer of her cultural moment, in the 1890s Fuller grew into her role as the embodiment of Art Nouveau, a style of art, architecture, and design noted for its use of organic forms and a whiplash line. Its subjects frequently were dedicated to women and flowers. Art Nouveau would prove a perfect context for the tenuous, swelling and contracting forms of Fuller's dance. In actuality, she was a consummate synthesizer, uniting the graceful, somewhat balletic skirt-dancer's steps popular in American and English music halls with the swirling linear elegance of Art Nouveau. In her Serpentine and Lily dances she translated that style's attenuated curvilinear ornament and its moving ornamental line into theatrical performance, while retaining its essentially two-dimensional motion. Dancing, she became a sensuous, intangible creature who could metamorphose out of the completely darkened background into plant, butterfly, flame, cloud, or mere shadow (1892; fig. 107). A writer of the day described her thus:

> at the back of the darkened stage, the indistinct form of a woman clad in
> a confused mass of drapery. Suddenly, a stream of light issued apparently

from the woman herself, while around her the folds of gauze rose and
fell in phosphorescent waves, which seemed to have assumed, one knows
not how, a subtle materiality, taking the form of a golden drinking cup,
a magnificent lily, or a huge glistening moth.[7]

And poet Stéphane Mallarmé, whose Symbolist circle formed the literary
counterpart of Art Nouveau, brooded on mysterious natural transmogrifications
Fuller enacted. After witnessing one of her performances in 1893, Mallarmé
wrote admiringly, "From her proceeds an expanding web—giant butterflies and
petals, unfoldings—everything of a pure and elemental order."[8]
Even at rest, Fuller displayed to American artists the living embodiment of
Art Nouveau principles. John White Alexander (1856–1915) became the leading American exponent of Art Nouveau, especially during his ten-year stay in
Paris beginning in 1891. In *Repose* (1895; fig. 108), White worked with a strong,
sweeping line, posing a figure—long thought to be Fuller—stretched languidly
along the length of a divan. She is dressed in creamy white with black accents,
her abundant draperies creating a graceful rhythm of shapes that become nearly
abstract in their fluidity. The artist's idealization of his subject, typical in both
his figures and portraits, does not immediately reveal her identity, but the *Paris
Lantern*, in reproducing the image, suggested to readers that *Repose* depicted
Fuller, just then the toast of Parisian nightlife.[9] While Alexander's decorative
treatment of her is typical of the then-current taste in American art for passive
females posed in domestic settings, the dancer herself was anything but passive. Thanks to her own artistry and prodigious energies, whatever repose Fuller
enjoyed was momentary; as a dancer she defied the period's ideology of separate spheres that granted to men the active public domain while women reigned
over the home and cultural activities.[10] Instead, Fuller bridged those spheres: rising from her couch, she enfolded the future within her voluminous draperies and
sailed across the threshold of an astonishing celebrity.
At this point, a further assessment of Fuller's relationship with the visual arts
is in order. More than any other performer of her era, she captured the imagination of visual artists, whose representations of her in sculpture, painting, and
prints attempted to capture this "magician of light." As with Isadora Duncan,
it is nearly impossible to count the number of visual images inspired by Loïe
Fuller, but she became a subject for at least seventy artists of various nationali-
ties. Her long residence in Europe made her an attractive and accessible subject
for many artists, but perhaps it was Henri de Toulouse-Lautrec who best understood that Fuller had made of light a veritable new participant, not merely an
enhancing effect—in the dance. He watched her onstage and responded strongly
to the effects of light and color, to her use of veils augmented by blasts from electric fans, and to the aura of mystery that lent poetic charm to her performances.
In her *Fire Dance*, Fuller performed on a pane of glass lighted from beneath, an
innovation in indirect lighting acclaimed as "greater than Bayreuth" and the primary inspiration, it was said, for Toulouse-Lautrec's lithograph of her. Printed in
color in an edition limited to fifty, the impression was later hand-finished by the
artist, who applied a metallic substance after the final inking of the sheet (1893;

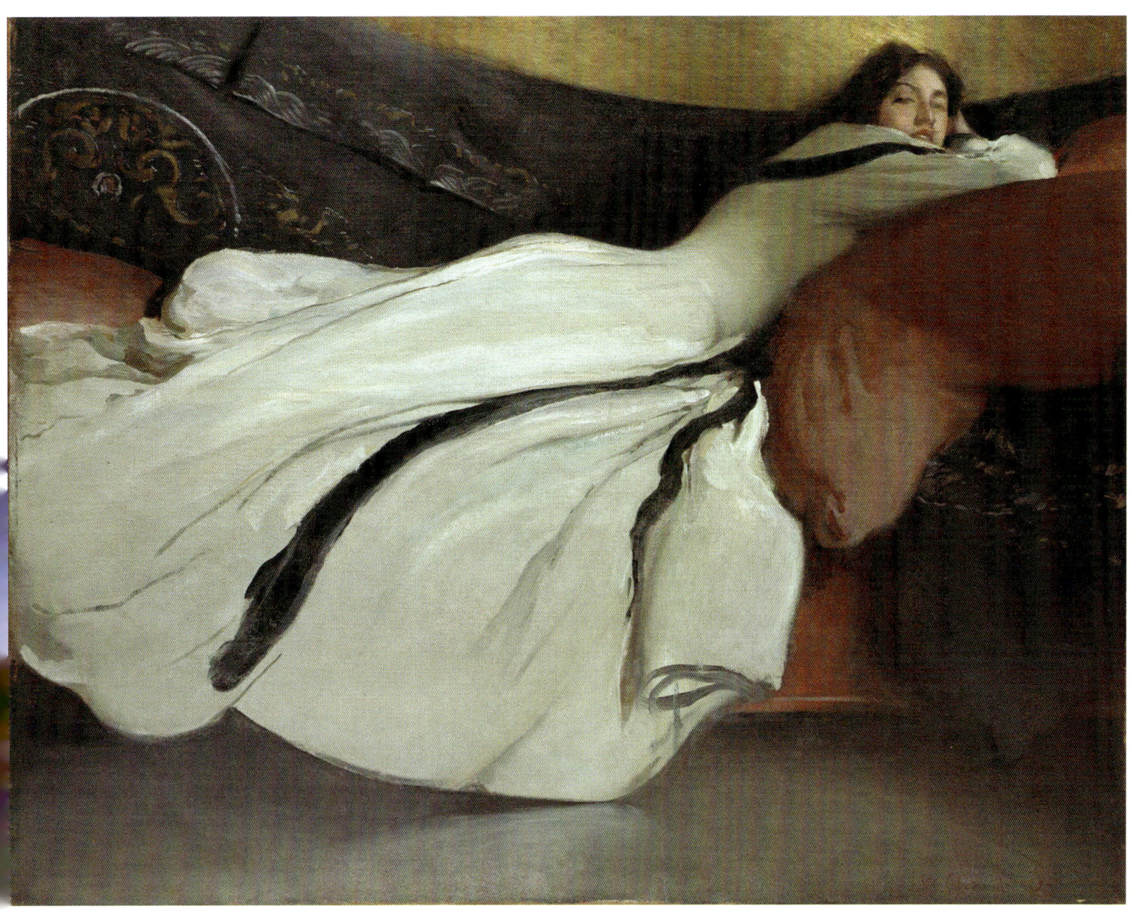

**Figure** 108 John White Alexander, *Repose*, 1895, oil on canvas, 52 ¼ × 63 ⅝ inches. (Metropolitan Museum of Art, New York, Anonymous gift, 1980, 1980.224; image © The Metropolitan Museum of Art/Art Resource, New York)

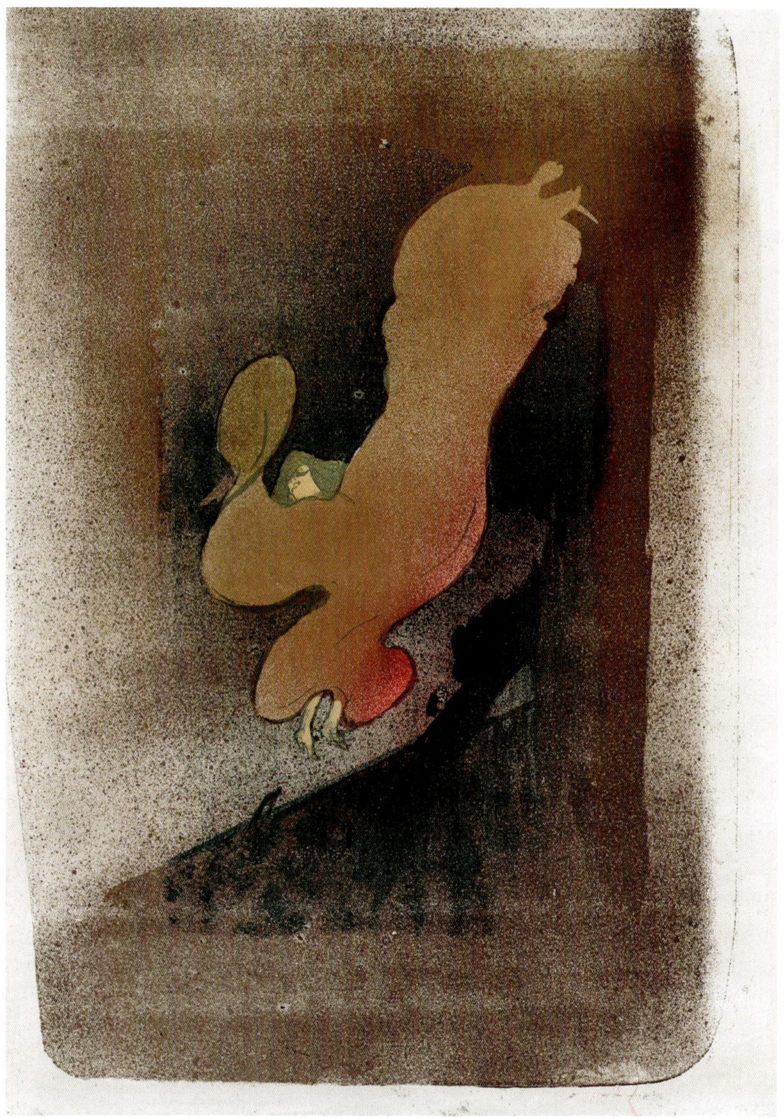

**Figure 109** Henri de Toulouse-Lautrec, *Miss Loïe Fuller*, 1893, lithograph in brown-mauve, blue-gray, curry yellow, red and gold on cream wove paper, 14⁹⁄₁₆ × 10¼ inches. (Art Institute of Chicago, The Joseph Brooks Fair Collection, 1942.20; photo © The Art Institute of Chicago)

fig. 109).[11] In this lithograph Fuller seems to float, borne aloft within the flat colored curves of her vaporous costumes. Toulouse-Lautrec's prints call forth a kind of Symbolist ephemerality, but as well—and perhaps more importantly—evoke the complex, changing light effects that became Fuller's hallmark. Colorists flocked to study her unprecedented effects. American painter Julius Rolshoven (1858–1930), then working in Paris, recalled, "At the Folies Bergère artists turned up night after night to study colour combinations as revealed by Loie Fuller— endless whirling draperies set off by a seeming black background bewitched the eye—Loïe Fuller's influence on pure colour seekers was undoubted." Soon, Rolshoven noted, "[paintings inspired by] Loïe Fuller hung in all sizes upon the [Salon] walls—her influence made her the colour Queen of that period. The great secret had been disclosed by an American girl."[12]

In 1900 the audacious "colour Queen" commissioned architect Henri Sauvage to design a new theater for her at the Paris Exposition Universelle. The structure fully embraced Art Nouveau design, with a door-framing relief emulating Fuller's flowing draperies and—floating above the entrance—Pierre Roche's over lifesize sculpture of Fuller, seeming to catch each breeze as she swirls. Inside, besides a stage, Fuller installed work by French artists such as Roche, Gallê, and Gérôme, all of whose subjects represented or referred to the dancer herself (fig. 110).

Auguste Rodin's images of Fuller were also exhibited in her theater that year, recognizing their long and close relationship. Fuller and Rodin shared an interest in gesture and a sophisticated rhetoric of the body. And both had taken a conventional genre and transformed it into something unexpected. Fuller cultivated Rodin's friendship over several decades and actively sought his interpretation of

her dance in sculpture, requesting from him first a figurine. Rodin had called Fuller a "lovely modern tanagra," referring to the Hellenistic Greek figurines, mostly of women, then especially popular as the topos of the dancer. That work was apparently never produced, but Rodin did sculpt a bronze *Head of Loïe Fuller*, unfortunately now lost. In turn, Fuller strove to advance Rodin's career in the United States, arranging his first American exhibition at the National Arts Club in New York in 1903, a show combining pieces owned by Fuller and others borrowed from the sculptor. After the National Arts Club exhibition, some of Rodin's pieces went on to the Metropolitan Museum. Fuller was thus responsible for introducing American audiences to Rodin's work in plaster, bronze and marble.

Although Fuller had never seen an art exhibition before her arrival

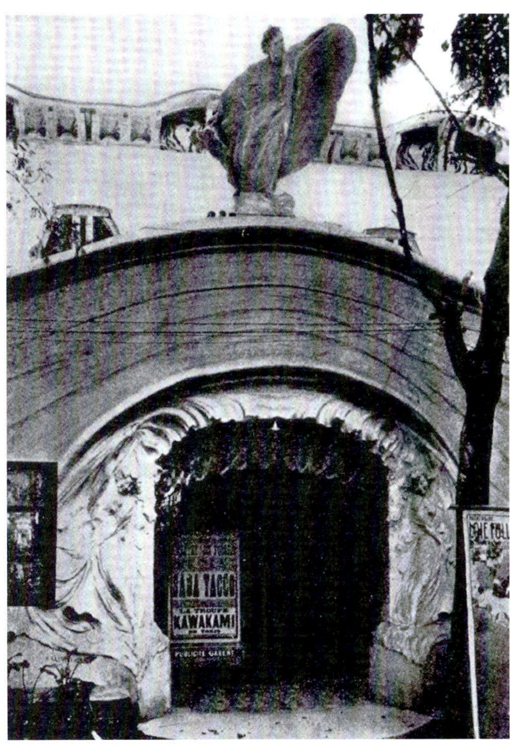


**Figure 110** Henri Sauvage, architect, Théâtre Loïe Fuller, Paris, 1900.

in Paris at age thirty, she responded powerfully to the visual arts. Eventually, her efforts would help to establish two new American museums, the California Palace of the Legion of Honor in San Francisco (opened 1924) and the Maryhill Museum in Washington State (opened 1940), both of which contained works of art by various French artists, including Rodin.[13]

Not least, Fuller became an exhibiting artist herself, combining her interest in light and fabric to develop acclaimed textiles. Beginning before the turn of the century Fuller had taught herself to dye or paint cloth so that, when performing outdoors, she could replicate in daylight some of the effects achieved by artificial colored light in the theater. Through her use of cold light by luminous salts, she anticipated the later invention of luminescence. As early as 1896 she had visited Thomas Edison's New Jersey laboratory, where he demonstrated his fluoroscope (a predecessor to the x-ray machine) that used phosphorescent salts. As scholar Rhonda Garelick reports, Fuller was immediately struck by possible application of the salts to her costumes: "This curious stuff all aglow . . . held me spellbound," recalled Fuller. "It suddenly occurred to me that if I could have a dress permeated with that substance it would be wonderful. I asked Mr. Edison if the salts would retain the luminousness when the lamp was gone. He hadn't thought of that so we tried it and lo and behold the light remained."[14] After experimenting with various processes, Fuller arrived at a technique of painting the salts on the fabric in droplets, which glowed onstage when struck by spotlights. Offstage, other varieties of her painted silk panels served as wall hangings in prestigious homes, where they were noticed by museum curators, including those in the decorative arts section of the Louvre. They invited Fuller to exhibit her work there in 1924, two dozen pieces gathered into a "Retrospective Exposition, 1892–1920" showcasing her studies in "Form, Line and Colour for Light Effects." Her softly tinted or stained designs were also adapted by designers of wallpapers, lampshades, and cushions.

By that time Fuller had long regarded herself as an artist in her own right, one whose primary medium was light. She basked in the artistic regard shown her by critics and pressed on with her efforts to learn the secrets of coordinating light and color. In statements such as the following she likened her vision to the process by which artists become colorists: "I began in utter ignorance of what effect of one color on another was, and had to learn as a painter does what colors gained by union, and what colors were ruined one by the other."[15] Through such statements Fuller was helping to construct her own mythology as an artist of light and color. And, like many artists of her era, she borrowed freely from various arts to create crossover sensory effects. "I seek," she told an interviewer, "to create a harmony of sound, light, and music. . . . Music is the joy of the ears. I want it to be also a feast for the eyes and, with that aim, to make it pictorial, to cause it to be *seen*."[16] Fuller was, in fact, regarded by her peers as a synaesthetic artist.[17] In the future, she expected that the harmonies, tones, and rhythms of light could be played on an instrument.

Critics listened, and many concurred that there was something of both the musician and the painter in Loïe Fuller. The dancer encouraged those correspondences, and she continued to invent new visual enhancements. Working as electrician, set designer, choreographer, and dancer, she amazed her audiences with what would today be called "special effects." Covering her stages in black velvet, she designed unprecedented kinds of projected stage lighting to produce high aesthetic voltage: calcium and incandescent lights, optical tricks achieved with mirrors and revolving disks, colored glass lanterns and gels. In short, Fuller's visual artistry lay in her use, if not invention, of many aspects of modern stage lighting, achieved above all by that protean technological miracle, electricity.[18]

For a 1907 performance with 120 participants at the Paris Hippodrome, Fuller created an entirely new effect. She set up slide projectors in front of a thin white gauze curtain hung just behind the footlights, sending pictures through the gauze onto a thick white curtain at the back of the stage. One critic commented that in her new kind of ethereal, projected scenery "La Loie Fuller has put into practice her theory of the orchestration of light; indeed, she plays what are literally chromatic scales, harmonizing multifarious hues. With the imagination of an artist and a poet, in her six tableaux she paints pictures by means of light."[19]

When a respected art critic such as Louis Vauxcelles (who had first used the terms "Fauves" and "Cubism") acclaimed Loïe Fuller, he also looked to painting for an apt metaphor to describe what she did. In an effort to distinguish Fuller from Isadora Duncan (whose reputation drew alongside Fuller's about 1914), Vauxcelles turned to the vocabulary of the visual arts: "Isadora sculpts. Loie Fuller paints," he insisted. "It is useless to compare them."[20] This is an important distinction, one that addresses both the style and the relative plasticity of each dancer's forms—Fuller's highly ephemeral, Duncan's fluid but more solid and studied. Vauxcelles ultimately decided he preferred the pictorial effects Fuller achieved through abstract forms and seemingly spontaneous movements. For her part, Duncan also acknowledged Fuller's pathbreaking innovations: "All the magic of Merlin," exclaimed Isadora. "What an extraordinary genius! No imitator of Loïe Fuller has ever been able even to hint at her genius!"[21] The savvy Fuller, by encouraging her dance to be likened to visual art, had raised it to a realm far above the accessible, popular spectacles of her early days at the café-concert. Although, in order to make a living as a dancer, she would continue to perform in both dance halls and more rarefied venues, she had secured a reputation (in France, at least) as a legitimate artist, the first American dancer abroad to do so. That European adulation, especially when interpreted in visual images that crossed the Atlantic, would encourage American artists to respond more fully to dance.

One of Fuller's last choreographic achievements took place at the 1925 Decorative Arts Exposition in Paris, which heralded the introduction of the Art Deco or *moderne* style. For the opening gala Fuller conceived a new kind of performance, a hybrid of visual art and dance staged by her company on the massive staircase of the Grand Palais. Titled *Sur la mer immense* (On the mighty sea), it was performed to the piano accompaniment of Debussy's *La Mer.* The effect was an abstraction of the sea itself: "Stretched over the stairs was a tremendous expanse of silk cloth, hundreds of square feet of it. Underneath, invisible, the girls held up the cloth and manipulated it while projectors threw light of varying color and intensity upon it. The effect was fluid drapery, a silken sea that rose and fell, rolled and ran, seethed and foamed."[22] In her early performances, Fuller had danced as a Symbolist-inspired abstraction of Woman—ethereal, vague, tantalizing. By 1925 she had transferred that abstraction to one of nature's greatest forms, the scope, grandeur, and unceasing dance of the sea itself.

Fuller's achievements in breaking old choreographic molds and paving the way for modern dance have been debated (there were those who said what she did was not truly dance), but there can be no doubt about her imaginative and technical mastery of the changing effects of light on the moving body, all set to important music. Regardless of whether she herself could dance or mime, nearly everyone agreed with the reviewer for *L'Echo de Paris*, who declared as early as 1895 that she had "the gift of playing with electricity." In that technological sense we see a second way, beyond her personification of the spirit of Art Nouveau, to consider Fuller's expression of an immediate cultural moment through dance. Was it a French or an American moment? Critic and novelist Joris-Karl Huysmans found Fuller's special effects typical of her native country. After seeing her dance he confided to his journal, "Mediocre dancing. After all, the glory goes to the electrician. It's American." What Huysmans did not acknowledge, or perhaps did not know, was that Fuller herself was the originator of the lighting effects. On her tours back to the United States, American journalists were quick to claim her spirit, "La Loie off the stage is a cheerful, blue-eyed, soft-voiced creature, frank, honest and real, devoid of affectations, full of imagination, and extremely American."[23] As American, perhaps, as fireworks, as its sublime scenery, or the grandest of its human gatherings. To a writer for *Metropolitan Magazine* she was "a spectacle that is scarcely equalled by rainbows, torchlight processions, Niagara Falls, or naval parades."[24]

Successful as she was in Europe, Fuller clung consciously to her own American identity, always retaining her citizenship, even invoking the useful, if limiting, stereotypes of her nationality. She saw in herself and other Americans a kind of vitality and enthusiasm often cited by cultural observers. She predicted that American women would be "the leading dancers of the future" because they possessed a "freedom of spirit . . . lacking in those abroad."[25]

In a sense, that insistence on change as a starring element is precisely what swept Fuller's dance out of the languor of the fin-de-siècle and into the modernity of the twentieth. Her Symbolist-inspired ephemerality merged with a more deliberate, prosaic—and yes, mechanical—change that brought a new kind of immediacy to her dance. Poetic in its own way, Fuller's innovative lighting only elevated her in the eyes of her admirers. To them she became "the Symbol of Art itself, a fire above all Art itself, a fire above all dogmas." Eventually, few would question her art, just as—by the 1920s—no one questioned the presence of machine subjects in painting. If Fuller introduced the presence of the machine to dance performance, she was following the celebrated path laid down by Monet in his interiors of Parisian train stations, filled with the ennobled, shimmering belch of locomotives. Fuller's breakthroughs with light place her dance in a new realm—that of the momentary, the machine-oriented, the technologically modern. Perhaps it is that very periodicity—being unmistakably of her moment—that allowed Fuller's reputation to fade after her death. She is less well remembered today than Isadora Duncan or Ruth St. Denis, despite the fact that those three made up America's first generation of important solo dancers. Each in her own way redefined the role assigned to the body in dance, but no one belonged more determinedly than Fuller to her own cultural moment, largely through her use of technology.[26]

# Social Dance
## *Visual Artists Take the Pulse of Twentieth-Century America*

Social dance, a kind of conversation between bodies, has often been celebrated, as well as inevitably altered, when seen through the bending lens of artistic representation. At the turn of the twentieth century, American artists looked to their own cultural lineage, as well as to European precedents, for ways to explore the expressive potential of social dance. The Impressionists, for example, had often enlisted the material capabilities of paint to express physical sensations, and especially the antic immediacy of the dance. Renoir's *Le Bal à Bougival* (1883; fig. 111) portrays a kind of sun-dappled Eden, where dancers swirl in a working-class paradise.[1] Renoir choreographed an idyll of urban leisure and outdoor pleasure, paced to the soft scrapings of dancing feet under the trees. In tune with his era, Renoir captures Baudelaire's passing moment, but his dancers belong as well within the epic embrace of social dance in every era.

If today we see bright, glancing movement in the swirling patterns of Renoir's waltz, we should remember that that dance was not always viewed so benignly. When first introduced in the late eighteenth century as a reaction against the affectations of the minuet, the waltz's close bodily contact between couples made it seem vaguely dangerous. But before long, taken up by the bourgeoisie, the waltz became a perfect subject for artists such as the Impressionists, who focused on the leisure activities of the middle class. The French had their airy *balance valse*, a slower, gliding variant of which became the Boston waltz.

As communications improved, dances spread more rapidly and brought dramatic changes in the look and execution of social dance. Long after the shock value of the waltz dimmed, newer dances took on the mantle of the suggestive or outrageous. Wildly popular vernacular dances demonstrated modernity's redesign not only of painting, sculpture, and fashion, but of the human body itself, reconfigured to move in new and daring ways. Typically, the new jazz-based dances of the twentieth-century lacked bodily contact between participants. Instead, dancers swung their shoulders, moved their hands gesturally, and vibrated their legs. Watchers, including visual artists, saw the bodies turn, twist, and bob, disrupting expectations and keeping the traveling gaze in thrall. In the Black Bottom, for example, dancers slapped their hands on their backside, pushing their bodies forward through the pelvis. Dancers of both the Black Bottom and the Charleston moved the body as if it were one long tube, with hinged segments and flailing extremities. The Charleston kept knees close together, with feet

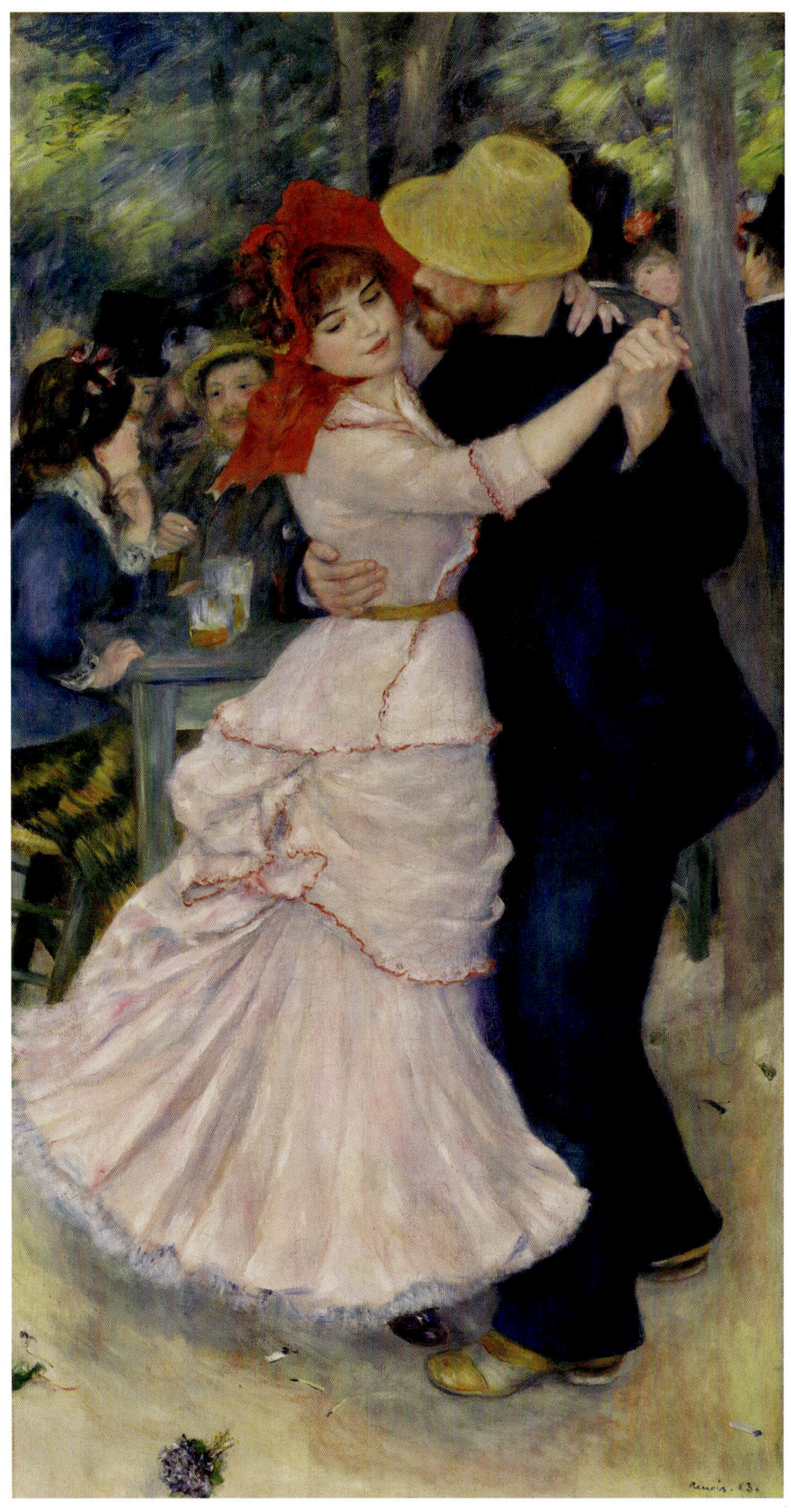

**Figure 111** Pierre-Auguste Renoir, *Le Bal à Bougival*, 1883, oil on canvas, 71 ⅝ × 38 ⅝ inches. (Museum of Fine Arts, Boston, Picture Fund, 37.375)

twisting out wildly, while arms flapped oppositionally or described Egyptian-type movements. Geometric, tube-shaped dresses enhanced the new angular separation of the body into parts (a reminder of what Nijinsky had done in theatrical dance performance). Jazz Age flappers, seeming to represent the restlessness, abandon, and daring of their era, made the Charleston the rage throughout the United States. Photographs from the 1920s gather into a single image the flailing motions of multiple arms and legs animated by the sweet-hot wail of a saxophone.

Simultaneously, as the dances spread all over the Western world they carried the seed of American culture, a culture that, ironically, had assimilated many forms of imported dance and made them seem American. The 1920s introduced a period of unprecedented collaboration between elite and popular culture. As Ann Douglas has argued, it was an era when anything was "capable of popularization."[2] Thus, melding ballet with classical dance was an inevitable effort. One classic example of the incorporation of social dance styles into the broader range of American dance is seen in the efforts made by Lincoln Kirstein to Americanize George Balanchine, with whom he cofounded the New York City Ballet. In 1934 Balanchine choreographed a ballet called *Alma Mater*, one of the pieces that introduced his new choreography to American audiences.[3] With sets and costumes by John Held Jr., the artist whose watercolors and illustrations expressed the quintessential spirit of the Jazz Age, Balanchine's new ballet proved a veritable catalog of American types, behaviors, and social dances in full vogue. Lincoln Kirstein set the tone in the program notes he wrote for a performance of *Alma Mater* in Hartford, Connecticut:

> Crowds at the stadium entrance hail the half-back piled on his admirers' shoulders. Flappers dash up for autographs; posed against the fence a photographer snaps his portrait. Snake dance is a rah-rah bacchanal; not even the goal-posts are left standing. The villain in a coon-coat, his charger a bicycle-built-for-him and his cock-eyed girlfriend, encounters the hero and socks him as he plucks daisies for her. We are transported to a rag-time dreamland.[4]

In America, social dance helped the country cast off solipsism, introversion, and an outworn delicacy to embrace a new physiology, pulsing with dynamism and striving variety. Artists who interpreted social dance, at least the best of them, learned to invest vernacular idioms with a timeless eloquence. On the other hand, and paradoxically, social dance representations posed a deliberate challenge to "high" art through that selfsame introduction of deliberately vernacular, even vulgar visual language. The very banality of popular dance, steeped in humanity, ensured its recurrent newness in art.

Aided by the phonograph and (after 1920) radio, couples everywhere tried the new dance steps. Social barriers eroded with the growth of popular dancing establishments, where the curious came in droves. Americans, formerly content to sit and watch exotic and remote spectacles, were brought to their feet and propelled onto the dance floor by the tango, turkey trot, and bunny hug.

Photographer Arnold Genthe wrote of the curiosity about American social dance shown by the celebrated classical dancers Anna Pavlova and Mikhail Mordkin during their visit to San Francisco about 1910. Pavlova, despite her ethereal grace onstage, was no hothouse aesthete. She adapted quickly to the mixing of cultural levels in America and within a few years would dance her *Sleeping Beauty* sandwiched between circus acts, an ice show, and drill teams at New York's vaudeville Hippodrome. In San Francisco, Genthe reported that "Pavlova wanted to see the new dances she had heard so much about—the Turkey Trot, the Texas Tommy and the Grizzly Bear."[5] At one of the crowded dance halls on the city's "Barbary Coast" the Russians first watched, then made their way to the dance floor where, incognito, they "began to feel out the barbaric rhythm with hesitant feet. Gradually they were carried away by it and, oblivious to their sordid surroundings, they evolved, then and there, a dance of alluring beauty. Gradually, one couple after another stepped aside to watch, forming an astonished circle at the edge of the floor. When Pavlova and Mordkin had finished, there was a moment of silence, followed by wild bursts of applause. . . . This incident has always seemed to me a thrilling example of the power of great art."[6]

Clearly there was significant curiosity and performance crossover between social and theatrical dance early in the century.[7] Certain dances lent themselves to both performance and participation, among them the tango. From its birthplace in the brothels and bars of Buenos Aires, the tango found its way to Europe. In 1907 Nice advertised the first tango contest, setting in motion a rave that by 1912 swept the social dancing world in France. In the latter year a dancer called Guerrero introduced the Tango at the Marigny Theatre on the Champs Elysées, Paris. Instantly it became a sensation. Observers described it as "a new and startling dance . . . a curious mixture of composure and frenzy, and at first acquaintance [the tango] seems full of complications. [Guerrero's] rendering of it is said to take away the breath of the English and American tourists who fill the popular music-hall among the chestnuts of the Champs Elyseé [*sic*]."[8] Like an epidemic, the tango infected prewar France. It was impossible to know whether people danced in spite of the threat of war or because of it.

Soon the tango's rhythms crossed the Atlantic, propelled by its torrid reputation as "a vertical expression of horizontal desire." Indeed, poet and art critic Guillaume Apollinaire described it as "that marvelous and lascivious dance which seemed born upon a Transatlantic luxury-liner."[9] In New York and Los Angeles, elegant hotels invited dancers to "tango teas," sedate affairs where professional couple dancers demonstrated the new steps.[10] Elie Nadelman's *Tango* (c. 1920–24; fig. 112) is one of his modish and witty sculptures integrating urban sophistication with the chaste, almost taxidermic forms of American folk art. Nadelman made at least seven sketches leading up to *Tango,* his dancing couple changing positions many times before they found their final frontal convergence. Always, Nadelman's preliminary drawings were based on his refinement of the curving line, which he then orchestrated into harmonious figures. "Here is how I realize it," he wrote of his approach to drawing. "I employ no other line than the curve, which possesses freshness and force. I compose these curves so as to bring them in accord or in opposition to one another. In that way I obtain the life of

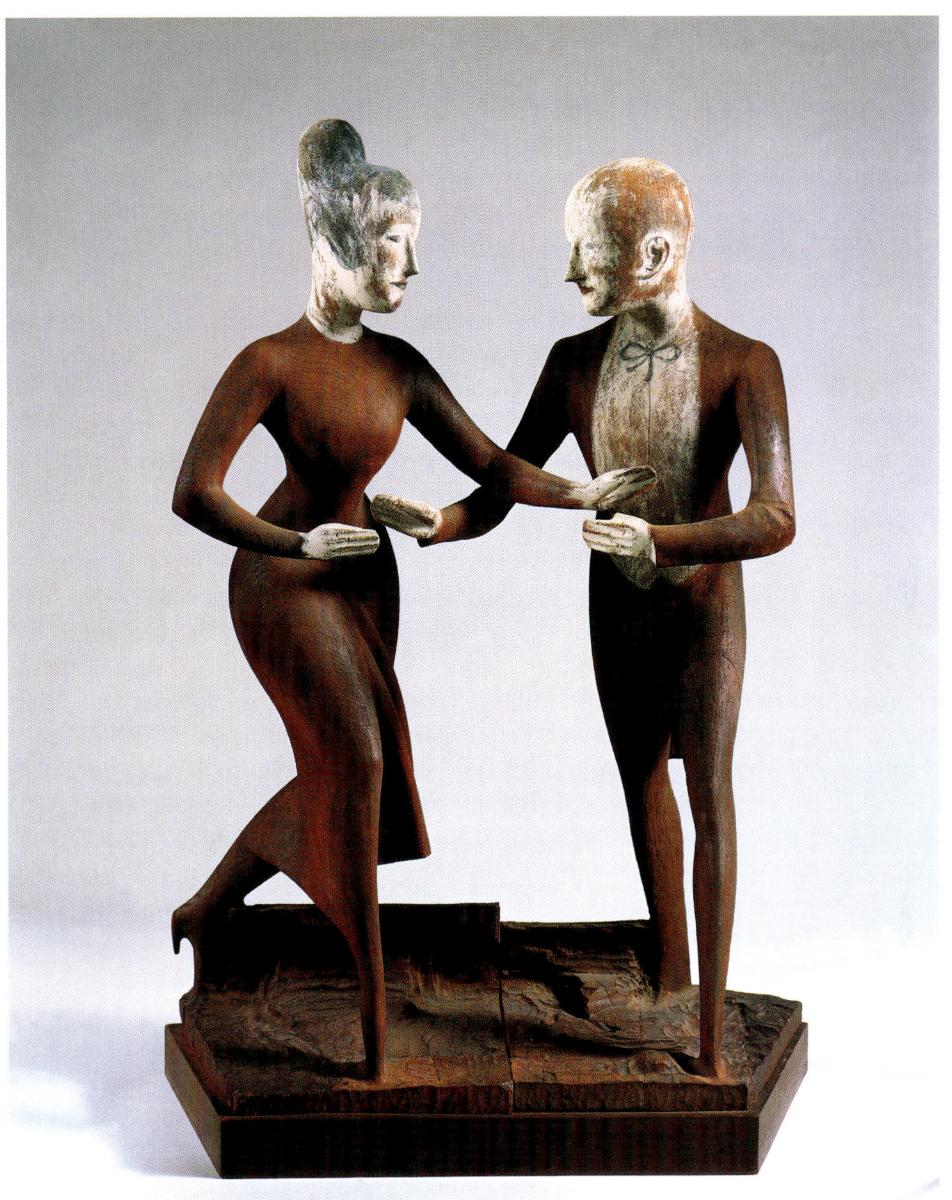

**Figure 112** Elie Nadelman, *Tango*, c. 1920–24, painted cherry wood and gesso, 35 ⅞ × 13 ⅞ inches. (Whitney Museum of American Art, New York, Purchase, with funds from the Mr. and Mrs. Arthur G. Altschul Purchase Fund, the Joan and Lester Avnet Purchase Fund, the Edgar William and Bernice Chrysler Garbisch Purchase Fund, the Mrs. Robert C. Graham Purchase Fund in honor of John I. H. Baur, the Mrs. Percy Uris Purchase Fund and the Henry Schnakenberg Purchase Fund in honor of Juliana Force, 88.1 a–c; photo: Jerry L. Thompson; art © Estate of Elie Nadelman)

form, i.e., harmony."[11] Next came a plaster model, with delicately particularized features of heads, hair, and costume. Finally Nadelman produced the definitive sculpture in wood and gesso, flattening and smoothing ears and hair and monumentalizing the figures. Their stiff fingers approach, but do not touch each other, creating a tense, almost fatalistic duet. So closely did Nadelman observe the dance that he invented, over the course of twenty years, a distillation of the significant arrested pose within a transient craze like the tango. In their high degree of finish, Nadelman's dancers project a formal wholeness, a classical self-sufficiency as objects of visual pleasure and material culture. Yet for all their serenity, Nadelman never lets us forget their incipient movement, which invites the viewer's imagination to anticipate and to "complete" the work as an active, participatory gesture of looking. In social dancing Nadelman saw a behavioristic portrait of his era, and his tango dancers serve even now as a monument of their decade.

Besides Pavlova, many other theatrical dancers were tempted to try the intricate new steps of the tango, and it soon migrated from chic ballrooms to Hollywood sound stages, where such luminaries as Rudolph Valentino released its libidinous heat. Ruth St. Denis, in an effort to compete with the fast-paced participatory dances luring crowds away from her concerts, added stylish numbers to her routines, one of them an unlikely combination of the tango and Cakewalk, danced to the music of Victor Herbert. Even the ethereal Isadora Duncan felt the tango's tug. At a party following one of her performances at the Metropolitan Opera, Duncan saw a young man she recognized "the most famous tango dancer in the Argentine." She summoned him to her side, and they proceeded to electrify the room with an impromptu version of the erotic, sensational dance.[12] Although no visual records survive of Pavlova, Mordkin, or Duncan dancing the tango, the fiery Argentine dance engaged a number of other American artists to represent its rhythms in solo or couples, on stage or in social settings on crowded dance floors.

American Beatrice Wood (1893–1998) took up the tango, both in practice and in visual expression. Her stylized watercolor *Tango* (c. 1923–25; fig. 113) features an urbane couple, all angular arms and legs, pasted against each other like paper dolls and moving horizontally in the stereotyped tango slink. Perhaps the woman is the glamorous scamp Wood herself, for she was a tango enthusiast during her years in Paris. "I became a very fine tango dancer," she recalled. "It is just the most dreamy experience you can have. . . . [Your partner] holds you close and you dance as one person in this wonderful sensuous music."[13] For the young American, it was a heady period, suffused with the arts, especially dance. Besides the tango, Wood also learned Russian folk dance, taught her by Anna Pavlova's own choreographer. She attended the 1913 premiere of the Ballet Russe's *Le Sacre du Printemps*, met Nijinsky (as well as Pavlova) and nearly became a professional dancer herself. But just as Wood's dancing began to bring professional offers in Paris, her mother—scandalized that her daughter would consider such a debased occupation—quashed that budding career. Instead Beatrice turned to acting, even while continuing to consort with dancers such as Isadora Duncan, for whom she created tie-dyed fabric for costumes.

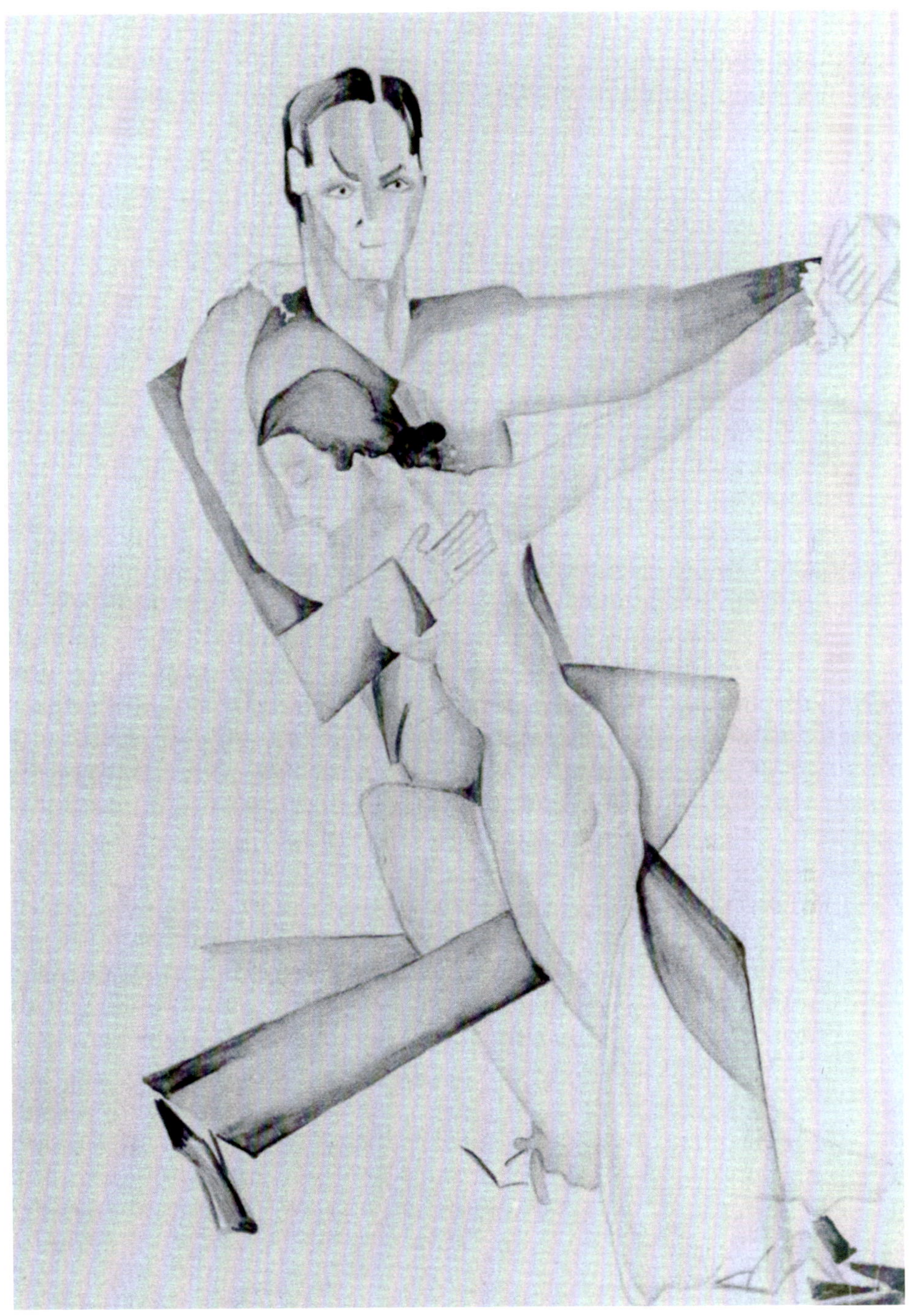

**Figure 113** Beatrice Wood, *Tango*, c. 1923–25, pencil and watercolor, 17 ⅝ × 13 ⅞ inches. (courtesy Beatrice Wood Center for the Arts/Happy Valley Foundation)

Long after Wood's return to the United States, subjects of the dance continued to appear in her drawings. By 1916 she was part of the motley international band later known as the New York Dadas, an avant-garde circle centering around Marcel Duchamp and Walter and Louise Arensberg. Duchamp encouraged Wood's efforts at drawing, at first "scrawls and little horrors, but [Duchamp] patiently looked at them, pointing out the bad and the good."[14] Wood became deeply involved in the irreverent New York Dada movement, participating in its "little magazine" *The Blind Man* and designing a poster advertising the "Ultra Bohemian, Pre-Historic, Post Alcoholic Blindman's Ball" (1917; fig. 114). Wood's strutting, insolent stick figure—"lost in a mad dance," as her lover Henri-Pierre Roché described it—thumbs its nose at the world. The spirit, both piquant and vaguely jaded, is quintessentially Dada, a portent of the riotous event itself. On the fateful evening Wood donned her elaborate Russian folk costume brought from Paris and stepped gingerly onto the floor. "Dressed as a muzhik," recalled Roché, Wood "opened the ball with a Russian peasant dance, arms crossed, knees bending, valiantly kicking out her tiny boots before her. Her playful eyes, her smile, rewarded with great ovation."[15]

The Blindman's Ball, held in May 1917, was one of a cluster of bohemian costume balls inspired by the Parisian Left Bank tradition of Quatre-Arts Balls. Radical journalist Floyd Dell had initiated the trend in 1914 with balls he called "Pagan Routs" held in Greenwich Village as fundraisers for *The Masses* and the Liberal Club. Many other bohemian dances followed, featuring outlandish costumes, body paint, and a generally rebellious counterculture spirit. In an unsurpassed example, Emma Goldman hosted the "Red [Revolutionary] Revel," during which she, dressed as a nun, demonstrated a new dance step she called the Anarchist's Slide. Together, the mix of dance, artists, and radical politics raised the mischief quotient in this era of New York Dada.[16]

As they searched actively for new creative directions, dancers, visual artists, and writers found in modern social dance the potential for translating matter and energy into art. Machine imagery was one means of siting motion in the moment, and even of dictating the emotional level of poetry, painting, or dance. Resourceful artists found ways to introduce machine synergy into many kinds of representation. As Lewis Mumford remarked in his essay "Machinery and the Modern Style" (1921), the new art exhibited "the characteristic achievements of technology by which our daily activities have been molded into a hundred new patterns."[17] In *Manhattan Transfer* (1925), his definitive literary portrait of the modern urban experience, John Dos Passos looked back to the eve of World War I, when his young characters "talk not of dying but of being a nurse or war correspondent, and then dance. Here the life seems animated—for what could be more animated than a dancer."[18] But as they dance, outwardly defiant in the face of war, fear propels Dos Passos's characters into a mechanistic, joyless ritual; animation lapses into brittleness. This is dance recast in a weirdly military cadence:

> "Get up on your toes and walk in time to the music," says Ellen. "Move in straight lines that's the whole trick." Her voice cut the quick coldly

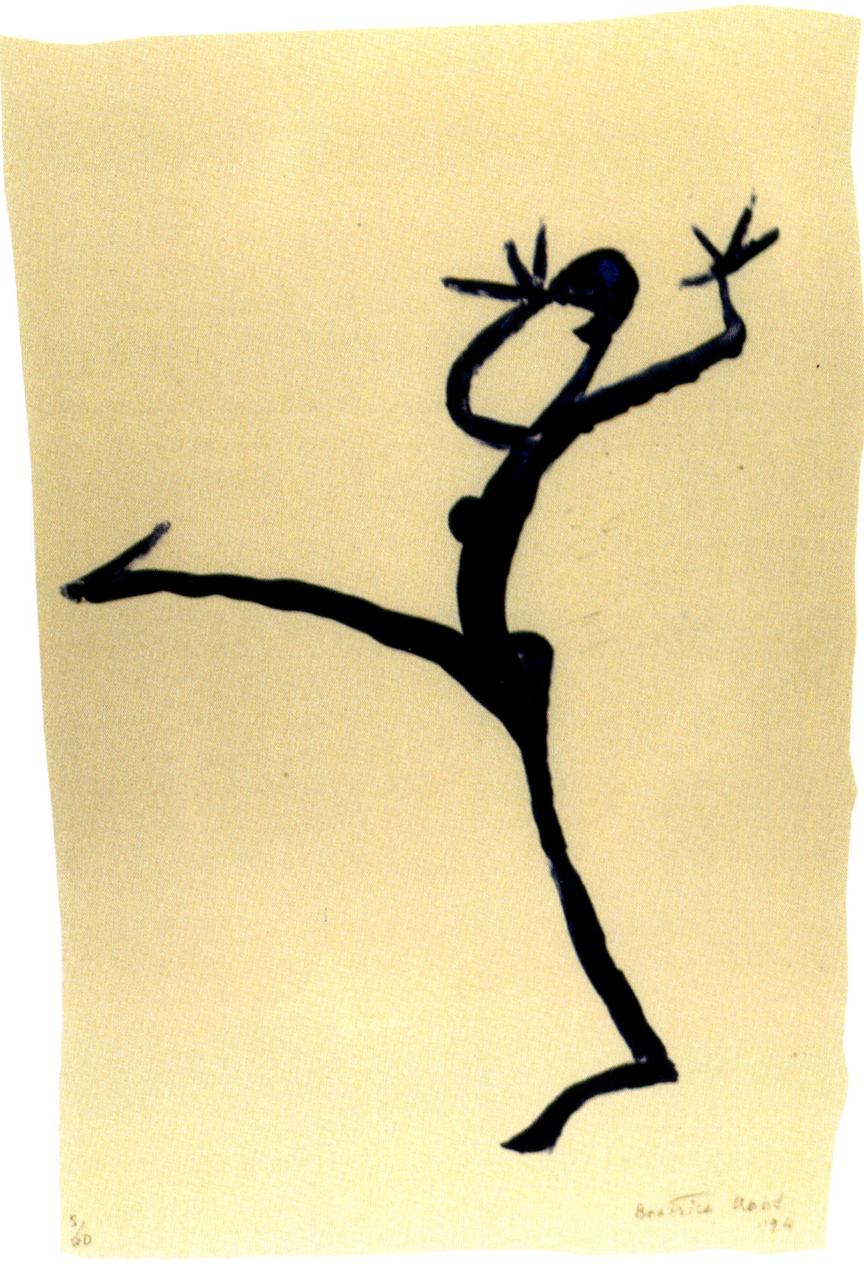

**Figure 114** Beatrice Wood, poster for Blindman's Ball, 1917. (courtesy Beatrice Wood Center for the Arts/Happy Valley Foundation)

like a tiny flexible sharp metalsaw. Elbows joggling, faces set, gollywog eyes, fat men and thin women, thin women and fat men rotated densely around them. He was crumbling plaster with something that rattled achingly in his chest, she was an intricate machine of sawtooth steel whitebright bluebright copperbright in his arms.[19]

Here, dance registers the emotional temperature of a generation on the brink of war. In another passage from *Manhattan Transfer* Dos Passos uses social dance once more, this time to explore simultaneity, to accelerate the stream of consciousness before time destroys a fragile moment. In a poignant compression of midday courtship, peppered with fragments of pseudo-exotic food and music, a second couple dances urgently, as if reality will end when the song does: "Noon sunlight spirals dimly into the chopsuey joint. Muted music spirals Hindustan. He eats fooyong, she eats chowmein. They dance with their mouths full, slim blue jumper squeezed to black slick suit, peroxide curls against black slick hair."[20] In step with the pace of his streetwise New Yorkers, Dos Passos's dancers repeatedly create vivid verbal tableaux, injecting magic into otherwise drab lives.

During the same year, F. Scott Fitzgerald's *The Great Gatsby* presents dance as an occasion of memory. When Daisy and Gatsby take to the floor in a "graceful conservative fox-trot," Fitzgerald conjures a scene, like others in the book, intended to summon for the reader a visual picture, a fragmentary moment within a larger tale comprised—in modernist fashion—more out of such bits and pieces than from a sustained linear narrative. If Fitzgerald's characters are defined (in part by dance) as essentially conservative, artist Peggy Bacon's (1895–1987) are anything but. In her frenetic *Dance at the League* (1919; fig. 115), Bacon's knot of costumed participants range from Lincolnesque to clownish to neo-odalisque. Some artists' images of dancers are profoundly indifferent to them as individuals. What sets Bacon's dancers apart is their specificity: typical of her satirical prints, this crowded scene includes incisive caricatures of recognizable persons, likely her own colleagues from the Art Students League, where she studied between 1915 and 1920. Inspired by masters such as Daumier, and using hatching and patterns reminiscent of the German Expressionists, Bacon creates a rollicking dance scene, a kind of gallery of human types. Cloaked in the semi-anonymity of costumes and suffused with the almost palpable reek of alcohol, Bacon's dancers reveal their most uninhibited selves. In the center of the levity a man raises a chair menacingly above his head, a gesture that transforms Bacon's theme from lighthearted romp into a penetrating look at the proximity of hilarity and violence within the human character.[21]

In the same year, and perhaps inspired by the same occasion as Bacon's dance scene, Guy Pène du Bois (1884–1958) painted his *Costume Dance* (1919; fig. 116). Pène du Bois, an urban realist who had studied with Robert Henri and Kenneth Hayes Miller, creates a very different mood. Pène du Bois paints just three dancers, none of whom actually dances, or even moves, for that matter. Two look away from the spectator, while the center figure, in clown costume and makeup, stares out absently, her face a mask of pale impassivity. Missing entirely are the variety and hilarity of Bacon's scene, here replaced by heavy, volumetric forms, carefully modeled to accentuate their roundness. Pène du Bois paints a psychological moment of quiet isolation amid gaiety, an irony predicting his later satirical works and carnival subjects in which figures became almost robotlike.

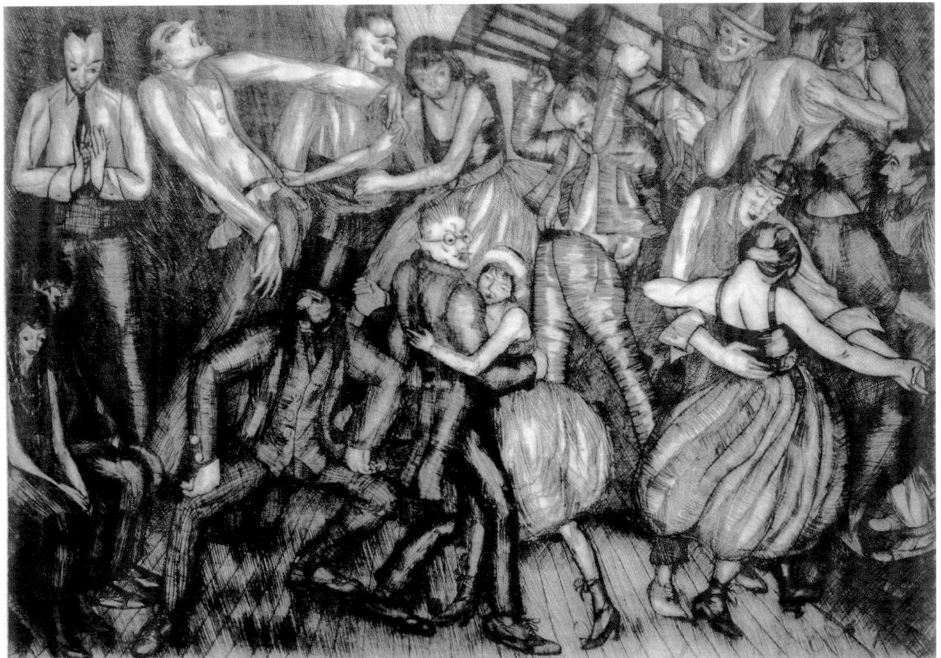

**Figure 115** Peggy Bacon, *Dance at the League*, 1919, drypoint, 7 × 10 inches. (photo courtesy Juley Collection, Smithsonian Institution)

Equally incisive but decidedly more ghoulish is George Bellows's *Dance in a Madhouse* (1917; fig. 117), which exists as both a drawing and a lithograph. Bellows (1882–1925) was a painter associated with Henri and the Eight. Always attuned to social causes, Bellows here uses his considerable talents to illuminate the plight of the mentally ill. Bellows observes a collection of individuals, dancers, and onlookers, whose emotional states range from euphoria to despair. Like Bacon, Bellows caricatured his dancers, but his manner is markedly Goyaesque. The subject is based on Bellows's visits to his old friend Socks Raymond, with whom he had played baseball as a youth in Ohio. Raymond had suffered a

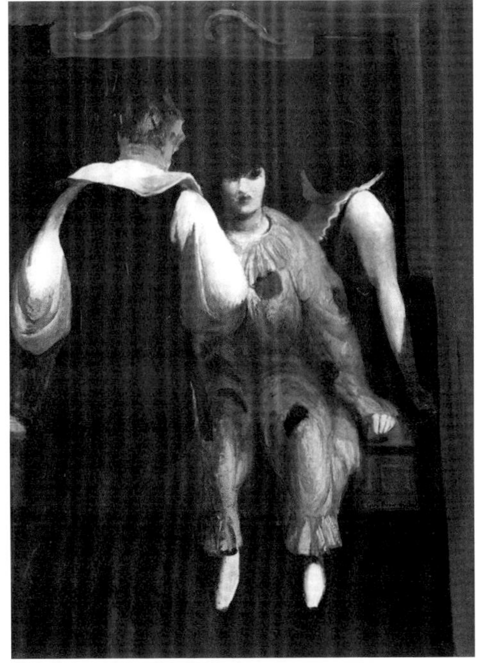

**Figure 116** Guy Pène du Bois, *Costume Dance*, 1919, oil on panel, 19 ¾ × 15 inches. (Dallas Museum of Art, Chester Dale Estate, 1963.171)

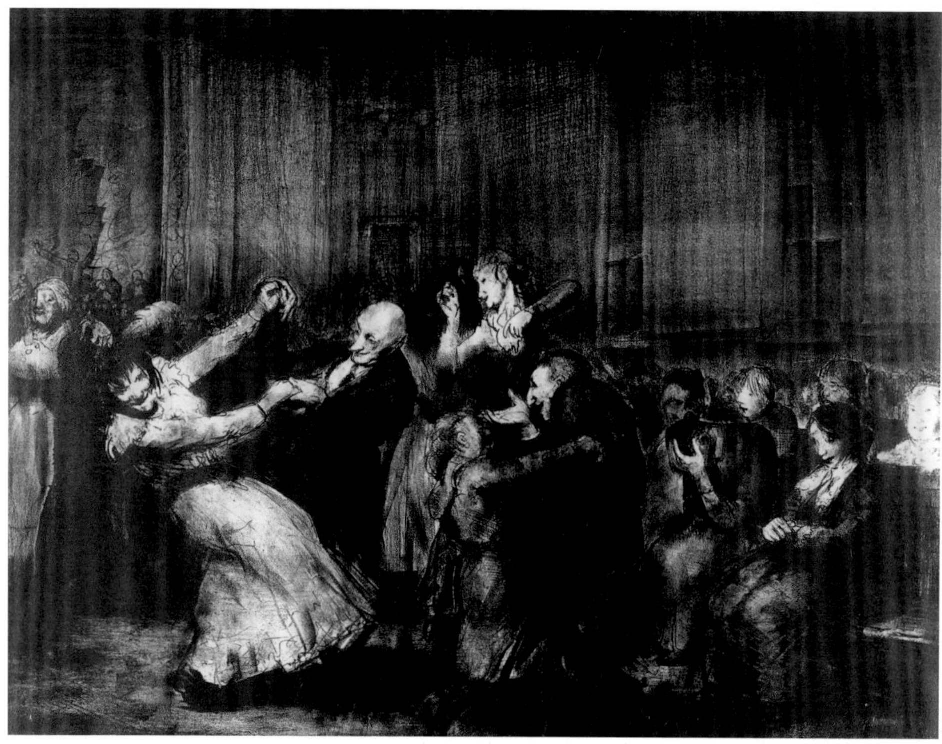

Figure 117 George Bellows, *Dance in a Madhouse*, 1917, lithograph on oriental paper, 18 ½ × 24 ⅛ inches. (photo courtesy Juley Collection, Smithsonian Institution, PPJ-6673)

mental breakdown and was confined to the State Hospital in Columbus. Bellows described his memory of eerie visits to that "Madhouse":

> For years the amusement hall was a gloomy old brown vault where on Thursday nights the patients indulged in "Rounds Dances" interspersed with two-steps and waltzes by the visitors. Each of the characters in this print represents a definite individual. Happy Jack boasted of being able to crack hickory nuts with his gums. Joe Peachmyer was a constant borrower of a nickel or a chew. The gentleman in the center had succeeded with a number of perpetual motion machines. The lady in middle center assured the artist by looking at his palm that he was a direct descendant of Christ. This is the happier side of a vast world which a more considerate and wiser society could reduce to a not inconsiderable degree.[22]

# American Vernacular
## *Visual Art and the Dancing Mechanized Body*

## Modern Architecture as Dance: John Marin and the Dancing City

John Marin (1870–1953), who lived in Europe from 1905 to 1910, returned to New York to find a city alive with change. Elevated trains rumbled, subways shook the ground, and new skyscrapers stretched overhead to unprecedented heights. To Marin, such pulsing energies were proof of life—"pushing, pulling, sideways, downwards, upwards, I can hear the sound of their strife and there is great music being played." In time to that monumental music the whole metropolis moved: "Thus the whole city is alive; buildings, people, all are alive."[1] As Marin wrote those words in 1913, he was in the midst of drawing and etching Cass Gilbert's just-completed Woolworth Building, one of the skyline's most dynamic, soaring forms. Of those animated interpretations, Marin's *Woolworth Building [The Dance]* (1913; fig. 118) is the liveliest, an edifice seeming to bend and sway on its very foundations, while the surrounding sky pulses with graphic energies. Marin inscribed one of the edition to his friend Alfred Stieglitz, who he knew shared his excitement in the dynamic dance of the city. Not yet on hand in New York, but already well known to Stieglitz and, through him, to Marin, were Marcel Duchamp's recastings of the dancing body in an architectural idiom: "[*Nude Descending a Staircase*], commented Duchamp, "is not a typical nude, but an architectural nude. Imagine the different planes that begin to move; for example, the buildings of walls that begin to dance, to rise up, instead of remaining safely fixed in place."[2]

In the spirit of Duchampian play, Marin's high-spirited Woolworth Building frolics on its foundations. As one critic wrote, Marin's "great building seems to begin to join the dance in which all New York is swinging away."[3] Like the ten-cent stores on which the Woolworth fortune arose, Marin's cavorting edifice refuses the serious demeanor of most swaggering skyscrapers. Its owners and designers might be embroiled in the deadly serious business of pursuing fortunes, but Marin's dancing Woolworth building capers playfully on the visual scene, as if to say "I've arrived!" Marin made his buildings engage actively with their surroundings: in his hands metal and masonry became major performers in a new kind of urban choreography, dancing out their aliveness as mechanical–human hybrids, matching their own pulse to the systole and diastole of the city. Marin's

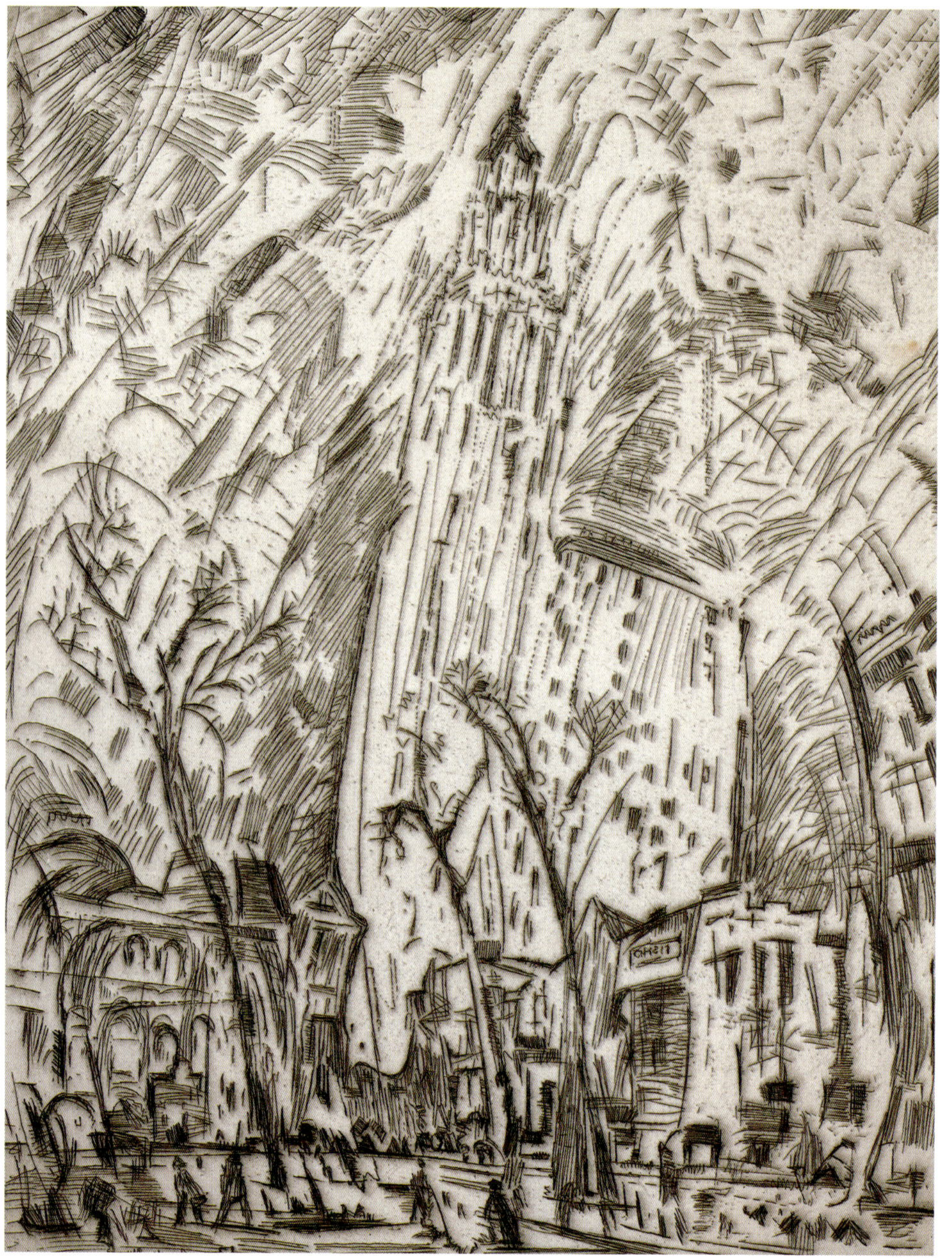

**Figure 118** John Marin, *Woolworth Building [The Dance]*, 1913, etching on white laid paper, 13 × 10 ½ inches. (Art Institute of Chicago, Alfred Stieglitz Collection, 1949.906; photo © The Art Institute of Chicago)

dancing buildings set his own imagination in motion and, as he explained, "the more they move me the more I feel them to be alive."[4]

Across the Atlantic, Picasso made New York skyscrapers dance in the towering costume of the American Manager in the 1917 Satie-Cocteau ballet *Parade*. For New Yorkers at home, the whimsical notion of buildings dancing came closer to literality in the celebrated 1932 Bal des Beaux Arts, when the city's skyline—or at least its major architectural landmarks—arrived as costumes with tall headpieces. The most dramatic was the inimitable Chrysler Building, worn by its flamboyant designer William Van Alen. Supporting on his head the seven-tiered groined vaults of its fantastic finial, it is difficult to imagine Van Alen actually dancing at the ball. Still, a grand ball scenario was magnificently suited to this celebration of American skyscraper architecture, especially to Van Alen's bravura with detail, statuary, finials—an exuberance celebrated as full flowering of an authentically native style.[5] Just a year later, as if in response to Van Alen's or Marin's dancing skyscrapers, New York showman Busby Berkeley would make Manhattan skyscrapers sway to a musical beat, propelled by invisible dancers, in his hit movie musical *42nd Street* (1933).

Manhattan's skyscrapers were seen as an epic defiance of the laws of gravity, thrusting upward in an unprecedented display of masculine power and ingenuity. Finding—as architectural critic Sheldon Cheney did—"beauty in the naked uplift of steel and concrete," a kind of romance had to be invented to embrace that beauty.[6] And where there is romance, there is usually dance: on parapets or bare girders hundreds of feet above the street, dancers were hired to perform for the camera, in one case staged against the Chrysler Building tower (1930s; fig. 119). It is a whirl of joy atop this new American icon, a dance of skyscraper-crazy American confidence in a future of resplendent capitalism. All that prodigality would soon be swept away in the

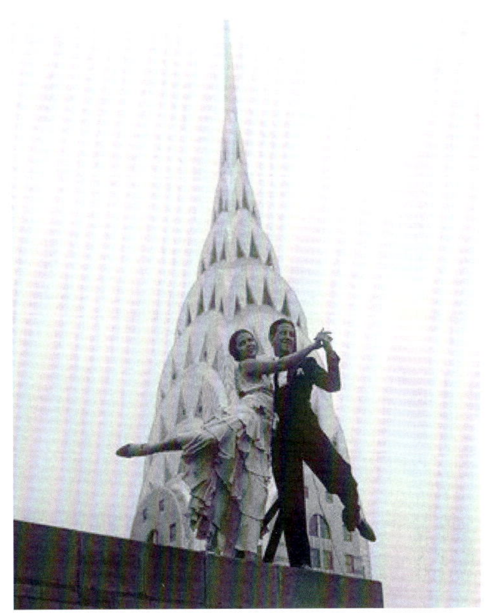

**Figure 119** Anonymous, photograph of couple dancing in front of Chrysler Building tower, New York, 1930s. (private collection)

wake of Black Monday and the tsunami of the Great Depression. The frenetic dance of the American economy—seemingly unstoppable in the 1920s—faded to moribund silence in the vacant, echoing corridors of capitalism's overbuilt cities.

## Futurism: Dance's Dynamism Crosses the Atlantic

The Italian Futurists, whose work constituted their nation's major contribution to modern art in the early twentieth century, sent shock waves through European and American art circles. From its beginnings, Futurism was widely discussed in America as well as in Europe. Illustrated reports of their exhibitions in France, England, Germany, and Holland were published widely in the United States, and their activities were followed by avid American artists. Although the Futurists chose not to exhibit as a group in the 1913 Armory Show, they assembled a broad range of their work for the 1915 Panama-Pacific International Exposition in San Francisco. Of the exposition's many participants, both American and European, the Futurists were by far the most avant-garde—therefore the most discussed—in an essentially conservative field.[7] Writing in the show's catalog, Umberto Boccioni called for an art of "absolutely modern sensation," which explored "the particular rhythm of each object, its inclination, its movement, or to put it more exactly, its interior force."[8] In other words, the peculiarly Futurist obsession was to animate even the inanimate, bringing alive objects, such as machines, that were stubbornly inert. Little wonder that dance, inherently linked to rhythm, sensation, and interior force, was featured prominently at the exposition, both as subject for the Futurists and in theatrical performance.

On hand were Loïe Fuller and her dance troupe performing with an eighty-piece symphony orchestra. The *San Francisco Call* declared it a bonanza for the arts in their city:

> La Loie Fuller's first appearance in America at Festival Hall last night was a triumph. Before a crowd of fully 3500, including the city's foremost art lovers, the world famous danseuse and her company of pretty girls interpreted musical masterpieces in the dance, presenting new terpsichorean creations. In color effects, revelry, spirit and art the dances charmed the large audience, winning great plaudits for the artists.[9]

San Franciscans perhaps did not fully recognize the cultural cutting edge on which both Fuller and the Futurists were dancing. In Paris the year before, Fuller had presented a mixed-media piece set to the musical pyrotechnics of Stravinsky's *Fireworks,* a performance described as an "orgy of color, light and sound." That same year, the Ballets Russes's Diaghilev commissioned Futurist Giacomo Balla to create the mise-en-scène for another performance of *Fireworks* by his own company. The result was a culmination of the aspirations of Futurist theater. Borrowing ideas from Fuller's recent production, Balla "filled the stage with disturbing crystalline forms, beams of colored light, coral formations, symbols of the infinite . . . aerodynamic symbols . . . all projected onto a black backdrop illuminated from behind with red rays."[10] At San Francisco, where Fuller's own inventions again took center stage, audiences could experience an unprecedented avant-garde mélange of painting, dance, and music. Among the exposition's hundreds of temporary buildings was its tallest, a forty-three story "Tower of Jewels" covered by colored glass "jewels" shimmering in the Pacific light. Spotlights were also used to spectacular effect—thousands of them illuminating the exposition buildings—while forty-eight colored searchlights aboard a barge in San Francisco Bay hurled their beams at the night sky.

Between that light extravaganza, the luminous performances of Fuller, and the visual pyrotechnics of the Futurists' canvases, exposition-goers glimpsed a future of unlimited technological promise. Exhibiting separately within the exposition, but sharing an interest in "color effects, revelry, spirit and art," Fuller and the Futurists scored stunning successes in San Francisco in 1915. The painters were given their own gallery and exhibited a total of fifty works. From there, the influence of the Futurists radiated outward as American artists saw and responded to the new work. Reports, manifestoes, and commentary were splashed across the pages of many a little magazine, periodical, and newspaper. And in an exhibition the following year—the Post–Panama Pacific Exposition Exhibit at San Francisco's Palace of Fine Arts—American artists left out of the conservative 1915 show made a splashy appearance, including Arthur B. Davies's Futurist-influenced dance murals, discussed below. It was the beginning of an ironic riposte to the Futurists' early cry of "Burn the museums!" At San Francisco their work opened the floodgate for dynamic movement in modern American art, movement bodied forth triumphantly in images of the dance.[11] What had exploded on the West Coast echoed in New York with a 1917 show at Stieglitz's Gallery 291, some twenty-five paintings, drawings, and pastels by the dance-intoxicated Futurist Gino Severini. His work, and the origins of Futurist dance, warrant a closer look here.

Filippo Marinetti (1876–1944), the Milanese editor and poet, was Futurism's sire. In 1909 he published his "Foundation and Manifesto of Futurism" in a Paris newspaper. Marinetti railed against all that was old, dull, safe, and "feminine," exhorting his countrymen to thrill to unfettered energy, modern technology, and the "masculine" experiences of war and full-throttle speed. Two years later Milan saw the publication of the "Technical Manifesto" of Futurist painting, whose five signers vowed to express "our whirling life of steel, of pride, of fever, and of speed." Building on the fragmentations of Analytic Cubism and the sequences within time-lapse photography, the painters chose various subjects to capture the emotion and dynamism of the modern experience. Painter and sculptor Umberto Boccioni (1812–1916), for instance, chased the pulse of the modern industrial city, while Giacomo Balla and Carlo Carra sought to extract from Cubism the ability to construct complex spatial organization without sacrificing clarity in their paintings.

Those Futurist affinities for the pulsing dynamisms of the modern city are well known, but there were other rhythms and sensibilities these artists wanted to isolate. Not least among them was the kinetic energy, glitter, and unabashed beauty of the dance in Futurist art, a subject not yet well explored as a force in and on American art. In Paris, the Futurist presence seemed a catalyst for artistic ferment of all kinds. Critic Carl Van Vechten saw in Nijinsky's choreography for *Le Sacre du Printemps* (1913) a deliberate attempt to emulate the style of the Futurists in painting.[12] And Marinetti alluded to dance when he declared that the Futurists were "going to the war dancing and singing," words that anticipate his whole "Manifesto of Futurist Dance" (1917). In this tongue-in-cheek document he declared, "We must imitate with gestures the movements of motors, pay assiduous court to steering-gear, wheels, pistons, prepare the fusion of man and machine."[13] The hybridized man–machine was pure Futurist hyperbole, but Marinetti's wild homologizing looks ahead nonetheless to the robotics of the future. In the meantime, Marinetti championed the strutting energies of the

African American Cakewalk, gave qualified praise to Nijinsky and Duncan, and lauded the electrified conjurings of the "magician of light," Loïe Fuller.[14]

Dance proved an amenable subject to the radical Futurists for several other reasons. In particular, they chose to emphasize process rather than things, and (crediting Henri Bergson's writings) they touted the power of intuition to synthesize sense and memory into a coherent "simultaneity." Combined with their expressed wish to downplay the isolated human figure in favor of its entire "surrounding atmosphere," and to incorporate the "harmony of the lines and folds of modern dress," the dynamic processes of dance proved eminently suitable to certain of the Futurists, especially Gino Severini.[15]

Severini (1883–1966) settled in Paris as early as 1906 and began painting patterned compositions with elements derived from Divisionism and from Vuillard. In subjects based on street life and crowds, Severini seemed less interested than the others in Futurism's vaunted taste for violent action and mechanical speed. He also eschewed polemics, for the most part, preferring formal preoccupations to the evocation of force. For the 1912 Futurist exhibition in Paris, he produced a huge canvas of Parisian dancers and a crowd, *Pan Pan at the Monico* (now destroyed). In this and subsequent canvases, Severini revealed his interest in nightlife and in the city's simultaneous interplay of sight, motion and sound.

In quick succession Severini produced a series of dancers to extend the success of his much talked-about *Pan Pan*. He recognized that such subjects—usually individual female dancers—would enable him to find energy within the figure and explode it outward, yet with a fluid, lyrical quality sited in the *idea* of dance itself. While his colleagues explored the human figure as athlete or street rioter, Severini sought in milder abstractions of dance forms what he called "the pictorial rhythm of an ideal world."[16] For him, dance approximated that ideal world, where the rhythmic element is built in, not overlaid. Severini explored dance's intrinsic fluidity just at the time when the Parisian Cubists were introducing ever sharper geometry into their compositions. In *The Obsessive Dancer* (1911, private collection) he paints two women, each holding a cat. Apparently they are the same figure, seen sequentially, rendered in a charming patchwork surface of divisionist dots. There is little to suggest the movement of the dance. But that would soon change for Severini. The next year, in *Blue Dancer* (1912, private collection), Severini's internal lines curve with the rustling rhythms of the dance, while multiple gesturing hands, flashing sequins, and varied tones of blue enliven the whole. In Severini's *Second Dancer (White)*, the movements of the "chahutteuse," the high-kicking cancan dancer, call for a more breathless, staccato conveyance of the dance's furious pace. Here the feet, instead of the hands, are repeated multiple times. Knees, ankles, skirts—all are active elements in the high kineticism of the café dancer.

Having compared the pictorial rhythms of individual dancers, Severini turned to even more complex compositional questions. His large *Dynamic Hieroglyphic of the Bal Tabarin* (fig. 120), painted in Italy during the summer of 1912, forces the issue of synthesizing abstract rhythmic forms and addresses the Futurist desire to paint—as Marinetti advocated—the "whole of its surrounding atmosphere." Although one female dancer again predominates—this time with

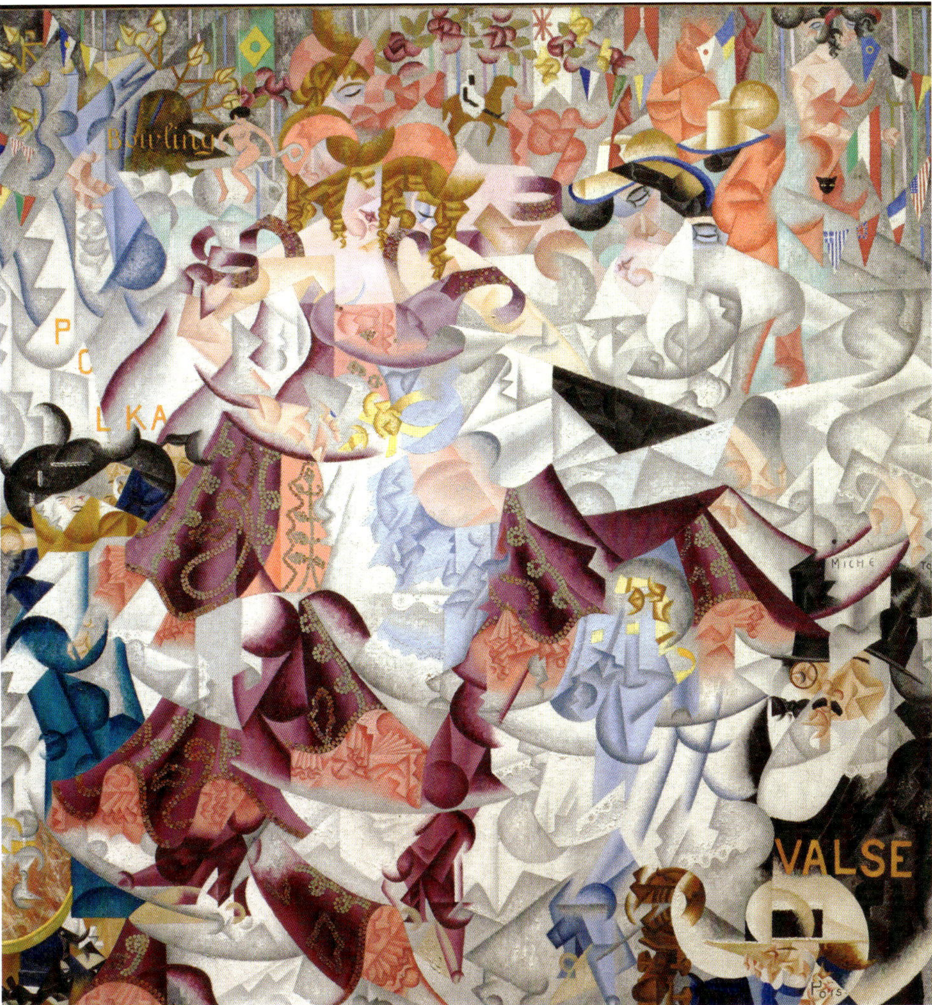



**Figure 120** Gino Severini, *Dynamic Hieroglyphic of the Bal Tabarin*, 1912, oil on canvas with sequins, 63 ⅝ × 61 ½ inches. (Museum of Modern Art, New York, acquired through the Lillie P. Bliss Bequest; image © The Museum of Modern Art/Licensed by SCALA/Art Resource, New York)

blond hair, bows, curls, and a flurry of petticoats, many other figures crowd the periphery of the dance floor. It is as if the artist has constructed a sensory composite of remembered dances, evidenced in the jumpy typography of the words "polka" in the upper left and the ordered "valse" in the lower right, lettered across the slick form of a monocled, top-hatted man. The waltz and polka were still the standard ballroom dances of the day, soon to be challenged by the exotic imports from North and South America en route to Paris. In Severini's composition chaos reigns, but it is intentional chaos, designed to preserve the freneticism frozen in a remembered glimpse of a Parisian dance floor.

In the next two years Severini further extended the complex faceting of forms and surface typography he initiated in *Bal Tabarin*. Knowing (as the

Cubists had recently discovered) the viewer's inclination to read words in paintings, he created new compositions from street life featuring metro and bus signs. And he constructed a "free-word" drawing called *Serpentine Dance* or *Sea=Dancer*, which was published in *Lacerba*, in July 1914. Such onomatopoeic elaboration transforms dance—here, Loïe Fuller's Serpentine dance—into a violent, exploding wartime battle of words. But he interspersed such experiments in the Futurist literary theory of analogies within an ongoing series dependent upon light, color, and what he called "the plastic analogies of dynamism," a kind of charged connection between the self and motion of things outside the self. Light and the flickering surface of the sea were the apparent sources for two new paintings, *Dancer=Sea+Vase of Flowers* (1913–14, private collection) and *Dancer=Sea* (1913–14, private collection). Joshua Taylor suggested that in these works the sensation of sunlight over sparkling water likely reminded Severini of the rhythm of the dance.[17] Sequins are the seemingly insignificant element that sets up the visual equation. Sequins signify the dancer, so that even when the figure disappears in *Dancer=Sea*, the equivalency is maintained: sequined fabric=dancer=flashing surface of the sea. Moreover, the sequins draw attention (like words or signs) to the painting's surface and, perhaps most significantly, their small round shapes are a reminder of Severini's roots in the divisionist tradition.

Seen retrospectively, Severini's dance paintings thus form a highly logical progression, from the near-literality of *The Obsessive Dancer* to the more cryptic blue and white dancers to the flashing *Bal Tabarin* and the near abstraction of *Dancer=Sea*. In the latter painting the artist had begun to explore the radiating power of light, a visual inquiry he would press forward by returning to an active divisionist surface in such works as *Spherical Expansion of Light (Centrifugal)*, 1914. Dancers had proved a useful formal and metaphoric vehicle for Severini's conceptual and perceptual studies of motion in painting.

In the San Francisco Panama-Pacific Exposition of 1915, Severini showed no fewer than four studies for *Sea Dancer*. He also exhibited three versions of a work he titled *Forms and Color: Tone in the Argentine Tango*. The latter works, based on the recently introduced Latin rhythms of the tango, gave artists exciting new syncopations to explore visually. In the same exhibition Carlo Carra showed *Form of a Dancer in Circular Movement* and *Synthesis of a Music Hall*, while Umberto Boccioni exhibited *Muscles in Quick Motion* and Giacomo Balla presented *Dynamic Rhythm*. Among the Futurist works shown, there are nearly a dozen other titles that might well refer to dance. It is clear that dance subjects were of utmost value to the Futurists in their explorations of kinetic movement. The well-known American critic Christian Brinton, writing about the Futurist section of the exhibition, noted, "The distinction between Cubist and Futurist is that the former strives to express volume in the most elementary fashion known to human concept, while the aim of the latter is to create upon canvas the sensation of ceaseless, synchronous motion. The one is static, the other kinetic."[18]

The presence of the Futurists at the 1915 Panama-Pacific Exposition, with their avid interest in visualizations of dance and music, coincided tellingly with Ruth St. Denis's inclusion, in her 1915–16 concert tour, of *The Spirit of the Sea*, a work featuring an undulating blue cyclorama with a line of waves two feet high. Hauntingly akin in mood to Severini's *Sea Dancer*, it proved St. Denis's most popular dance and stayed in her repertoire for a decade, still performed when Loïe Fuller, for the 1925 Paris Decorative Arts exposition, introduced her own sea piece, discussed above. The year 1915 also saw the opening of a dance school founded by Ruth St. Denis and Ted Shawn in Los Angeles. At Denishawn, the principle of music visualizations would become a cornerstone of their practice. It involved portraying music in both movement and choreographic form, a fusion soon adopted by Denishawn student Doris Humphrey. Later famed for her choreographic skills, Humphrey used the visualization theories she had learned at Denishawn, turning them into highly evolved abstractions of choreographic form. Like the Futurists, she remained fascinated with the interrelationships of volumetric patterning, of force channeled into systematic abstraction. It may have been this refined engineering of dance that in the end lessened Humphrey's appeal. Although the equal of Martha Graham as a modern dance innovator in the 1930s, her theoretical inclinations appealed less to audiences than the dramatic force generated onstage by Graham. Perhaps for that same reason, few visual artists chose Humphrey as subject, while many portrayed Graham.

## Visual Artists and the Dance of the Machine

Severini's *Dynamic Hieroglyphic of the Bal Tabarin* (fig. 120, above) would make a profound influence on another Italian-born painter whose career took shape in the United States. Naples-born Joseph Stella (1877–1946) first immigrated through Ellis Island to New York in 1896. After studying with William Merritt Chase at the New York School of Art, Stella specialized for a time in magazine illustration, documenting social conditions in industrial areas. Discouraged by the social inequalities he witnessed, Stella decided to forsake his adopted country and sailed back to Europe. During a two-year stay in Italy Stella gained first-hand knowledge of the Venetian Renaissance masters, but began to long for an environment in which to pursue his own artistic inclinations. Paris beckoned, and he settled there in 1911. The French capital throbbed just then with the energy of the artistic avant-garde, which in 1911 was filled with the competing visions of Fauvism, Cubism, and Futurism. Robert Delaunay's Eiffel Towers danced through the Frenchman's canvases; rhythmic movement swept through many another modernist land- or cityscape.

Of the modernists Stella encountered in Paris, the most outspoken were the Futurists, savvy enough to publish and exhibit regularly in the French capital. On hand regularly was Severini, resident in Paris in those years, who befriended the young Stella. Whether encountering their statements in Italian or English, Stella could scarcely miss the Futurists' aggressive verbiage, much less their aggressive style of painting. In their canvases Stella glimpsed a vision that might, at last, be suited to the energy of America. And Severini's dance paintings, especially the *Bal Tabarin*, showed Stella how to deal with the fragmentation, visual anarchy, and explosive force of the modern city. Stella decided to give New York another try, returning in 1912 and joining the circle around Alfred Stieglitz at Gallery 291.

A bus ride to Coney Island pointed Stella to an American version of the frenetic nightlife Severini had captured in his blazing cabaret images. The lights and the delirious excitement of the great amusement park opened Stella's eyes to an American fantasy of pleasure-seeking after dark. In his *Battle of Lights, Coney Island, Mardi Gras* (1913–14; fig. 121), Stella's wheels and strings of light form dizzying patterns of energy. Powered by the modern miracle of electricity, they burst forth from the Tower of Lights, the Ferris wheel and the spiraling roller coaster. Across Stella's canvas the lights swoop and spin, like the reflected images of dancers in the park's mirrored dance halls, all caught up in a visual orgy of unprecedented wattage. Of his *Coney Island* Stella remembered, "I built the most intense dynamic arabesque that I could imagine, in order to convey in a hectic mood the surging crowd and the revolving machines generating for the first time, not anguish and pain, but violent dangerous pleasures."[19] Stella's choice of the word *arabesque* is especially apt, given its double meaning. It is first an intricate pattern of interlaced lines, which his *Coney Island* shows in spades. But an arabesque is also that characteristic, bending dance posture with arms and legs extended in opposite directions. Close inspection of the canvas reveals fragmented bodies of dancers moving with the pulse of the amusement park's dance hall bands. The dance metaphor is equally appropriate here, for Stella's painting (likely a remembered homage to Severini) takes the Futurist vision of dance several steps beyond anything envisioned by the Europeans.

Returning to the second part of Stella's statement, it is the "revolving machines" that perform and become the dance. He rightly credits them with opening a door to reckless levels of unprecedented pleasure. While he did not characterize those new thrills specifically as sexual, Stella's pulsating, dancing lights carry that kind of energy as well. Just as physical dance is often possessed of a erotic element, Stella's electric dance alludes clearly to a new kind of libidinous energy—taut and machine generated—promising, as he said, "violent, dangerous pleasures." It was an idea with a future beyond Futurism. At a time when overt reference to human sexual intercourse was an American artistic taboo, machine metaphors served in a subversive fashion. In New York Dada, Francis Picabia, Man Ray, and Marcel Duchamp would launch a blatantly erotic-mechanical style, culminating in Duchamp's unparalleled apotheosis of machine-love, *The Large Glass* (1915–23, Philadelphia Museum of Art). Industrialized popular culture was thus poised to create a cultural convulsion of unprecedented magnitude. For the newly minted vocabulary of the modern industrial age, the language of dance offered new idioms for the visual artist.

The machine, in the labor it performs, functions as an abstract surrogate for the human body and its work. It is an association that has survived over time and across far-flung cultures. Folkloric or newly invented variants of the automaton have figured in many artistic projects, from *Coppelia* to the *Ballet Mécanique* to Nijinsky in *Petrouchka*. And vestiges lingered in the stark movements of Balanchine's later plotless ballets, pairing sounds and steps in ways

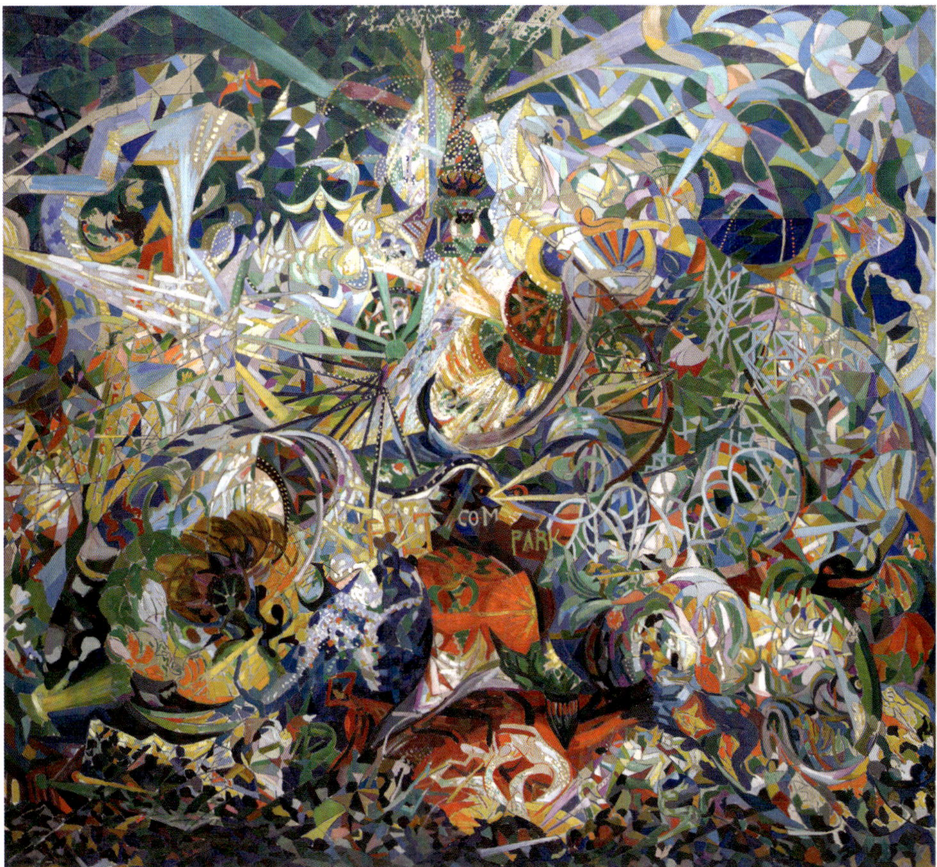

Figure 121 Joseph Stella, *Battle of Lights, Coney Island, Mardi Gras*, 1913–14, oil on canvas, 76 × 84 inches. (Yale University Art Gallery, New Haven, Bequest of Dorothea Dreier to the Collection Société Anonyme)

detractors saw as rigid and mechanical. Precisely the point, came the rejoinder: by placing his choreography within the aesthetic frame of visual modernism, those mechanical movements and gestures fit comfortably into certain expressions of modernity in the visual arts, notably Dada. As machine abstraction penetrated ever deeper into the visual arts, it often addressed the conditions of modernity Norman Bryson has named:

> Looking at the world built by abstraction, the subject sees reflected back not the rhythms of the body but the rhythms of the machine, and above all the three great, hammering rhythms of the first machine age: fragmentation (in bursts, spasms, jerks, pulses); repetition (the first precise repetitions, since the body repeats only approximately); and velocity (the trio of trains, cars, planes).[20]

Translated into the language of the body, these new movements inspired both dancers and visual artists to rethink human movement and structure. On stage or on canvas, the body, retooled as an assemblage of parts, might move in more insistently mechanical ways. Even Martha Graham, whose sources were often in humanist disciplines, acknowledged that machine culture was responsible for "a characteristic time beat, a different speed, an accent, sharp, clear, staccato" in her work.[21]

In the machine-derived work of Stella, Duchamp, and Picabia, we recognize that dance, as much as visual art, contributed to the transatlantic proliferation of modern culture: both mediums dealt with ways of reconceiving space and time. In this case, as in many others, it was often European visitors themselves who could speak with frankness and objectivity of America's unique cultural potential. Francis Picabia—a wealthy heir with a weakness for fast cars—when interviewed in the *New York Tribune* in 1915, explained that "since machinery is the soul of the modern world, and since the genius of machinery attains its highest expression in America, why is it not reasonable to believe that in America the art of the future will flower most brilliantly?"[22] Picabia (1879–1953), of Cuban and French descent, was a close follower of cultural movements across the Atlantic. In Paris during the early years of the twentieth century, he and his wife, the musician Gabrielle Buffet-Picabia, moved in avant-garde circles and immersed themselves in the life of the city, where she observed "a real madness for dancing in all levels of society." Given that ambiance, it is not at all surprising that in the months preceding their 1913 arrival in the United States to attend the Armory Show, Francis Picabia produced several paintings that explore new views of human movement through parallels between dance, music, and visual abstraction. His *Danses à la Source I* (*Dances at the Spring I*) (1912, Philadelphia Museum of Art) makes reference on one hand to the old union of the dance with nature, fecundity, women, and water, a well-traveled theme in famous earlier works by masters such as Ingres and Bouguereau. Picabia's *Dances* borrows those old affiliations with ancient ritual, but its more immediate source was a peasant dance seen at an outdoor festival during the Picabias' honeymoon near Naples.

Picabia sensed that the subject of dance could become a lightning rod for the whole issue of abstraction, a subject he wanted very much to engage. Treading on the edge of parody with the nineteenth-century academic painters, he turned abruptly in 1912 to face a new direction in which he glimpsed creative daylight: Picabia decided to marry the new visual language of Cubism to experiments in representing motion. Just as Duchamp's nude was not merely posed on, but in the act of descending a staircase, so Picabia's two cubist women in *Dances at the Spring* move as well. As dancers, they engage in significant movement, which lends visual credibility to pictorial space. More, they represent a survival of the figure, or at least its traces, in an era defined by steady negation of narrative, figuration, and readable pictorial space.

Following *Dances at the Spring,* Picabia made two more dance-related paintings in 1913, both shown at Stieglitz's Gallery 291: *Star Dancer with Her Dance School* (1913; fig. 122) and *Star Dancer on Board a Transatlantic Steamer* (1913, unlocated). Even as his style evolved, Picabia found the subject of the dance adaptable to different formal means; the last-named work is less figural and cubistic than his previous two, and it forecasts the artist's affinities with

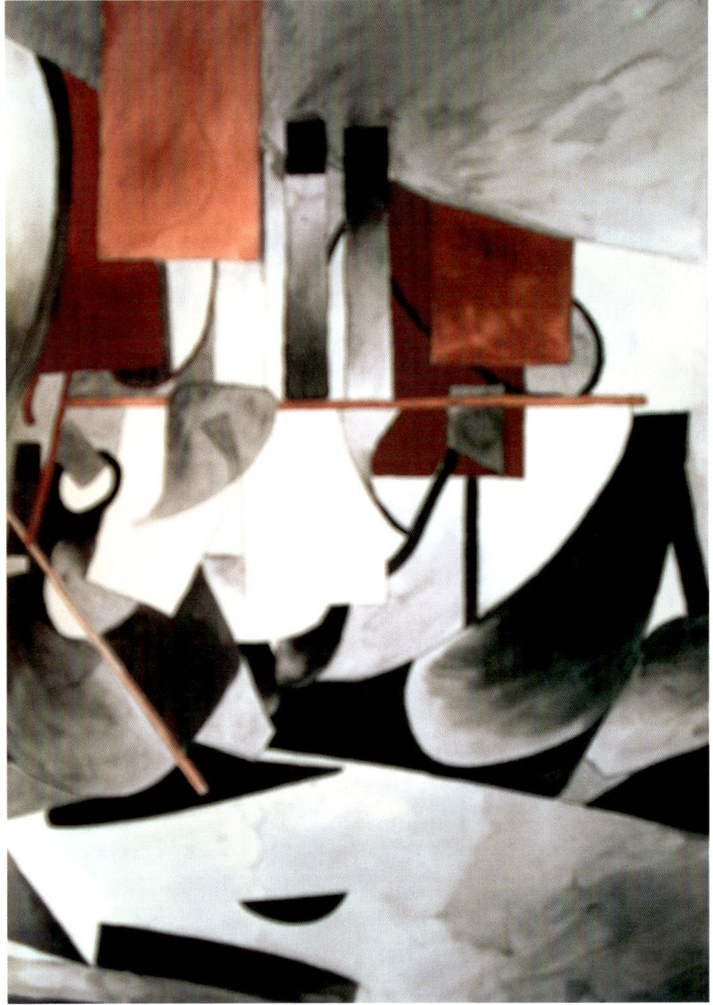

Figure 122 Francis Picabia, *Star Dancer with Her Dance School*, 1913, watercolor on paper, 22 × 30 inches. (Metropolitan Museum of Art, New York, The Alfred Stieglitz Collection, 1949, 49.70.12; image © The Metropolitan Museum of Art/Art Resource, New York)

the linear elements and geometries of Duchamp's *The Large Glass*. Dance and dancers continued to engage Picabia during these years. The model for his *Star Dancer* paintings was Stacia Napierkowska, a popular dancer bound for an American tour when the Picabias encountered her aboard ship. Picabia reportedly portrayed Napierkowska in the first of his machine-inspired "object portraits," *Mechanical Expression Seen through Our Own Mechanical Expression* (1913). Schematically, the drawing made reference to the dancer as an x-ray emitting tube, encoding a reference to her sexually charged dancing.[23] A few years later Picabia had a tempestuous affair with Isadora Duncan, which further confirmed his role linking the world of dance and the riotous company of the New York Dadaists.[24]

Picabia's and Duchamp's figure-based abstractions anticipate the Cubist dancers Arthur B. Davies (1862–1928) would soon begin painting. Davies, one of the chief organizers of the Armory Show, was a sometime muralist whom the collector Lizzie Bliss commissioned to decorate her music room in 1914. It was a large project, thirteen panels in all, for which Davies painted Cubistically conceived seated or standing figures. Emboldened by the critical success of those murals, the artist next undertook several new ones, this time with the figures engaged in dance. Originally titled *New Numbers, Decoration, Dances,* Davies's mural glows with intense color, its bodies and gestures painted in abstract, rhythmic curves (1914–15, Detroit Institute of Arts). Retitled *Dances,* the mural was exhibited at the Montross Gallery in 1915, from which the adventurous collector John Quinn purchased it. Later (1927) the work was acquired by the Detroit Institute of Arts for the highest price that institution had yet paid for an American painting. A smaller version called *The Dancers* (later retitled *Day of Good Fortune*) (c. 1914; fig. 123) was equally successful as a Cubist dance composition and was again purchased by Lillie Bliss. Davies's cubist dancers are less abstracted than those of Picabia, free and uninhibited in their nudity, yet memorable more for their color patterning than their sensuality. Davies continued to use the dance as a frequent subject in those years, making dance drawings shown at Macbeth's gallery in 1915 along with many dance sculptures by various artists. A New York critic commented, "The most successful and gratifying interpretation of the dance is not that of the sculptors, but it is to be found in the color sketches of Arthur B. Davies. . . . The flashes of pure color are used with thrilling effect to intensify the rhythm."[25]

Davies also tried his hand at sculpture, producing a number of dance works in wood and bronze. Of the former members of the Eight, Davies was alone in moving, in the wake of the Armory Show, into abstract oils and three-dimensional subjects. The dance had given him another plane on which to imagine, a way in which to explore the fusion of Cubism, Futurism, and Synchromy.

The French moderns in the Armory Show also influenced another emerging abstractionist, Man Ray (1890–1976). Born Emmanuel Radenski in Philadelphia, Ray studied with Robert Henri and became a regular visitor at Stieglitz's Gallery 291. His friendship with Duchamp gave impetus to his Cubist inclinations and fostered an interest in movement, whether fluid, graceful, or spasmodic. Predictably, dance entered his visual vocabulary, no doubt because it provided an infinitely variable metaphor for movement. At the beginning of 1915, Ray later recalled, "I changed my style completely, reducing human figures to flat-patterned disarticulated forms."[26] Then he saw a vaudeville performance (the kind of popular-culture immersion Henri advocated) in which a dancer performed in the glare of bright floodlights, balanced precariously on a tightrope stretched over the heads of the audience. That performance would inspire the most significant painting of Man Ray's early years, *The Rope Dancer Accompanies Herself with Her Shadows* (1916; fig. 124). Back at his studio after the vaudeville show, the artist made a number of sketches to fix the dancer's movements. Instead of rendering her naturalistically (as Whistler had in his portraits of the skipping-rope dancer Connie Gilchrist, discussed in chapter 9).

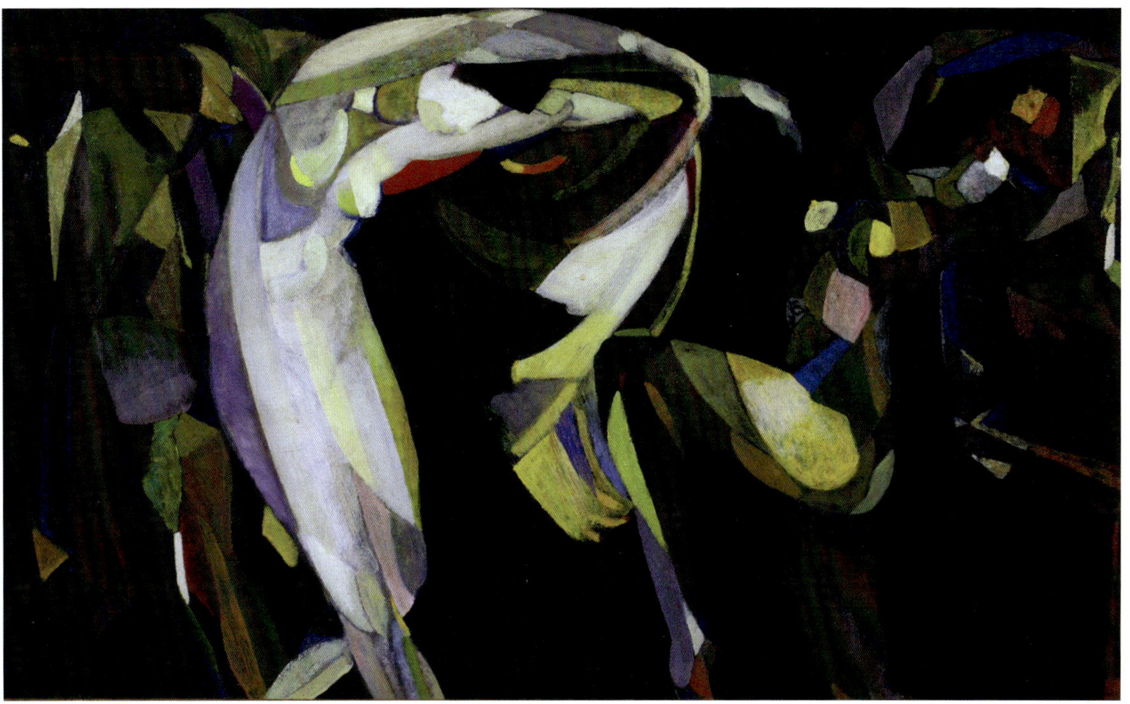

**Figure 123** Arthur B. Davies, *Day of Good Fortune [The Dancers]*, c. 1914, oil on canvas, 18 × 30 inches. (Whitney Museum of American Art, Gift of Mr. and Mrs. Arthur G. Altschul, 71.228)

Man Ray opted for a kind of mechanomorphic animation, a choice perhaps influenced by his recent resettlement from rural New Jersey to a bustling neighborhood in Manhattan. In that new urban environment, the artist later recalled, he decided to turn "away from nature to man-made productions. . . . With my new surroundings in a busy and changing city, it was inevitable that I change my influences and technique."[27] As Francis Naumann explains, Man Ray explored color possibilities for *Rope Dancer* by snipping shapes from brightly colored construction paper.[28] Attuned in Dadaist fashion to the fortuitous role of chance, he then discarded those cut shapes in favor of the random abstract scraps littering the studio floor. Ray played with contrast and placement, anchoring whimsy in overlapping configurations, then painting the result on his six-foot canvas. "Scrapping the original forms of the dancer, I set to work on the canvas, laying in large areas of pure color in the form of the spaces that had been left outside the original drawings of the dancer." Lest she disappear altogether, Ray reinserted the dancer as a crystalline star shape at the top, a composite form constructed from Ray's original rope-dancer sketches and tethered by ropes to her "shadows" below. As he would later say, "the shadow is as important as the real thing," which reality can be inferred as Ray's remembered experience of the performance itself transferred to canvas.[29] Once the artist lettered its title along the bottom, he pronounced himself delighted: "The satisfaction and confidence this work gave me was greater than anything I had experienced heretofore, although

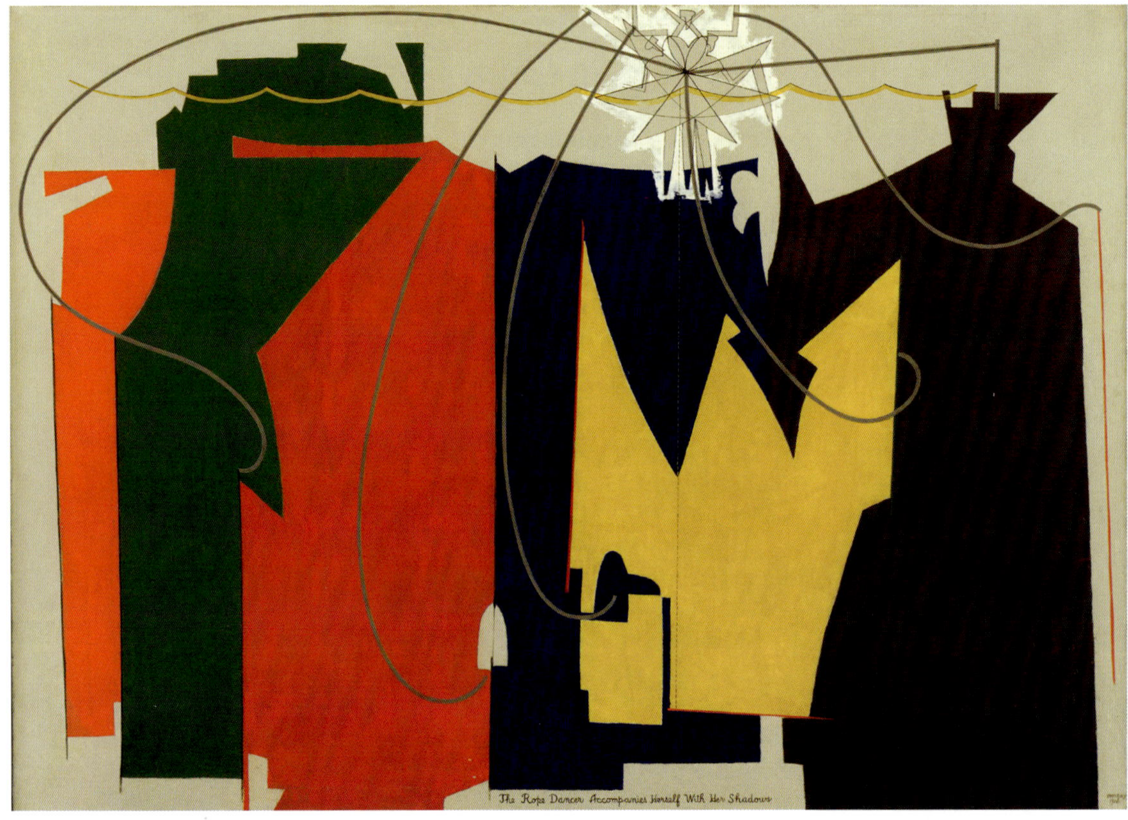


**Figure 124** Man Ray, *The Rope Dancer Accompanies Herself with Her Shadows*, 1916, oil on canvas, 52 × 73 ⅜ inches. (Museum of Modern Art, New York, Gift of G. David Thompson, 33.1954; image © The Museum of Modern Art/Licensed by SCALA/Art Resource, New York)

it was incomprehensible to any of our visitors who saw it." Suspended high up near the studio skylight, Man Ray's bright canvas, like its eponymous dancer, was tied only loosely to realism, more closely allied to a new Dadaist analysis of the mechanics of motion, the optical properties of color, and the experience of volume, space, and determined flatness. When Stieglitz saw the *Rope Dancer* exhibited at the Independents Show in 1917, he recognized its importance, commenting on the nearly blinding power of its optical vibration.[30]

At the Independents' Show and elsewhere in New York, Man Ray and Duchamp collaborated on Dadaist activities; through his French friend the American gained access to the latest writings of Dadaist painters and poets in Europe. That contact introduces another way—admittedly subtler and more speculative—in which Man Ray's *Rope Dancer* may be considered. Jean Arp, writing in 1915 for an exhibition catalog preface, discussed the distinction between artists who copy nature and those who wish instead to produce, not merely reproduce. "To reproduce," wrote Arp, "is to imitate play-acting, tight-rope dancing." By contrast, Arp praised "works [that] are constructed with lines, surfaces, shapes, and colors." In this sense, Man Ray's *Rope Dancer*, painted just a year after Arp's catalog preface and with it in mind, addresses Arp's dichotomy between production and reproduction, seen retrospectively as modern art's deepening crisis of representation. The artist who merely reproduces teeters like a dancer on a tight rope, creating only shadows (in a Platonic sense) of objects or of nature. Here is a new, abstract metaphor in art: the painter as dancer, engaging in a kind of conceptual acrobatics. He or she must choose among the realities oscillating before the eye, searching to find some kind of larger subject—shapes and colors, Arp insisted—to replace the reproducible object. Teetering, dizzy with possibility, is Man Ray himself, working with the larger idea to test Arp's insistence that ultimately, "Art, however, is reality and the reality of all should triumph over the particular."[31] The dance here serves the irreverent spirit of Dada, that anti-art movement which challenged and redefined art itself.

Yet another clue to an alternative interpretation of the *Rope Dancer's* iconography may lie in a contemporaneous verse by American poet Witter Bynner about Isadora Duncan. In 1913 Duncan's two young children had drowned near Paris in a tragic auto accident. The following year her newborn infant had lived only a few hours. These losses plunged Duncan into an abyss of grief, assuaged only by her beloved dance students, whom she kept nearby whenever possible. As Bynner wrote (*Opus 1*, 1916),

> More desolate than they are Isadora stands,
> The blaze of the sun on her grief;
> The stars of a willow are in both of her hands,
> And her heart is the shape of a leaf. . . .
> Till light comes leaping
> On little children's feet,
> Comes leaping Isadoran—
> And the white stars beat
> Their drums.

It is possible that those young dancers, surrogates for Duncan's own lost children, are the "shadows" beneath the blazing sun- or star-shaped dancer at the top of Man Ray's painting. The artist began with an experience of a real-life dance spectacle, but he has spun from it a web of dazzling iconographical possibilities. *Rope Dancer* is a composition suggestive of multiple meanings, and is capacious enough to hold them all in poetic suspension.

Within a few years Man Ray turned his efforts in another direction, engaging the twin energies of dance and machine and introducing newly complex metaphors. The mechanomorphic body, which began as a benign fantasy, now assumes a grimmer potential: the machine may also be cast as the body's negative or dark side—a fascinating, even dangerous concept when machines have a semblance of life. If the mechanized machine/body is the human "other," that notion, when taken to its extreme, harbors the dread that the machine might assume control, might generate a world of machine forms, disrupting traditional human values. Man Ray flirted with that darker side of machine energies. *Danger/Dancer ILXT* or *L'Impossibilité* (1920/1972; fig. 125) was, like

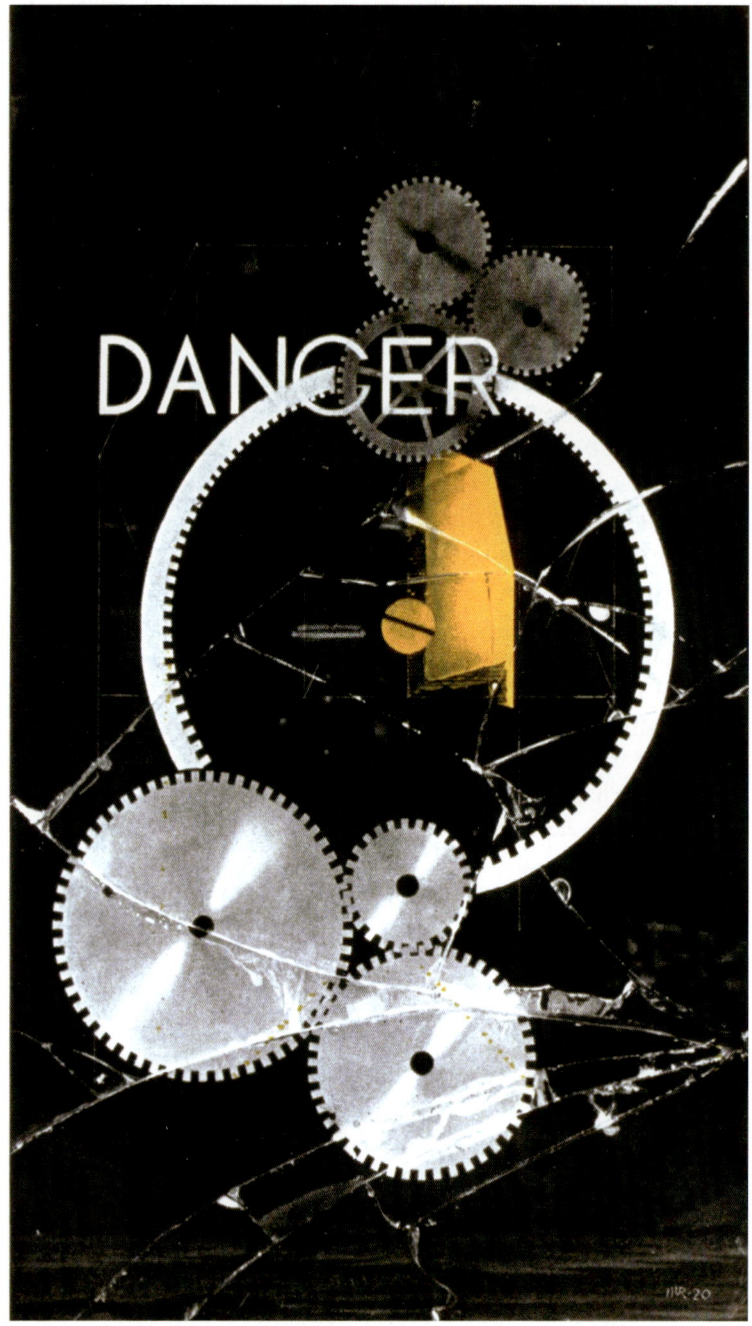


**Figure 125** Man Ray, *Danger/Dancer ILXT* or *L'Impossibilité*, 1920/1972, photolithograph, 23 ⅜ × 15 ³⁄₁₆ inches. (University of Michigan Museum of Art, Gift of the Marvin Felheim Collection, 1983/1.212)

his *Rope Dancer*, inspired by the turns and twists of a dancer performing in a local musical. Across his new painting the artist inscribed the word "DANCER," but his letter "C" looks very much like a "G," hence the deliciously dual title. Are dancers also potentially dangerous in their gyrations? Might they capture the viewer as menacingly as a machine's cogs might entrap an unwary hand? Asked to assemble the interlocking gears that appear in this painting-on-glass, a mechanic told Man Ray that it was an impossible, nonfunctional arrangement, accounting for the third aspect of the title. Produced in part with the airbrush (Man Ray's means of applying paint in hands-off, mechanical fashion), the fragile glass support cracked and was repaired by the artist (like Duchamp's *Large Glass*). *Danger/Dancer* is a painting that emits energy and frustration, both mechanical and libidinal. Within it lies an implicit recognition often at the heart of Dada's caustic anxiety: that humanity's hubris sometimes dooms its machinations to failure. Perfection eludes the artist as surely as Perpetual Motion (a title used previously by Man Ray) defies the dancer and the machine.

Curiously, the same year Man Ray completed *Danger/Dancer*, an unforeseen thing happened: the artist surprised himself by learning to dance. Berenice Abbott, then a sculptor but later a prominent photographer, offered to teach him, and in doing so opened to him a new world of artistic expectation. What had simultaneously engaged and eluded him suddenly became possible. In fact, recalled Man Ray, "[T]here was nothing to it. I had a sense of rhythm, [Abbott] said—that was all one needed. I was elated—all the arts that had seemed beyond me were now within my grasp; photography, dancing, everything was possible."[32] Dancing gave Man Ray a liberating answer to the siren call of rhythmic movement in human and machine performance. Its effects would linger into the artist's Surrealist years. For his silent film *Emak Bakia* (1926–27) Man Ray created a visual montage, alternating sequences of legs dancing the Charleston with a hand strumming a banjo. According to the artist, such cropped and disjointed clips, projected with a syncopated jazz accompaniment, were designed to enhance the film's dreamlike irrationality and automatism.[33]

## Dances with Chance, Dances with Deliberation: Calder and Mondrian

Alexander Calder, who had used dance as a motif in his witty wire sculptures of Josephine Baker (discussed in chapter 2), found continued inspiration in the expressive possibilities of individual and group movement, action that encouraged yet another departure—this time into more abstract kinetic pieces. After Miró and Mondrian saw Calder's *Circus* in the 1920s, he was invited to their Paris studios. At Mondrian's, he recalled, "I thought at the time how fine it would be if everything there moved."[34] So Calder proceeded to make moving "Mondrians," painting geometric forms in primary colors and attaching them to hand cranks or motors. His *Dancing Torpedo Shape* (1932) set into motion a white square, a blue disk, and a red cylinder. That Calder thought of these oscillating shapes as dancelike is telling; clearly he was not after mere mechanized movement, but a kind of lyrical grace, however machine derived. He explored that potential for grace in a 1936 motorized sculpture, *Dancers and Sphere*, constructed from sheet metal, wire, and wood. "With a mechanical drive," Calder explained, "you can control the thing like the choreography in a ballet." Eventually Calder yearned for even more rhythmic, varied movement, the kind produced by air currents and wind.

For Martha Graham, the sculptor was able to engage his creative kineticism in a pairing with dance. She recalled,

> Alexander Calder had a primitive and startling idea about space the uses of the stage. Calder's pieces moved. He designed the pieces for my ballet *Panorama*, which premiered in Bennington in 1935. The next year, for *Horizons*, he created a set of mobiles and stabiles, which had to be manipulated from the sides, by two dancers. This was new for the dance and we wanted to make clear to the audience the role of the dancers as opposed to the role of the set. We placed the following in the program notes:
>
> The "mobiles" designed by Alexander Calder are a new conscious use of space. They are employed in *Horizons* as visual preludes to the dances in this suite. The dances do not interpret the "mobiles" nor do the "mobiles" interpret the dances. They are employed to enlarge the sense of the horizon.[35]

In Calder's mobiles, as Marcel Duchamp first called them, the sculptor learned to exploit his own fascination with the elements of change and surprise, testing new shape relationships and compositions created by movement. "When everything goes right," said the sculptor, "a mobile is a piece of poetry that dances with the joy of life and surprises." But the innovative use of three-dimensional kinetic sculpture could pose its own set of difficulties for the dance, at times seeming to compete with the dancers themselves. Graham ultimately decided that Calder's sculptural forms for *Horizon*—blocks among which the dancers moved, augmented by spinning spirals and circles—were less than successful. Perhaps they engaged too assertively with the temporal element intrinsic to dance, encroaching on a domain normally reserved to the body. In any case, they remained, in Graham's mind, incompletely integrated into the movement of the dance itself. She never used Calder again. Still, for the sculptor, dance in all its variations remained a vital, inventive metaphor in his work. At his death, Calder's friend James Johnson Sweeney mused, "The dancer is gone but the dance remains."[36]

Both in Europe and later in the United States, the Dutch painter Piet Mondrian (1872–1944), who had already inspired Calder, eventually wove dance into his own visual compositions. Best known for his attempts to paint universals through dynamic oppositions of horizontals and verticals, Mondrian also focused closely on the dual forces of matter and spirit through his study of Theosophy and Hegelian dialectics. But there was another, earthier side to Mondrian. For all his philosophical erudition, the artist was a devoted, if idiosyncratic social dancer, who practiced, performed—and even painted—the new

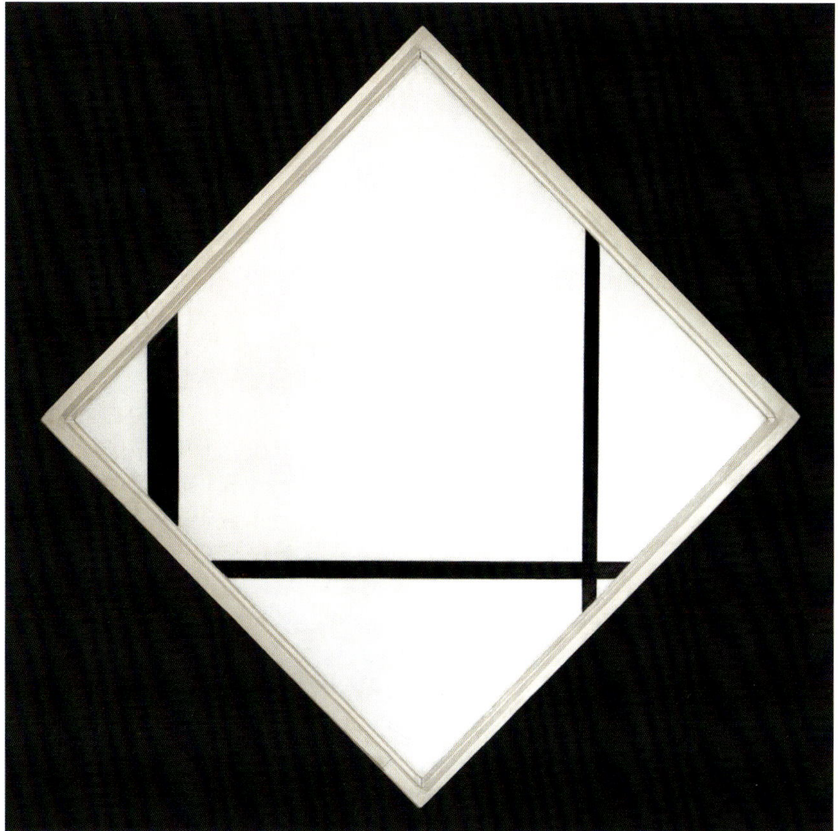

**Figure 126** Piet Mondrian, *Fox Trot A*, 1930, oil on canvas, 30 ¾ × 30 ¾ inches. (Yale University Art Gallery, New Haven, Gift of the artist for the Collection Société Anonyme)

dances. As a friend recalled, Mondrian "took lessons in such modern steps as the fox-trot, tango, etc. Whatever music was being played, however, he carried out his steps in such a personally stylized fashion that the results were frequently awkward and rarely satisfactory to his partners. . . . His own devotion to danc-ing . . . preoccupied him most."[37] Mondrian's idiosyncratic moves were, in fact, deliberate expressions of his resistance to rhythmic sameness. He tried to explain it in his writings, likening oppositional rhythms in dance to the Neo-plastic prin-ciples embodied in his paintings:

> Today the dance, the dance which has some subtlety, as well as the music, to which, or rather *against* which one dances, expresses a duality of two equivalent elements. The straight line is the plastic expression of this fact. In music, the various rhythms oppose each other, as they oppose the melody, and as the steps of the dance oppose each other.[38]

In 1930 Mondrian painted a work called *Fox Trot A* (fig. 126), which dem-onstrates, with just a few lines, new subtleties of rhythm and syncopation.[39]

By then, living in Paris, Mondrian had already discovered jazz, which he described as "this music bombshell."[40] Jazz and dancing became passions in his life, passions he tried to reconcile with his art and even with machine imagery. "In our time," he concluded, "rhythm is more and more accentuated, not only in art, but in mechanized reality and in the whole of life. Marvelously determined and full of vitality, it is expressed in real jazz, swing, and Boogie-Woogie music and dance."[41]

Throughout the 1930s Mondrian's search for a free and open rhythm led him to further exploration of the dynamic relationships between line and colored rectangles. Then, just ahead of the advancing shadow of war, Mondrian fled Paris for London in 1938, and after two years there sailed for the United States. He loved New York from the beginning. Working in studios on East 56th and East 59th Streets, the painter proceeded to find new rhythmic expressions for the city. During the war years the syncopations of jazz and dance held continued sway over his work, appearing in the break-up of his larger painted shapes into tiny yellow, red, blue, black, white, and grey ones, like notes in a chaotic urban musical score. In the spacings of the pulsing shapes in *Broadway Boogie Woogie* (1942–43, Museum of Modern Art, New York) one can almost feel the jerky, obsessive steps of the dancing painter along the gridded streets of Manhattan. In a sense, this late work reprises Mondrian's beginnings as a landscape painter. However abstract his designs became, they reflect his unflagging concerns for readable gravity and bodily balance. Always, Mondrian danced to his own tune, played in the gap between the vernacular and the absolute.

Mondrian's painted representations of a dancing city bring earlier ones, notably John Marin's dancing buildings, full circle. While both measure the living energies of a modern metropolis, Mondrian's are characteristically more restrained and subtle while Marin's—brash, frolicsome—unleash the cocky swagger of the new American century. Together they restate a compelling case for the adaptability of dance as a visual and rhythmic metaphor of modernity.

# Part Four

## Terpsichore Transformed

### Dance, the Liberated Body, and America's Artistic Revolutions

# 9

## Class, Vice, and the Revolt against Puritanism

As we have seen in previous chapters, dance in all its variety, from classical ballet to the explosive abandon of the Montmartre, gave nineteenth-century American audiences a wide range of dance performances appealing to the most educated or most vernacular tastes. The accolades granted to foreign dancers visiting the United States in the nineteenth century undoubtedly heightened American interest in dance but did nothing for those home-grown performers clamoring for artistic legitimacy. For one thing, they were hampered by the lack of a solid tradition of American theatrical dance. Missing were major theaters and opera houses, well-supported schools, and government patronage of the type afforded Europeans. Serious artistic dance could not develop without self-challenging artists, who must emerge from a larger enlightened urban elite, which was nonexistent or poorly developed before the twentieth century.

Perhaps a greater impediment to legitimacy was the taint of sexual license often assigned to nineteenth-century American dancers. For a few, that taint could be converted into commercial value: entrepreneurs bent on capturing the same effects that had titillated Samuel Clemens in Parisian dance halls billed many young Americans as vaguely French. Writes dance historian Olga Maynard: "The American dancing girls of the period had the worst of reputations, especially as the management believed in advertising them as Parisians, and had them masquerade under Gallic names, with the supposed Gallic reputation for amorousness. They were required not only to dance but often to sing, act, and support comedians, trained animal acts, or starred singers, in variety shows. Many of them worked in factories by day and danced in the *corps de ballet* at night."[1] In short, respectability was as hard to come by as professional training.

Whatever their personal virtues, dancers of all kinds tended to be painted with the broad brush of vice, in colors earned by a few notorious ones. At a time when actresses and dancers were only beginning to emerge from long associations with prostitution and the *demimonde*, exposing one's body to the public gaze gave most "respectable" women pause. In the most favorable light it required either strong moral or aesthetic conviction. At worst, the inferences were of moral laxity driven by ambition. Years later, Isadora Duncan still wondered, "What was it that made men at that time exclaim, 'I would rather see my daughter dead than on the stage?'"[2] The answer is plain: automatically categorized with prostitutes and hucksters, American dancers were trapped within the net of the demimonde.

Besides troubling moral issues, theatrical dance raised issues of class and social origins. Clearly, what has not been well reconciled, either in European or American visual art, is the outward veneer of glamor affixed to dancers in contrast to the gritty, class-based distinctions that separated them from many in their audiences. But that very distance seemed to engage some visual artists. In 1876 or 1877, American-born James McNeill Whistler, then living in London, painted the young dancer Connie Gilchrist, who had begun her career just two years earlier, at age twelve, as a skipping-rope dancer at London's Gaiety Theatre. Whistler portrayed her in that role, yet, immersed in his search for an art of purely aesthetic values, he designated the portrait as a *Harmony in Yellow and Gold: The Gold Girl—Connie Gilchrist* (c. 1876–77; fig. 127). Not long afterward, he painted her again in a different color mood as *The Blue Girl* (1879, Hunterian Gallery, University of Glasgow). Her fame enhanced by Whistler's portraits, Gilchrist found herself a dancer in demand. Propelled by her own charm as a performer, Gilchrist's future blossomed: she rose through London's ranks of light comedy and burlesque, finally shattering the class barrier completely when she left the stage in 1892 to become the Countess of Orkney.

Across the channel in France, another fourteen-year-old dancer engaged Edgar Degas, who exhibited his bronze *Little Dancer, Aged Fourteen* (1881) at an Impressionist show. Unlike Whistler's upwardly mobile Connie Gilchrist, Degas's ballerina was less fortunate. She has been identified as Marie von Goethem (b. 1865), a student at the Paris Opera Dance School and one of the myriad *petits rats* who swarmed back stage at the Opera Ballet. Von Goethem danced for a couple of poorly paid seasons in the company, during which time she posed for Degas.[3] Upon seeing his sculpture of Marie, with her eerily realistic gauze skirt and silk bodice, many observers thought she resembled something out of Mme. Tussaud's wax museum. Or worse. Parisian critics were divided: while a few in the avant-garde considered her "quintessentially modern," others called her a "monkey," and "a monster . . . [from] a museum of zoology." In short, she was condemned as aggressive and unappealing, redolent of all the imagined vices of her social class and lacking any of the redeeming graces of her profession.

For American viewers, the ironies were even more blatant: traditionally uncomfortable with seemingly undemocratic social distinctions based on class, Americans were unsure what to make of the dancers they saw performing on their own stages, and that ambivalence made them uneasy at times. The long flirtation between dance and art had not yet been legitimized in the minds of Americans, and dance had not yet achieved the status of Art with a capital A. Vexing questions remained: by what kind of alchemy could sweat, physical strain, and unrelenting practice be transformed onstage into seemingly effortless art? For decades, dance in America languished somewhere between mere entertainment and physical labor, as yet incapable of bestowing, guarding, or conveying cultural meaning beyond the pejorative.

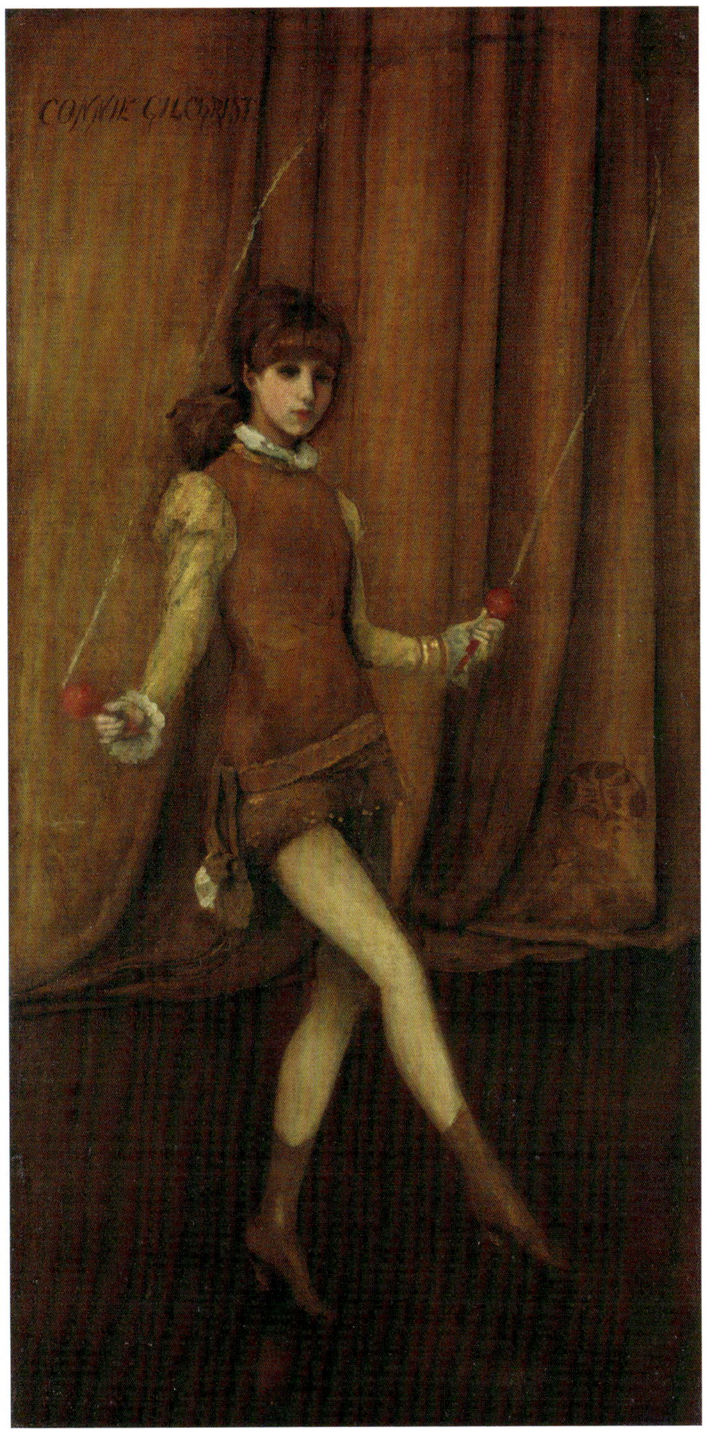


**Figure 127** James Abbott McNeill Whistler, *Harmony in Yellow and Gold: The Gold Girl—Connie Gilchrist*, c. 1876–77, oil on canvas, 85 ¾ × 43 ⅛ inches. (Metropolitan Museum of Art, New York, Gift of George A Hearn, 1911, 11.32; image © The Metropolitan Museum of Art/Art Resource, New York)

Things changed slowly. When American dancers traveled abroad at the turn of the twentieth century, the performers had to contend with stereotypes—hyperbolic definitions of American character rooted in the nineteenth century and conveyed in part through the American "types" made famous in paintings such as Bingham's riverboat dancers. Decades after Bingham's heyday, American dancers—male or female, black or white—performing on the continent raised expectations of unbridled exuberance, not subtlety. London critics took care not to "mistake this character, this American 'grit' and 'bluff' for beautiful art." As late as 1908 European critics were clearly caught off guard when a degree of refinement wafted east across the Atlantic. "Coming from America," wrote an astonished critic, "the young lady [Maud Allan] might have been expected to give an exposition of high-kicking, whirlwind, and cake-walk dances. But hers is the very antithesis of this sort of terpsichorean revelry. She is perfectly artistic and sylph-like in all her movements."[4] If delicacy had supplanted sheer bravado in American dance, what might that do to perceptions about the emerging (or declining) American character? Among other changes, might it signal the breakdown of an ideology of separate spheres, which had long given men free access to the public domain while keeping women's influence largely within the walls of her drawing room? It would remain for the new generation of dancers abroad, including Maud Allan, Loïe Fuller and Isadora Duncan, to begin to break down old stereotypes and to redefine the American character through performance as something much more complex and varied than previously thought. At home, in the meantime, Americans were only beginning to grope their way out of a cultural scene shrouded in the old fog of Puritanism.

Despite the proliferation of liberating influences in American culture, well into the twentieth century dancers and visual artists constantly came up against lingering cultural inhibitions surrounding the body, a legacy often attributed to the Puritans. When a dancer such as Isadora Duncan argued that dance could access the divine through movement, engaging both body and soul, Americans of puritanically self-righteous inclinations would have none of it. As dance historian Helen Thomas explains, Duncan "maintained that the puritanical distrust of the body, which had pervaded American life, made it virtually impossible for the majority of the people to treat her Dionysian celebration of the body in dance (and life) as anything more than smut."[5]

When it came to dance, most Americans fiercely resisted high-toned philosophical considerations. Even though neopaganism had suggested one new model for pleasure-seeking through the senses, America's cultural establishment still wore its old skin of Puritan morality. Generally, Puritan tradition held that art required moral content, without which it was inherently suspect. Some cultural historians have thought that Americans discarded that requirement in the Civil War era. But many others have disagreed. In the United States of the early 1900s, cultural nationalist writers sympathetic to modernism recognized—and lamented—a residual *puritanism*, by which they meant certain sexual and emotional restrictions inimical to a desired art of genuine feeling. In that view, no healthy creative life could emerge in the new century while the old puritanical character—built on materialism, industriousness, efficiency, and the intellectual life—yet survived.

The power of Puritanism, rooted in the seventeenth century and lingering into the twentieth, embodies one of America's oldest cultural paradoxes. It is this: a deeply humanistic sense is embedded in American consciousness—people stand at the center of its history, experience, and structure, and the public entertainments pursued by its people have long been fodder for visual artists. Besides, as John Martin pointed out, several other cherished American traits—individualism, functionalism, and anti-authoritarianism—were also attributable to the nation's Puritan and frontier legacies.[6] Yet when it came to the physical touch and embrace of dance, American painters and sculptors historically retreated from that aspect of the humanistic—a love of the sensuous life. The very physicality of dance created a distinct form of discomfort.

Van Wyck Brooks and Waldo Frank were among the modernist critics who called for an embrace of intuition and the defeat of corrosive inhibition in works such as Brooks's *The Wine of the Puritans* (1908). During that decade the New York anti-vice crusader Anthony Comstock was still actively working to censor art. Objecting to bare feet and gauzy costumes, he tried to ban the dancing of Loïe Fuller, Isadora Duncan, Maud Allan, and Ruth St. Denis, all performing during the 1909–10 season in this country.[7] Attempts to censor St. Denis failed, perhaps because of artistic representations of her, such as the sculpture carved just then by Gaston Lachaise (*Ruth St. Denis*, c. 1911, Museum of Modern Art, New York). By 1910, in spite of widespread uncertainties, it seemed that some Americans had begun to regard the new dance as artistic, beautiful, and "natural"—perennial saving graces in the American censorship wars. A jubilant dance critic crowed, "The nation which has been the most pitiably enthralled by the ideals of a decadent Puritanism has become foremost in this cult of physical beauty."[8]

The antipuritanical chorus was swelled by many artists, writers, and dancers who sought to embody the sensual and the sybaritic in their work. It was as if the old "A" Hester Prynne was forced to wear in Hawthorne's *The Scarlet Letter* might be ripped from her bodice and transformed into a new symbol: A for "Art," the tool for seeing beyond the restrictive dystopia of Puritanism. Isadora Duncan sang in that antipuritanical chorus; in fact, she was one of its major soloists. More to the point, she danced it. Her antipuritanical impulses, refusal of imposed limits, and dramatic abandon made Duncan a leader in challenging the certainties of the past, especially moral constrictions. The socialist writer Max Eastman saw her as a virtually unstoppable force for the liberation of American culture: "All who have escaped in any degree from the rigidity and prissiness of our once national religion of negation owe a debt to Isadora Duncan's dancing. She rode the wave of revolt against Puritanism; she rode it, and with her fame and Dionysian raptures drove it on."[9] Especially in Europe, Duncan embodied "a miraculous vision of sensual innocence, an incarnation of a pagan America, and an evocation of the glories of ancient Greece in a single body."[10]

For dancers as well as visual artists, there were continuing collisions with the legacy of Puritanism. As Wanda Corn has pointed out, a modern American ballet called *Within the Quota*, written in the 1920s by expatriate painter Gerald Murphy, included a Puritan in black top hat and frock coat among the cast of American types, who dance out the varieties of American experience for a young Swedish immigrant, newly arrived in the port of New York. Besides the dour Puritan, the young Swede's adventures include lighthearted encounters with a dancing millionairess, a "Colored Gentleman" vaudeville stepper, a shimmy-dancing "Jazz Baby," a cowboy, and a movie star. The finale brings forth a floor full of couples dancing the latest steps. All this in the mere eighteen minutes of Murphy's contemporary ballet, danced to the jazzy music of his collaborator Cole Porter. In synoptic fashion, Murphy makes dance define (and exaggerate) American character, from Puritanism forward, for European audiences.[11]

A decade later and in a far more serious vein, Martha Graham (whose path-breaking Americanist themes we first encountered in chapter 1) chose to study the paralyzing effects of Puritanism through the fluidity of dance, an irony she engaged with deliberation. Graham believed that dance reveals the mood of the times and of a particular society. Working from that premise, she scored her first popular success by challenging the Puritan ethic in her 1938 dance drama *American Document*. In that piece, which highlights various periods from American history, a key section called the "Puritan Episode" focuses on sexual repression in that early era. A narrator recited lines from the sensuous biblical *Song of Solomon* alternating that text with passages from sermons of the Puritan divine Jonathan Edwards—this while Graham and Erick Hawkins danced an intense "Love Duet." In one of its dance passages, Hawkins stood erect and resolute, while Graham slithered around his body down to his feet. Hawkins's rigid posture reminded at least one observer of a figure from an iconic American painting, Grant Wood's *American Gothic* (1930, Art Institute of Chicago).[12] So well known was Wood's painting (then and now) that it could serve as an instant visual analog for a certain Puritan-derived rigidity in the American character, a trait in stark contrast to the sinuous desire Graham's own movements conveyed. Barbara Morgan's photograph of that love duet captures and sharpens the tensions between its competing impulses (1939; fig. 128). She searched within Graham's choreography for the power and the key gestures that would illuminate Graham's inquiry into the conflicts surrounding Puritanical sexual repression. Carefully, the photographer studied Graham and Hawkins in rehearsals and performances before setting up a studio shoot. Morgan was an extraordinary photographer: tough, contemplative, highly sensitive to light and gifted in the organization of forms. She used dramatic lighting to accentuate the black-and-white costumes, and the hidden and revealed faces to augment the inherent tensions in Graham's piece. With her small Speed Graphic 4-by-5 camera, she moved about like a dancer herself, producing "artistic treatments" rather than mere publicity photographs.

During the six years of their collaboration, Graham and Morgan worked to position dance in the landscape of history, using it to enlarge an audience's historical awareness while illuminating particular social issues. Unabashedly, Graham wanted to help free Americans from the constraints of Puritanism, and her "Puritan Episode" shone a bright light on what she saw as a repressive

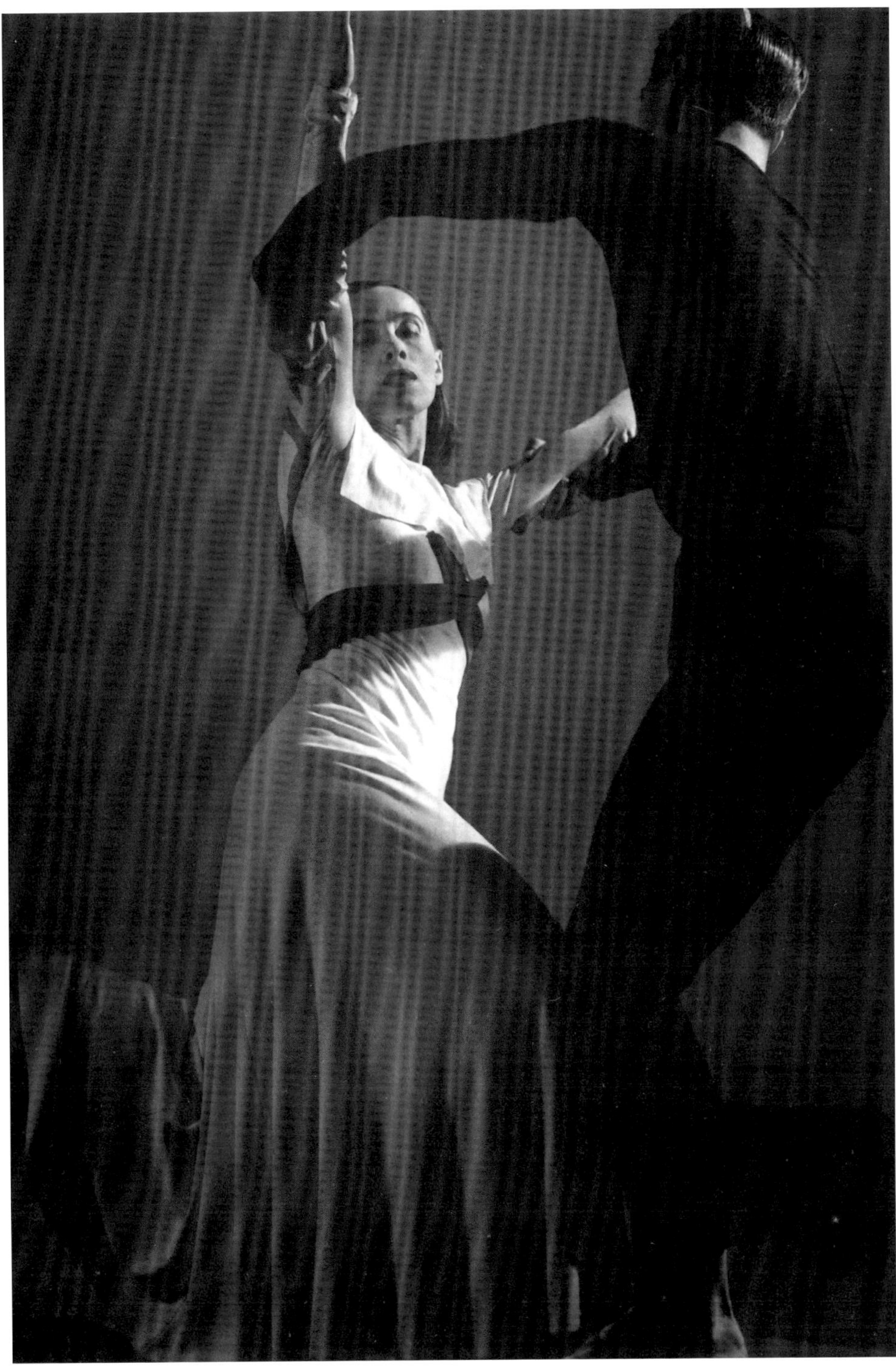

**Figure 128** Barbara Morgan, *Martha Graham and Erick Hawkins, Puritan Love Duet*, from *American Document*, 1939, silver gelatin print. (© Barbara Morgan, The Barbara Morgan Archive)

legacy. At the same time, the project suited her long-term goal of providing models for a modern avant-garde culture, one that turned outworn social convention on its head.

Looking back on the period, museum director Lloyd Goodrich summed up the liberating impulse at work among American modernists:

> In those pioneer days, modern art was not only a revolution in artistic language, it was a visual expression of a new spirit, challenging the outworn Puritanism of established American culture. It was a freeing of emotional expression from deadening inhibitions. It was a return to the deep physical and sensuous springs of being, to the joy of life.[13]

## Dance and the Modern Body: New Approaches to Identity and Visual Representation

If every historical period reinvents the muse in its own image, the twentieth century lost no time in harnessing a reborn Terpsichore to a whole array of issues surrounding cultural change in America. As part of a generational revolt expressed in literature, politics, science, and all the arts, modern dance conspired to overturn the certainties of the past and to advance new possibilities on all fronts. Nobody seemed certain where the new energies would lead, only that the arts promised powerful, if potentially subversive, cultural directions. A Saint Louis journalist in 1916 expressed a cautious optimism about the new dance, lumping it together with visual art and literature:

> Through all of that new artistic movement which generally presents itself as cubism, futurism, Max Reinhardt scenery, frank sex plays, symbolistic poetry and not least the art of dancing as diversely shown by Isadora Duncan, Ruth St. Denis and the Russians, there is a strong reach out for new truths.[14]

One of modernism's chief aims, according to the Viennese architect Otto Wagner, was "to show modern man his true face." In a sense, one sees dance producing a variant of that goal: the possibility of showing modern humanity its true *body*—a modern body reconfigured artistically and re-choreographed to reveal new expressive potential.

In the United States, various cultural threads were woven into the complex web of ideas surrounding the modern body. On one hand there was a widespread sense that the nineteenth century's supposed marriage of material and spiritual progress remained unconsummated. Americans saw much historical evidence that humanity's history of "progress" was far from a sustained linear trajectory, but instead looked more like cyclical processes of development and decline. Growing among American cultural critics at the turn of the century was a consequent disillusionment with capitalism's corrosive impact on community, family, craft, faith, and—in the excesses inherent within urban life—on physical well-being itself.[15]

In the minds of many Americans, well-being grew out of a life lived intensively, wrapping morality together with radiant physical and mental health. The late nineteenth century saw a rising interest in physical culture augmented by improved hygiene and notions of manly virtue woven together with patriotic concerns. The American cult of the strenuous life was preached by Theodore Roosevelt, who argued that in order to combat physical decline, much of life should be spent outdoors, where the body could not only move, but do so in fresh air and sunlight. Motion itself became a kind of virtue, supported by the larger beneficence of the healthful outdoors. Frederick Lewis Allen noted the proliferation of "schools of rhythm, hygiene, physical culture and correlated arts prancing among the sand dunes," a recasting of Rooseveltian "manly virtue" into a feminized realm.[16] Dance could indeed fit neatly into this vision of an active life, part of an evolving blueprint for a more liberated and enlightened society. Writes one dance historian, "By 1916 dance meant something very substantial to Americans. . . . Physical culture enthusiasts—the women who made their families take the fresh air, the men who did exercises—connected artistic dance to an ideal state of the body and therefore the soul."[17]

As a carrier of cultural change—even revolt—dance inevitably became a politics of the body. Sometimes it signaled broad change, sometimes a focused, gendered one. Early in the twentieth century, especially among women, dancing was a synthesis of two realms of self-expression, the physical and the artistic. It was an antidote to the boredom of factory and office work, which had replaced American women's former physical exhaustion from farm work. Floyd Dell, editor of the radical *Masses*, sited much social change in the body of woman: "It is to the body that one looks for the Magna Carta of feminism." And no one better embodied that spirit than Isadora Duncan, named by Dell's colleague Max Eastman as "the extreme outpost of the movement for woman's emancipation."[18]

## Duncan's Revolutions: Body, Movement, Politics

Although later critics have debated whether Duncan (widely recognized along with Maud Allan, Ruth St. Denis, and a few others as the "founding mothers" of modern dance) was producing work that undercut the period's gender norms, many in her own era had no doubts.[19] Unquestionably, Duncan was a profoundly revolutionary spirit, who proclaimed and practiced a new aesthetic of liberation. She danced always in the first person singular, with movements that were intimate, revealing, and determinedly "natural." She claimed among the far-flung sources for her dance the art of ancient Greece and the relentless waves breaking on California beaches. While preparing an essay called "The Dancer and Nature" she mused on women's movements in nature: "I've been writing about dance waves—sound waves—light waves—all the *same*."[20] Within the rhythms of nature she tried to locate the wellsprings of modern movement: "For hours I could stand quite still," she wrote, "my two hands folded between my breasts, covering the solar plexus. I was seeking and finally discovered the central spring of all movement, the creator of motor power, the unity from which all diversities of movement are born, the mirror of vision for the creation of the dance."[21]

In her efforts to provide a bridge between nature and "natural" movement, Duncan drew from longstanding philosophical obsessions. Enlightenment thinkers, at the dawn of the early modern era, conceived of dance as a universal medium of communication through the "natural" movements of the body, uncorrupted by constructed language. Since then, dance had been called upon repeatedly to figure forth the notion of natural movement, of liberated and authentic bodies.

One of Duncan's great sources of inspiration was the German idealist philosopher Friedrich Nietzsche. In his *Thus Spake Zarathustra* (1883), Nietzsche wrote famously, "I would believe only in a god who could dance. . . . Now I am light, now I fly, now I see myself beneath myself, now a god dances through me."[22] It was Nietzsche who formulated the modern understanding of a Dionysian–Apollonian divide within the human soul. On one hand, he saw a rational, disciplined Apollonian component based on the Greek god of light, music, and truth. On the other side, Nietzsche found a Dionysian delight in movement, a "strong, free, joyous action," a mood ascendant in Duncan's era, when visual artists often expressed the Dionysian experience by way of rich color, calling up depths of emotional or instinctual meaning.[23] Duncan herself said, "One can dance in two ways: 1. One can penetrate the spirit of Dance: to dance the thing itself, Dionysus. 2. One can contemplate the spirit of Dance and dance like someone who would be telling its story, Apollo."[24] As photographer Edward Steichen later recalled, "Her whole art of dancing was inspired by the Greek architectural friezes and the drawings on Greek vases. She was part of Greece, and she took Greece as a part of herself." Yet Steichen's own photographs of Duncan, made in 1920 at the Parthenon in Athens, depart radically from the Apollonian restraint of his 1903 studio photograph of her to convey a much more passionate, Dionysian flavor. Setting up his camera far enough away to capture the whole temple wall, Steichen posed Duncan against the sky visible between columns: "The idea," he recalled, "was that she was to do her most beautiful single gesture, the slow raising of her arms until they seemed to encompass the whole sky. She stood there for perhaps fifteen minutes, saying, 'Edward, I can't. I can't do it. I can't do it here.' But finally, after several tries, I saw the arms going up."[25] Steichen, who knew the dancer intimately, was able to capture on film an intensity distinctly Dionysian in character. His are perhaps the most artistic of any photographs ever made of Duncan (1921; fig. 129).

Duncan and other proto-modernists found through Nietzsche that human existence embodies a perennial tension between the stultifying weight of convention and the need to cast off that personal and collective inheritance to lose oneself completely in the transcendent moment, a state she found especially congenial to artists, musicians, and dancers. In Nietzsche's frame of mind, humanity desperately needed access to the tissue of connections between action and feeling, between intellect and the mythmaking powers present within every person. Dance, with its capacity to suggest the expansive range of human emotion and intellect, was seen as particularly suited to such explorations.

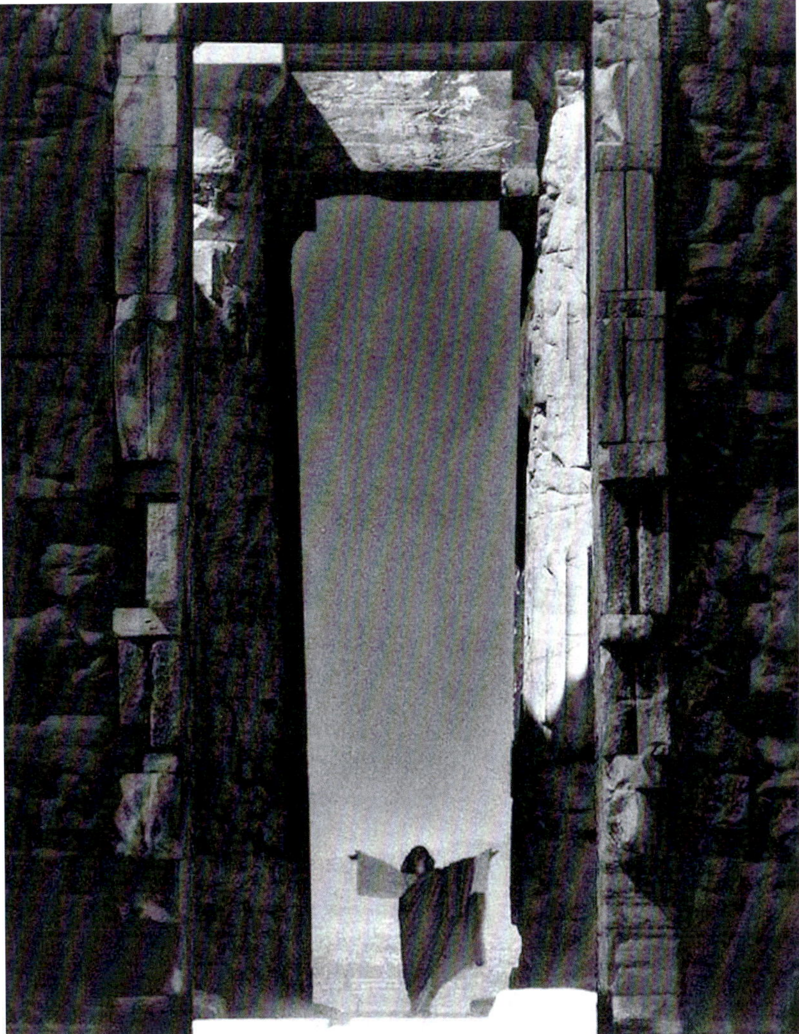

**Figure 129** Edward Steichen, *Isadora Duncan at the Portals of the Parthenon,* 1921, gelatin silver print, 13 ½ × 10 ¾ inches. (private collection)

Nietzsche also envisioned modern humanity as an evolutionary "bridge" to the future, specifically to a perfected "superman."[26] To many, Isadora Duncan personified that bridge—between a decadent Old World and a vital New one. Critic Janet Flanner credited Duncan with "fusing Zeitgeists."[27] If bridges were to be built between past and future, they must carry on them the traffic of change. Lurching and halting, the journey was often a bumpy one, creating critical and popular discomforts. Duncan's reputation as an advocate of the free, natural body seemed connected, in the minds of many, to her heretical views on love and marriage. In Germany, while dancing for a summer at the Wagnerian Bayreuth Festival (1904), she knowingly played the libertine before shocked visitors, whom she received lying on a sofa in a villa filled, as she described it, with rose-colored lamps and many low couches. There was not a proper chair in sight.

"The village people considered it a veritable witches' house, and described our innocent revels as 'terrible orgies,'" she recalled. In Duncan's mind, a crusade against convention was called for: "So here I was, a perfect pagan to all, fighting the Philistines."[28]

Onstage, what Duncan was fighting was nothing less than the venerable legacy of classical ballet, still the prevailing vocabulary of dance. In her mind the ballet represented all that was unnatural in dance. Performed on a proscenium stage, it features slender, lifted, extended bodies, small heads, and fully revealed legs. In seemingly weightless lifts and carries, balletic bodies come into frequent contact. "So distinctive is the 'look' of ballet," writes one analyst, "that it is probably safe to say that ballet dances graphically rendered by silhouettes would never be mistaken for anything else."[29]

Isadora Duncan was among those who lambasted ballet as antipathetic to the modern world, as well as to the modern body. "The real American type can never be a ballet dancer," she argued. "The legs are too long, the body too supple, and the spirit too free for this school of affected grace and toe-walking."[30] The contrast, explained Duncan, was like that between the "false" and the "true":

> The true dance is appropriate to the most beautiful human form; the false dance is the opposite of this definition—that is, that movement which conforms to a deformed human body. First, draw me the form of a woman as it is in Nature, and now draw me the form of a woman in a modern corset and the satin slippers used by our modern dancers. To the first all the rhythmic movements that run through Nature would be possible. . . . To the second figure these movements would be impossible on account of the rhythm being broken and stopped at the extremities.[31]

Duncan's own dynamic physicality, with its unprecedented freedom, drew the curious as well as the converted to her. Artists marveled at her forward-arched or backward-swept torso, and at the way expressive movement seemed to flow from the center through her whole body. Unlike ballet movement, in which limbs often moved as peripheral and separate entities, Duncan's movement incorporated her whole form. Most of all, perhaps, artists took note of her bare feet, which—above all else—testified to the "natural" form of her steps. The toe shoe, formerly ubiquitous in European theatrical dance, sculpted the foot into an elongated crescent, while Duncan's bare foot (or the soft slippers or sandals she sometimes wore) exposed the foot's natural instep and allowed the foot to grip the floor firmly and to rise with flexible strength.

Duncan's arm movements were also profoundly new, and were widely copied. Choreographer Michel Fokine, as soon as he saw Duncan dance in 1904, began to integrate her broad, asymmetrical *port de bras* into his dances. And Anna Pavlova told interviewers that her fluid arm movements in *The Dying Swan* came from Duncan. It is hard to overstate the influence of Duncan's unorthodoxy on modern dance; it changed forever the entrenched vision of dancing. Soon after her first appearances in Saint Petersburg in 1904–5, Fokine's choreography for the women of the Russian Ballet began to incorporate the new "natural," non-balletic bodies, freed from corsets as well as toe shoes. The flowing draperies of the ancient Greeks, seen in sculpture and vase painting, were one source of Duncan's costuming. Another was the dress reform movement that, especially in her native California, owed a debt to the lingering influence of the British Pre-Raphaelite painters and their aesthetic of the natural.[32]

Alain Corbin said that when Duncan performed in Paris, "what her dancing really symbolized was the freedom to experience the body as something no longer external to the self."[33] And the writer Colette, who saw everything on Parisian stages, observed French women admiring Duncan, whom she called this "little naked creature in her veils." What astounded her female audience most was that the dancer performed unbound and unfettered, unlike themselves, who were still encased in corsets extending from armpit to knee. But Colette believed that most of the women watching Duncan were not ready for much freedom—physical or social—but desired, in fact, to remain bound. They were not prepared to contemplate the bombshell issues Duncan embodied, those involving feminism and sexual power. Added Colette, "I muse on how peculiar women are, watching all these ladies who applauded Isadora Duncan . . . let us not fool ourselves! They acclaim her but they don't envy her. They salute her at a distance, and they contemplate her, but as an escapee—not as a liberator."[34]

If the Parisian public had trouble with Duncan's radical ideas about the liberated body, their confusion and dismay were shared by Americans. Besides her radical approach to costume and movement, Duncan simultaneously dismantled old expectations about the dancer's use of onstage space and light. While that added to Duncan's appeal for many visual artists, most American critics, to say nothing of the public, were both uninformed and distinctly uncurious about the mechanisms and constructs of their own solo dancers. They seemed unable even to discern whether Duncan was classical (in some sense) or modern. As one dance historian explains,

> In America people failed to grasp that a dance was a construct in space and time, involving principles of composition as palpable as those in painting or sculpture. No one ever asked Isadora Duncan how she arranged the movements she danced with such apparent artlessness on the stage, or even where she got them. The mere fact that she and other dancers were moving through space and light, setting in motion poses resembling those of figures in classical paintings and sculptures, made the public too giddy to examine the art. Those figures were distant and mythological, and appropriately half-dressed. The dancers who imitated them were disturbingly alive in the here and now.[35]

To lead her through the miasma of cultural change and to offer some familiar points of reference to skeptical Americans, Duncan invoked the individualism of America's best-loved poet. "I have discovered," she announced, "the dance that is worthy of the poems of Walt Whitman. I am indeed the spiritual daughter of Walt Whitman." She particularly invoked his belief in self, his cultivation of spontaneous simplicity, and his refusal of imposed limits.[36] Whitman, whose gospel of nature and redeemed sensuality she devoured, infused Duncan with new reverence for the artistic aspects of every human soul. "I Hear America Singing," Whitman had proclaimed, expressing his ecstatic vision of a people attuned to the rhythms of their land. Borrowing Whitman's notion, Duncan hoped to enlist America's composers to write the great music to which a nation could dance. Following his lead, she titled her own 1927 broadside "I See America Dancing." In it, she declared that a new, modern body type, quintessentially American, required fresh dance forms. "Long-legged strong boys and girls will dance to this music in a striking upward tremendous mounting, powerful mounting above the pyramids of Egypt, beyond the Parthenon of Greece, an expression of Beauty and Strength such as no civilization has ever known. That will be America dancing."[37] Arthur B. Davies, whose work we have already encountered in two previous chapters, was a close follower of modern dance in general and Duncan in particular. According to his contemporaries, Davies made many superb drawings of Duncan, but most were destroyed in a fire in the artist's studio.[38] Still, her inspiration lingers in such works as Davies's *Hylas and the Nymphs* (c. 1911, New Britain Museum of American Art, New Britain, Conn.). In his *Dance—Uplift* (c. 1920–28, Metropolitan Museum of Art, New York), Davies adapted Duncan's sensuous, dreamily choreographed movements to the firmly drawn figures in his ethereal landscapes.

For her part, Duncan clung to her conviction, evident as early as her efforts (c. 1900) to enact Botticelli's Renaissance painting *Primavera*, that visual art and dance, form and movement, were inseparable partners. Each could nourish and reinvigorate the other. Duncan challenged American women, especially, to "learn beauty of form and movement through the dance. . . . With the movement of her body she shall find the secret of perfect proportion of line and curve. The art of the dance she will hold as a great well-spring of new life for sculpture, painting and architecture."[39]

## Duncan and the Dancing Child

Duncan's new dance would spring from the American earth, fertilized by classical principles of beauty, motion, and form. Its youthful practitioners would be at the center of her vision, children educated through the medium of dance. The goal was not intended to train dancers for the stage, but rather to enrich education through the arts. "Only that education is right which includes the dance," insisted Duncan.[40] She started a succession of schools with this mission, near Berlin, in Switzerland, in New York during years of World War I, and in Moscow after the Russian Revolution. If her schools fostered swarms of dilettantes, perhaps it was because her particular art could not be codified. Lessons at the Duncan Schools were unconventional, to say the least. She led by inspiration, hoping to instill in her pupils knowledge of the self while encouraging the imagination. Students were surrounded by the visual arts: reproductions of dancers on Greek vases, of small Tanagra or Boetian figurines, of dancing children by Donatello and Gainsborough. Images of dancing children, reasoned Duncan, meant "the real children of my school, moving and dancing in the midst of these forms, would surely grow to resemble them, to reflect unconsciously, in their movements and their faces, a little of the joy and the same childlike grace."[41] But Duncan also provided more active lessons in natural movement. Besides living among visual representations of dance, she sent the students out armed with sketchbooks. "Few of us had any knowledge of drawing or any ability," remembered one former student. "Now I understand that sketching was just a ruse to get us to concentrate on natural movement. Trees and grasses, bending in the wind carry a message for every dancer. If she is observant, and even if she isn't, the rhythm and pulse of nature are bound to affect her."[42]

Clearly, Duncan believed that the spontaneity of a child's dance could express an unbroken connection to nature. Her 1906 essay "A Child Dancing" was inspired by seeing her young niece dancing on the beach. "She dances," wrote Duncan, "because she is full of the joy of life. She dances because the waves are dancing before her eyes, because the winds are dancing, because she can feel the rhythm of the dance throughout the whole of nature."[43] The notion of children as models of free, spontaneous creativity was widespread in Duncan's day.[44] But the dancing child was not always portrayed as joyous. John Ruskin, William Butler Yeats, J. M. Barrie and many others saw the darker, richer, artistic possibilities of youthful dance buried within folklore, fantasy, and fairy tales.[45] Visual artists too saw the more ominous portents in dancing children. Duncan's joyous dancing niece has a tragic counterpart who appears in Arthur B. Davies's *Dancing Children* (1902, Brooklyn Museum of Art). In this moody painting, children dance gracefully in a wooded glade while one (meant to symbolize the artist's late niece) is led away into death. A child's life, Davies seems to convey, is not all merriment, nor is it consummate innocence. The critic Sadakichi Hartmann, writing of Davies, noted that "the thought which underlies all his work is to render childhood (the conventional emblem of purity) more sensuous," a task in keeping with the era's dawning understanding of the complex— even sexual, in Freud's interpretation—nature of children's lives.

That cultural complexity was further explored in a 1916 *Vanity Fair* article about the celebrated child dancer Virginia Myers, one of a series monthly aesthetic-dance-photography features in the magazine. Critic Hutchins Hapgood saw young Virginia as a representative of a childhood exuberance and freedom potentially imperiled by conservative authorities. She possessed a life force that, however vital, was also fragile and, without encouragement, subject to cruel extinction. In that view female children, especially dancing ones, took on the role of cultural canaries, whose survival seemed vaguely necessary to the cultural health of the whole nation.

The expectation of a new, even revolutionary era for America's art and its children kept dance linked with the cultural avant-garde. Duncan's highly visible linkage of the visual arts to dance and education brought her praise from a number of visual artists. In *Dionysion*, a publication of the Committee to Further the Work of Isadora Duncan, Robert Henri wrote of the beneficial effect of Duncan's teaching on children:

> Our hope in America for a great art and a great life depends upon the free development of our youth. . . . Children must be free. . . . We have commenced to give them free bodies, but we are still disciplining their spirits. . . . I was tremendously impressed one day in Isadora Duncan's Studio, by the look in the faces of the children. As they passed me in the dance I saw great dignity, balance, ease. . . . The true teacher is one who awaits with deep interest the first sign of the birth of the new spirit, seeing in every child a new prophet.[46]

Stepping into an imaginary circle of child-inspired creativity, writers and visual artists danced out their era's most utopian dreams. In *Exile's Return*, his important summation of the 1920s, Malcolm Cowley detected some widely accepted beliefs, the first of which was "salvation by the child," the notion that the young, allowed to flourish naturally, could remake the world through creative self-expression.

As I have already argued, dance—better than most mediums—seemed to express the dream of a modern liberated body, especially the female body. More than anyone else, Isadora Duncan embodied those ideals, and visual artists saluted her creativity with their own. While he did not specifically represent Duncan in visual form, Wassily Kandinsky, in addition to sharing her passion for children's creativity, praised Duncan for her understandings of the "primitive" sources of both modern art and dance. For Kandinsky, a synthesis of the arts held the potential for recapturing some primitive unity and for expressing singularly powerful sensory effects. And dance was thought to possess a privileged access to the primitive. Remember that Kandinsky had written, "The origin of dancing is probably purely sexual. In folk dances we still see this element plainly. The later development of dancing as a religious ceremony joins itself to the preceding [sexual] element and the two together take artistic form and emerge as the ballet."[47] Duncan's unique contribution, according to Kandinsky, was this: "Isadora Duncan has forged a link between the Greek dancing and that of the future. In this she is working on parallel lines to the painters who are looking for inspiration from the primitives. . . . The new dancing is being evolved as . . . the only means of giving in terms of time and space the real inner meaning of motion."[48]

Among those visual artists who did represent Duncan was Auguste Rodin, who linked her artistry to that of the sculptor: "It may be said of Isadora Duncan," noted Rodin, "that she attains sculpture and emotion effortlessly. . . . Suppleness, emotion, these high qualities, the soul of the dance, are her complete and sovereign art."[49] As noted earlier, Rodin drew and sculpted many dancers, but none challenged him more than Duncan. He sketched or drew her from memory, usually in repose, rarely in motion (*Isadora Duncan Dancing*, n.d. Georgia Museum of Art, Athens, Ga.). This emphasis he regretted later, despite his belief "that any attempt to seize one moment alone in progression was fatal to the illusion of movement."[50] For her part, just receiving the attention of Rodin—a sculptor widely acknowledged as among the greatest artists of his era—intimidated the

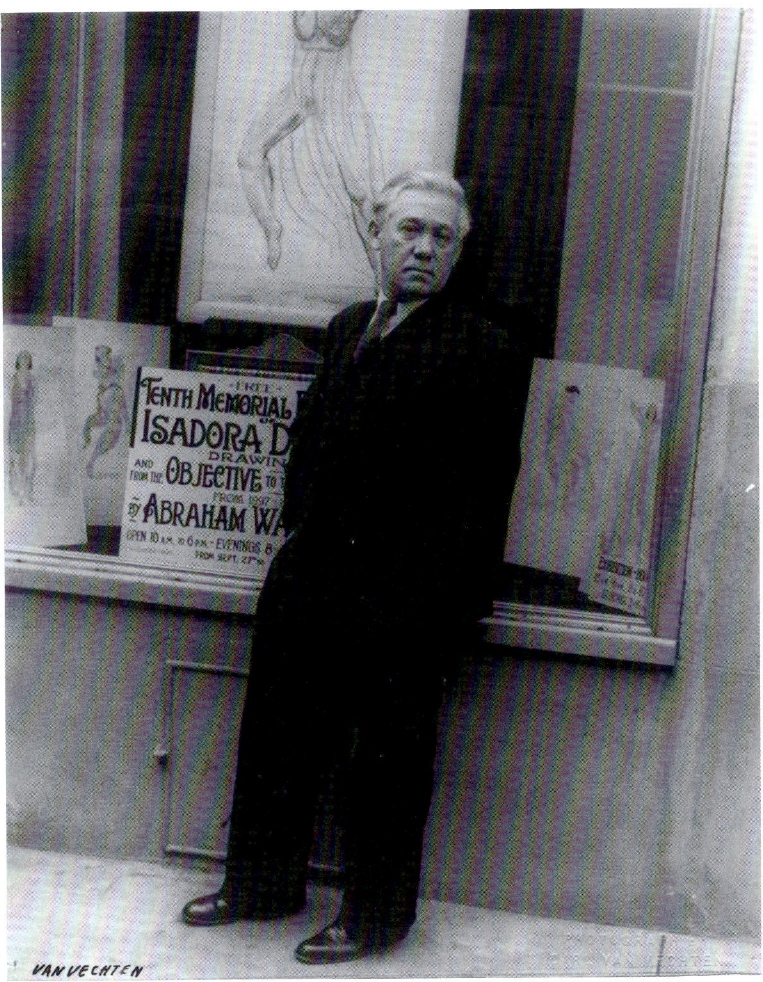



Figure 130 Carl Van Vechten, photograph of Abraham Walkowitz standing outside of the Isadora Duncan Memorial at the Shacht Gallery, 1931.
(from Abraham Walkowitz Papers, Archives of American Art, Smithsonian
Institution)

young Isadora, who likened him to the "very force of nature," a presence "too
great for me."[51]

Less reluctant than Rodin to bring Duncan's liberated movement to life
was Abraham Walkowitz (1878–1965). Russian-born Walkowitz met Duncan
at Rodin's studio in Paris and began a decades-long documentation, seemingly
of her every dance movement. Was ever an artist so riveted by the person and
performance of a dancer? Walkowitz (fig. 130) ultimately made thousands of
paintings and drawings of her (estimates range from five to eight thousand,
sold initially by the artist on New York's sidewalks for as little as five cents).
"I have done more Isadora Duncans than I have hair on my head," admitted
Walkowitz.[52] Of varying degrees of figural representation, some approach pure

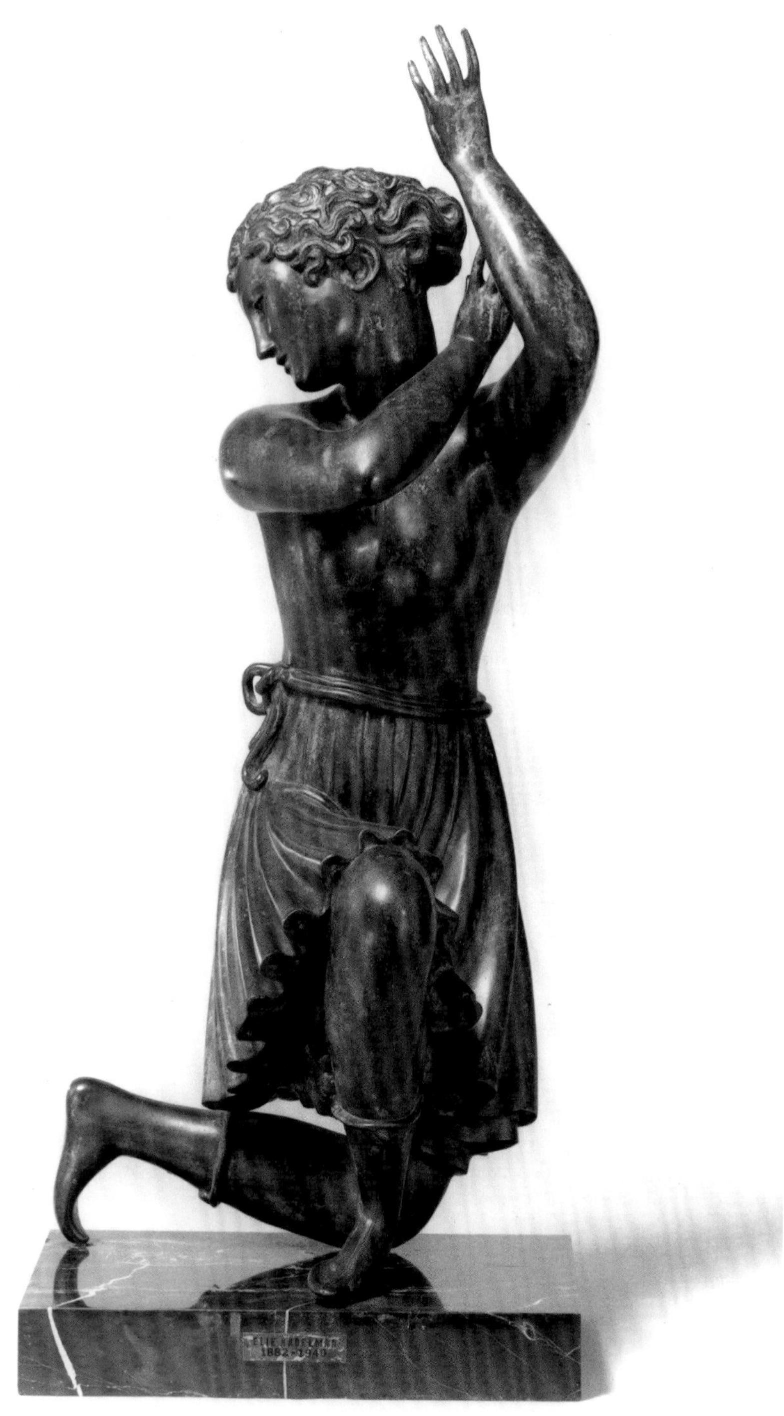

Figure 131 Elie Nadelman, *Dancing Figure [Kneeling Dancer]*, c. 1916–18, bronze on marble base, 31 ⅝ × 13 ⅞ × 11 ⅞ inches. (Smithsonian American Art Museum, Gift of Countess Helen Naselli in memory of Harry Wardman, 1972.168)

curvilinear abstraction, as when Walkowitz collapses her crouching shape into rhyming curves. For her part, Duncan would say to Walkowitz, perhaps prophetically, "You have written my biography in lines without words, I can pass on."[53] Here Duncan points to two unaccustomed roles for the visual artist, as biographer and amanuensis. Walkowitz, in his grand, decades-long attempt to "write down" or record Duncan, suggests the widespread fascination that surrounded her person and her movement. As her adopted daughter, the dancer Marie Theresa, wrote, "Sculptors and painters blessed her for the slightest bend of her head. She answered their searching eyes for dynamic line, contour, massive form, balance and statuesque completeness."[54] Walkowitz's images of Duncan capture that massive sense of force through bold, assertive line. When looked at in groups of images, what Walkowitz's synoptic portrait of Duncan ultimately reveals is that her dances were choreographed, not improvised; that they possessed patterns, gestures, and structure informed both by gravity and by naturally flowing movement.

Sculptor Elie Nadelman, encountered earlier as an obsessive observer of social dance, was moved as well by almost any kind of theatrical dancing—not only for authentic reproductions of historic movement styles, but for authentically plastic forms deriving from dance. His work paralleled Duncan's in their revolutionary embrace of both the ancient and the modern. Nadelman himself was a collector of Tanagrine fragments, owned dozens of books about antique figurines, and created a huge repertoire of plaster figures in the 1920s, most of them related to the dance. In that spirit, and perhaps in homage to Duncan, he turned (like her) to Greek art of the Praxitelean period. His bronze *Dancing Figure [Kneeling Dancer]* (c. 1916–18; fig. 131) is highly classical in demeanor and appearance, with the dancer's hair, profile, and draperies presented with an elegantly incised linear rhythm. Yet another Nadelman *Dancer,* reproduced in *The Dial* magazine in the 1920s, shows the artist moving away from classical restraint to a more Hellenistically inspired form. This dancer's voluptuous body sways and bends much more like a draped Tanagra figurine, to which artists such as Rodin had compared both Loïe Fuller and Duncan.[55] It is also a type Nadelman could have seen among the Tanagrine sculptures in the collections of the Metropolitan Museum of Art in New York. Nadelman's arbitrary, stylized grace was eminently suited to dance figures, whether in classically derived pieces or in his alternative, folk-art inspired mode.

As Duncan's star blazed across the cultural firmament, she trailed behind her yet another ntotion that would ignite audiences and artists in the United States—the idea that modern dance, along with modern art, functioned as revolutionary speech. War and revolution were simultaneously old and eerily current topics in the Armory Show era. Once hostilities broke out in Europe in 1914, Henri Rousseau's *Le Centenaire de l'indépendence* (1892, Getty Museum, Los Angeles), a poetic allegory in paint, would gain renewed currency in the person of Duncan. She created a transatlantic tour de force out of the French national anthem, the *Marseillaise,* when she performed it in 1915 at the Metropolitan Opera in New York. After long residence in France, Duncan sent her dance students, including the favored "Isadorables," to wait out the war in the safety of

New York. She soon joined them there, eager to express through dance her solidarity with the cause of French freedom and to rally American sympathy for her adopted country. Of her performance, she later wrote, "It was a call to the boys of America to rise and protect the highest civilisation of our epoch, that culture which has come to the world through France."[56]

Whether or not she knew Rousseau's *Le Centenaire* (discussed below), Duncan was clearly inspired by other French visual artists—by Delacroix (whose *Liberty* she evoked by baring her breast in performance *à la Marianne*), and by François Rude's sculpted *Marseillaise* (1833–36) on the Arc de Triomphe, the "Genius of War" exhorting the nation to battle. Strolling through one of the Right Bank's cultural districts, neither Duncan nor any other visitor to Paris would miss another public monument celebrating the dance: Jean-Baptiste Carpeaux's sculpture group *Spirit of the Dance (La Danse)* (c. 1867–69; fig. 132) on the facade of Charles Garnier's Second Empire neo-Baroque opera house. Dance's old history as domain of the unfettered emotion surfaced noisily in French public art in 1869, when Carpeaux's monumental figure group was installed. Parisians, long numbed by frozen academic allegory, were unprepared for Carpeaux's exuberant nude dancers. They too were allegorical, but fired with such energy and freedom that they threatened an unsettling thaw. The nude bacchantes, with a leering satyr in the background, dance around an androgynous winged "genius" of the dance. Upon its unveiling, scandal erupted in the salons and streets of Paris. A typical critic saw in Carpeaux's figures "The reek of wine and vice . . . their lascivious postures and cynical expressions provoke the beholders," concluding that the sculpture was "an insult to public morality."[57] Isadora Duncan, no stranger to scandal, may have had the wanton eroticism of the sculpture in mind years later when she frolicked wildly one night along the avenue de l'Opéra, described by an observer as looking exactly like Carpeaux's genius of the dance.

Compared to that impromptu street dance, Duncan's New York performances of the *Marseillaise* were far more somber, though no less exciting. Audiences thrilled to her upraised arms, extended in a broad gesture as if summoning the world to victory. The American critic Carl Van Vechten described the passion of Isadora's *Marseillaise* in a New York performance: "In a robe the color of blood she stands enfolded; she sees the enemy advance; she feels the enemy as it grasps her by the throat; she kisses her flag; she tastes blood; she is all but crushed under the weight of the attack; and then she rises triumphant with the terrible cry, *Aux armes citoyens*."[58] Duncan's dramatic fusion of politics, dance and powerful prototypes from the visual arts brought audiences everywhere to their feet; often, they climbed on their chairs and cheered. Carl Van Vechten wrote to Gertrude Stein of the war fever Duncan ignited in New York: "I tell you she drives 'em mad. The recruiting stations are full of her converts."[59]

By that time, Duncan believed firmly that dance could serve as an evolving blueprint for a more liberated and enlightened society. Her call for vengeance against tyrants, invaluable as wartime propaganda, made both dance and dancer immortal. Agnes de Mille, later famous herself as dancer and choreographer, remembered the climax of Duncan's epochal *Marseillaise*. Throwing the crimson robe over her shoulder, Duncan "stamped to the footlights and raised her arms

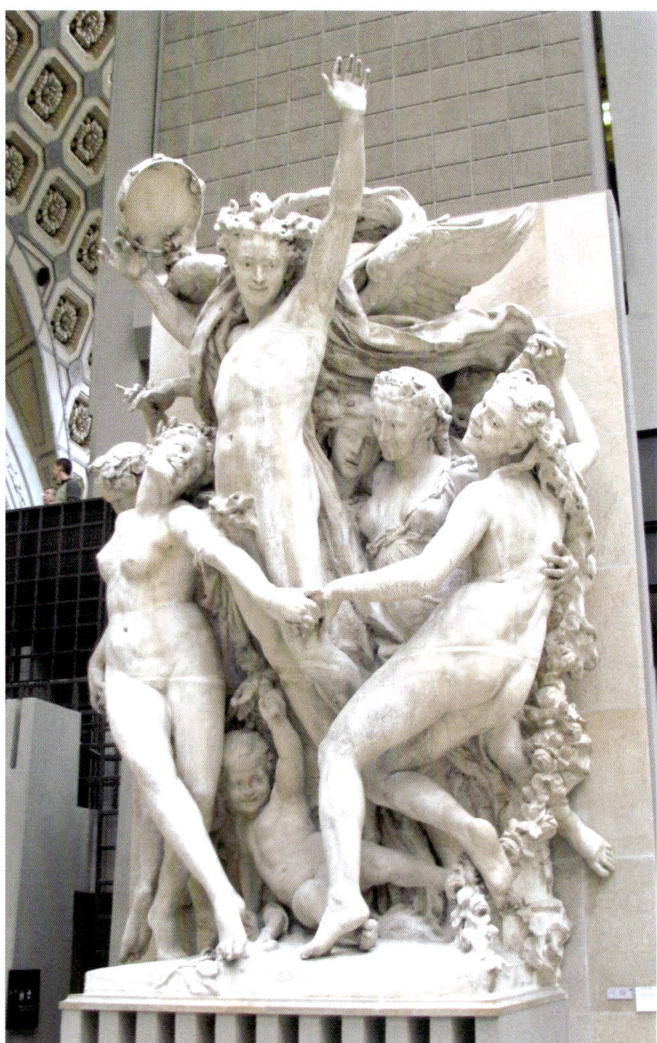

Figure 132 Jean-Baptiste Carpeaux, *Spirit of the Dance*, c. 1867–69, h. 13 feet 9 ⅛ inches. (original in Musée d'Orsay, Paris)

in the great Duncan salute. . . . This was heroic and I never forgot it. No one who saw Isadora ever forgot her."[60] By allying her performance with deeply imprinted images of revolution in politics and the visual arts, Duncan's dance took on a gravitas that eluded most staged efforts of any kind.

Visual artists were similarly struck by both the power and the poetry of Duncan's *Marseillaise*. Abraham Walkowitz, a Duncan acolyte since 1906, now drew her pausing as if in mid-march, chin and left knee lifted smartly, all drama and militancy. While not labeled as her *Marseillaise*, Walkowitz's watercolors of the subject can be interpreted confidently because of the blood-red tunic she wears and her poses in the characteristic mode she invented for the *Marseillaise* (c. 1916; fig. 133).

Arnold Genthe photographed Duncan in all the majesty of the climactic moment of the *Marseillaise*. German-born Genthe had started his career by making what he called "natural photographs" of San Francisco's Chinatown and its

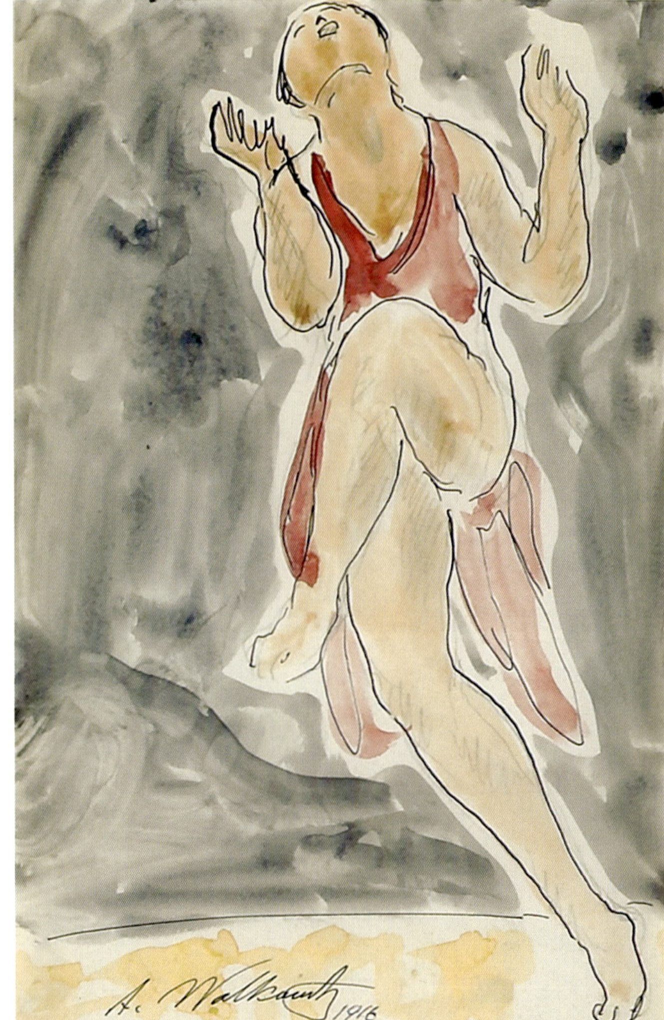

**Figure 133** Abraham Walkowitz, *Isadora Duncan Dancing*, c. 1916, ink and water-color on paper, 10 ¾ × 6 ¾ inches. (collection of Dr. Lawrence Lazarus)

1906 earthquake.[61] In 1910, with his move to New York, Genthe began to photograph many famous persons. He focused his lens on Duncan many times while she was in New York, later publishing a portfolio of twenty-four photographs of her.[62] As he wrote, "[Duncan] had always refused to have photographs made in dance poses. But when she discovered that it was possible to take pictures while she was in motion, she was eager to collaborate."[63] In Duncan, Genthe found a certain mythic quality. For her part, the dancer marveled at the psychological depth Genthe captured with his camera; if Walkowitz had captured every aspect of her physical self in his drawings, Genthe had found something deeper. "[Genthe] has taken many pictures of me," wrote Duncan in her autobiography, "which are not representations of my physical being, but representations of conditions of my soul, and one of them is my very soul indeed" (c. 1915–18; fig. 134).[64]

On both sides of the Atlantic Duncan's commanding presence continued to draw artists like moths to a flame. Poet Carl Sandburg, in fact, called Duncan

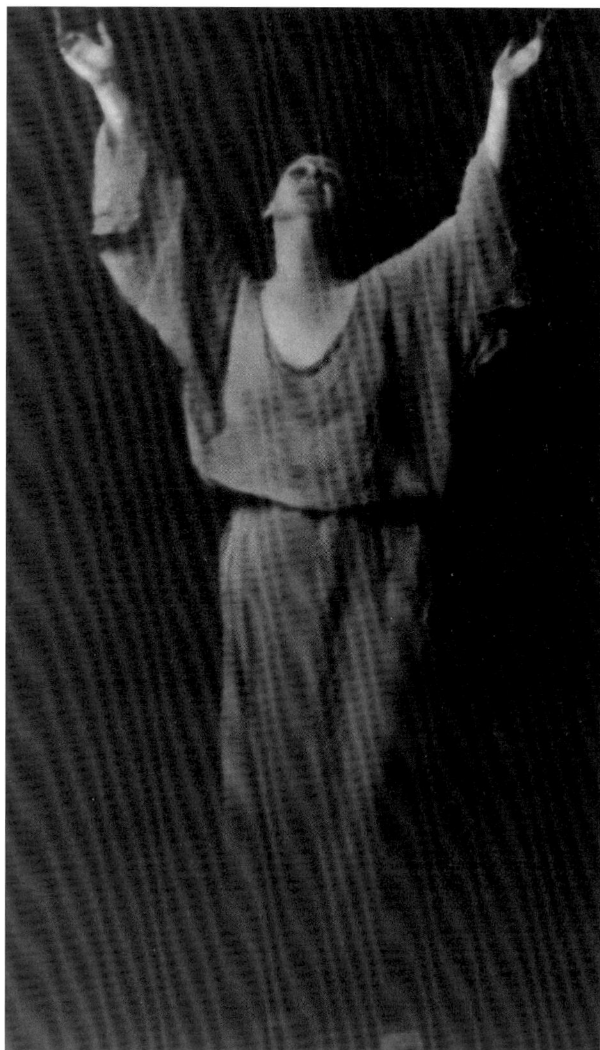

Figure 134 Arnold Genthe, *Isadora Duncan Dancing*, c. 1915–18, gelatin silver print. (photo courtesy Library of Congress, LC G422-7-9885)

"a flame sheath of flesh made for dancing."[65] One aspect of the attraction was that she made her creativity seem simultaneously difficult and effortless, perplexing and intriguing even the most sophisticated Duncan-watchers. Another of the talented American painters who encountered Duncan in Paris was Ernest Blumenschein (1874–1960), who matched his technique to hers, using loose, freely brushed strokes to suggest rapidity in her forward-striding movements (c. 1904; fig. 135). Blumenschein, who spent much time in Paris both before and after the turn of the century, studied there in 1902–8. Although his gouache is labeled, perhaps retrospectively, *Isadora Duncan, Paris Opera, about 1900*, it might well represent her 1904 premiere of Beethoven's *Seventh Symphony* at the Trocadero Museum, a role she would repeat in New York a few years later.

In a more abstract vein, Morgan Russell (1886–1953), who had seen Duncan perform in Paris after his move there in 1909, made a spare, linear drawing of her the following year (Seuphor collection, Paris). Russell looked to Renaissance

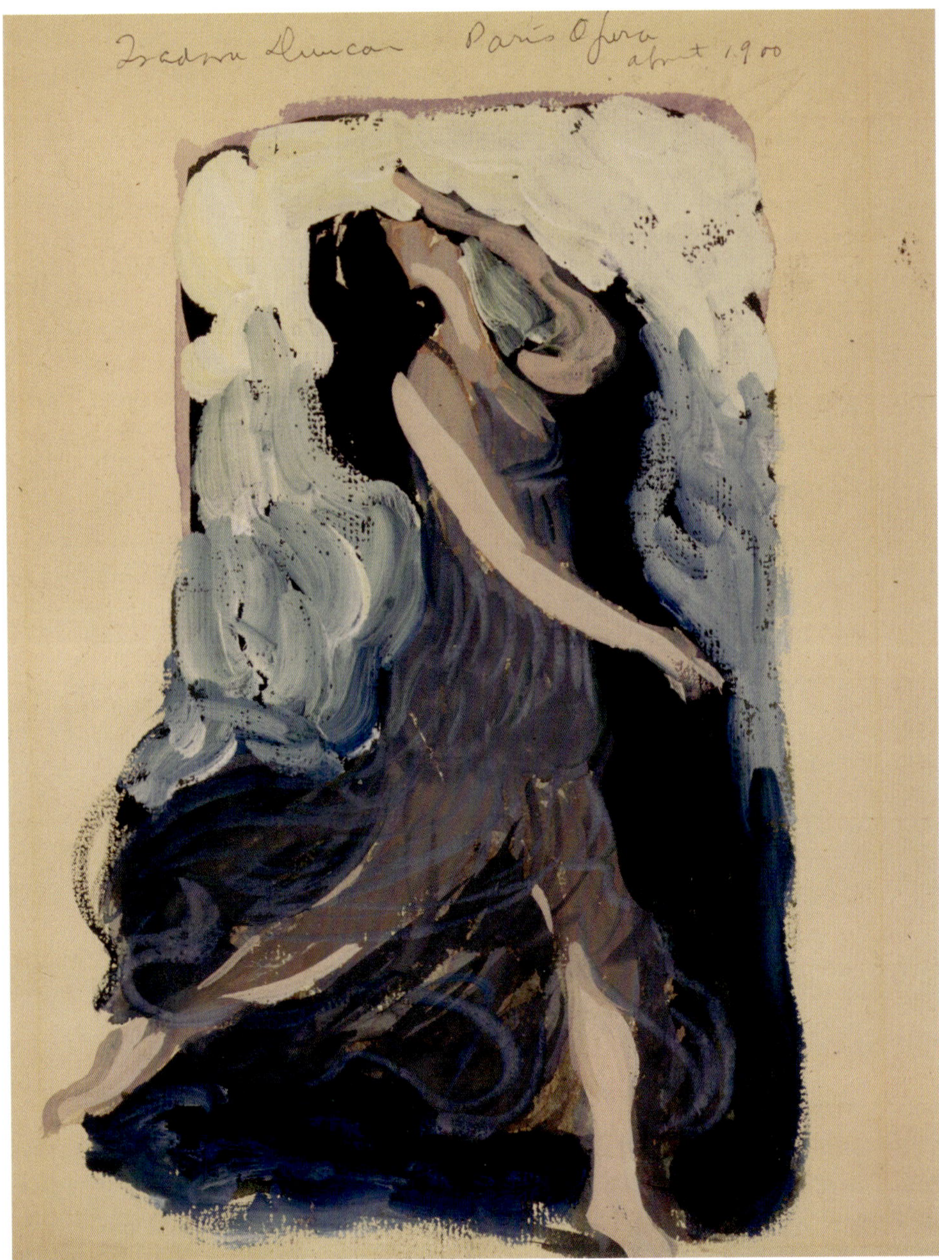



**Figure 135** Ernest Blumenschein, *Isadora Duncan—Paris Opera about 1900*, c. 1904, gouache, 9 × 5 inches. (New Mexico Museum of Art, Santa Fe, Gift of Helen Greene Blumenschein, 1964, 1629b/23D)

sculpture for firm, yet dynamic structure in this drawing, synthesizing Duncan's own sinuous motions with those of Michelangelo's celebrated *Dying Slave* (1513–16, Louvre, Paris). Along with other artists, Russell found that the fluid monumentality of Duncan's body and gesture could survive comparison, even interchange, with the powerful physicality of Renaissance sculpture. Elsewhere Russell would allude to music as the organizing principle in his abstractions, but here it was dance that triggered the brilliant chromatic energies of the brief but blazing visual experiments known as Synchromism.[66]

Morgan Russell was not the only artist inspired by the "statuesque completeness" Duncan's adopted daughter had noted. Painter John Sloan (1871–1951) likewise responded to Isadora, whom he regarded as part earthbound cultural primitive, part revolutionary. To him, Duncan's imposing physical stature only enhanced her mythic status. Writing in his diary in early 1911, Sloan seemed to be trying to figure out how Duncan's synergy worked:

> Dolly and I went to see Isadora Duncan. It's hard to set down how much I enjoyed this performance. Isadora as she appears on that big simple stage seems like *all* womanhood—she looms big as the mother of the race. A heavy solid figure, large columnar legs, a solid high belly, breasts not too full and her head seems to be no more important than it should to give the body the chief place. In one of the dances she was absolutely nude save for a thin gauze drapery hanging from the shoulders.[67]

In 1915 Sloan drew Duncan in her Marche Militaire for the cover of the radical magazine *The Masses*. He also made an etching of her, spotlighted on stage, hands waving gently overhead (fig. 136). Duncan turned thirty-eight that year, no longer sylphlike, and Sloan's rendering of her (unlike Genthe's portraits) resists idealization of the legendary dancer. In 1915, though "she lacked slenderness," recalled Sloan, "[Duncan] was still, in my opinion, the greatest dancer on earth."[68] The admiring artist produced a poster for her Dionysian performance with students at the Metropolitan Opera House.[69] To Floyd Dell, another social radical, Duncan had become "a curious combination of old washerwoman and Great Mother of the Gods."[70] There is indeed something faintly comical in this ponderous Isadora. Her maternally bulky body corresponds more closely to Janet Flanner's description of "a glorious bounding Minerva," than to sublime patriotic allegory.[71] Moving, Duncan reportedly overcame any figure faults, but visual artists could, at this stage of her career, seldom capture that transcendent grace.

Arnold Rönnebeck (1885–1947) was a German American artist who studied in Paris from 1908 to 1914. When he drew Duncan in 1912, he accentuated her imposing solidity as well as her flair for the dramatic gesture. In several watercolors from that year, notably *Andante* (1912; fig. 137), the dancer becomes almost a caricature of herself. Perhaps with a stylistic nod to Modigliani or to Elie Nadelman (both then working in Paris), Rönnebeck presents Duncan as an overripe Amazon with an attitude, an *artiste* taken more seriously by herself than by the painter.

In New York during her visits between 1915 and 1918, Duncan proved herself a very high-maintenance star. Her grand expectations for New York required substantial help from her American supporters. Besides Robert Henri, the committee established to further Duncan's American ventures would grow to include visual artists Paul Manship and Gutzon Borglum, as well as many other social avant-gardists: critic Mary Fanton Roberts, actress Ellen Terry, writers Theodore

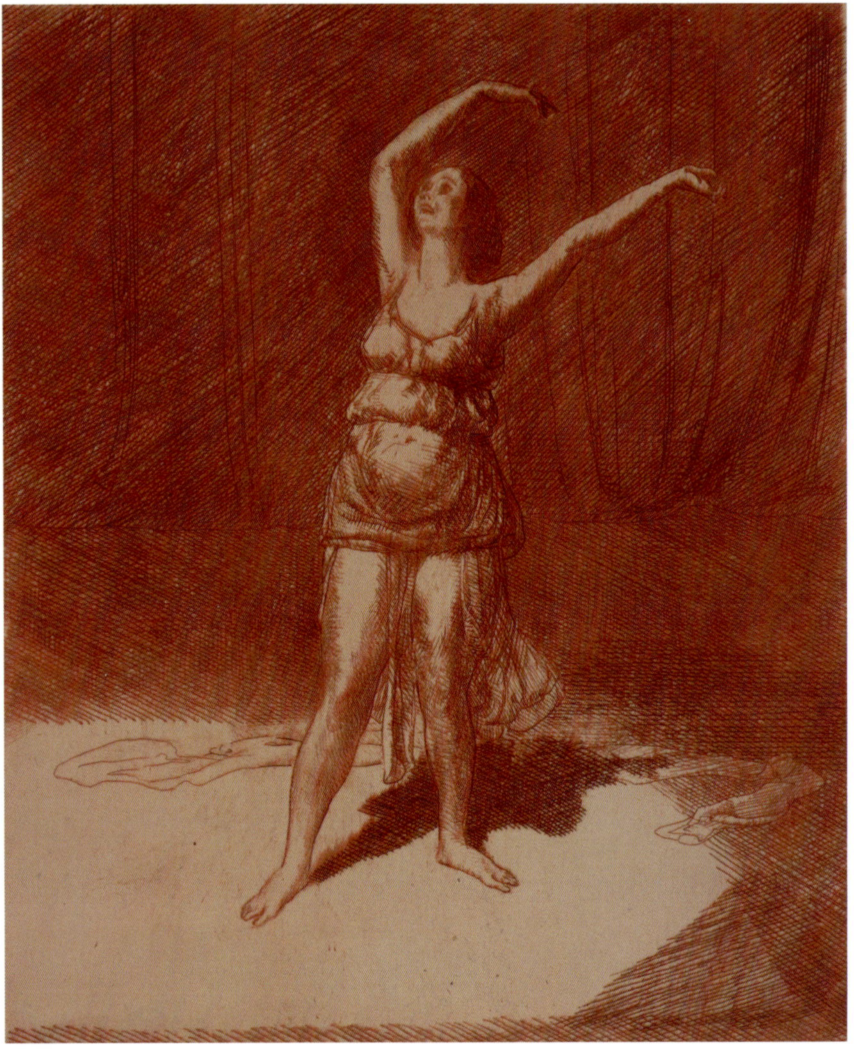

Figure 136 John Sloan, *Isadora Duncan*, 1915, etching on wove paper, 8 ½ × 7 ¼ inches. (New Mexico Museum of Art, Santa Fe, 369/23G)

Dreiser and Walter Lippmann, and anthropologist John Collier. Providing a unifying context for all of them was Mabel Dodge, whose Fifth Avenue salon gathered movers and shakers in all fields. As Dodge wrote to Gertrude Stein, she and the New York committee took on the "maddest project of getting [Duncan] the Armory, where she can teach a thousand unemployed people's poor children to *dance & feed & clothe them & charge rich people sums to come in & see her teach 'em. And we're going to get up some great out of door festivals for her. We're perfectly insane in our plans but sometimes insanity works."[72] This exuberance Duncan understood well, having flung her own energies in wildly disparate directions.

But Duncan could be arrogant and uncompromising in her artistic demands. To carry out her democratizing plans for dance, she envisioned nothing less

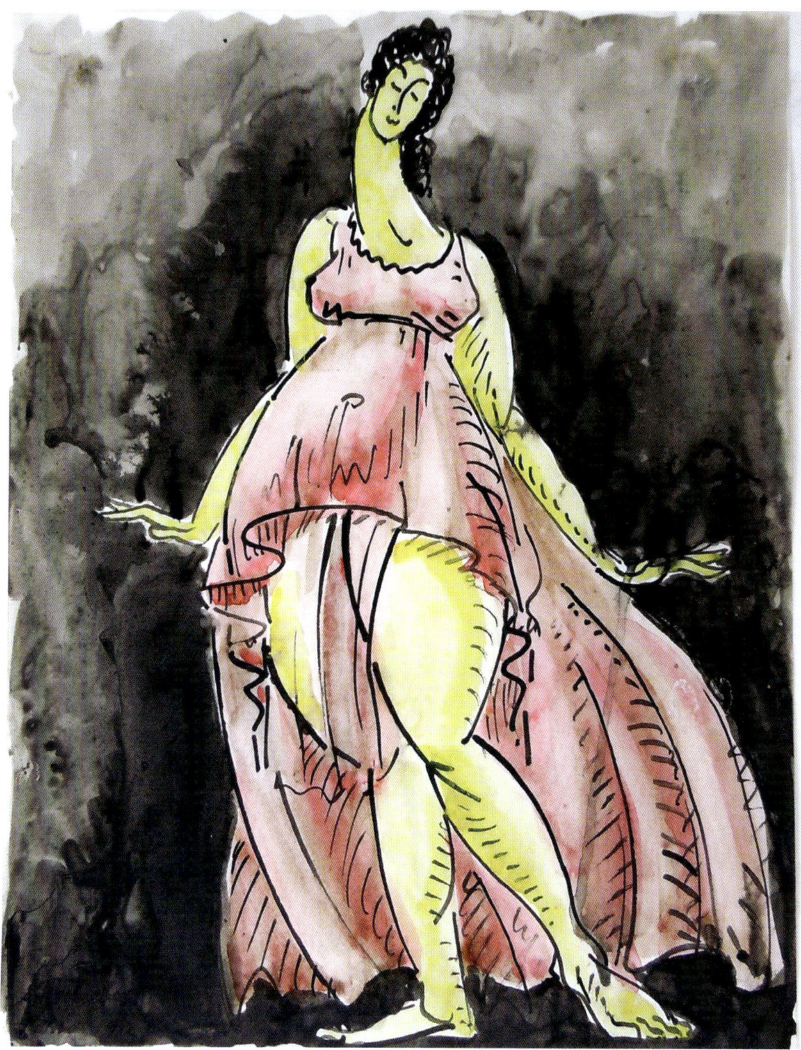

Figure 137 Arnold Rönnebeck, *Andante*, 1912, watercolor, 10 ¾ × 8 ¼ inches. (reproduced with permission of the Estate of Arnold Rönnebeck, all rights reserved)

than a new New York opera house seating six thousand people at a maximum charge of twenty-five cents per seat. Duncan's leftist politics offended some of her patrons, and she did little to soothe their feelings, denouncing America's elites as "crude, vulgar, cold, heartless, barren and inartistic."[73] Despite favorable reviews for the *Marseillaise* and certain of her other performances, some of her programs failed critically and financially. She ran up enormous debts and seemed to court animosity openly. "Of tact or self-control she had very little," said Arnold Genthe, "nor did she wish to have. She was the complete and willing tool of her impulses."[74] Somehow—familiar and famous though she became— Duncan preserved within her an enormous mystery, which abided always in a vast gulf between the woman's vaunted approach to dance and the dance itself. Duncan stretched credulity among artists and adoring audiences alike when she declared, "I hate dancing. I am an *expressioniste* of beauty. I use my body as my medium, just as the writer uses his words. Do not call me a dancer."[75] Could Americans really call her—with a straight face—a dance *expressioniste?* Little wonder that Duncan, worshiped internationally, also attracted her share of skeptics; some began to see her as unstable or—worse—mildly ridiculous. "Many Americans," writes one dance historian, "deplored her profligate Bohemianism, her open liaisons with men, and her two illegitimate children; moralists scourged her as an amateur indulging in the most shameless kind of self-advertisement."[76] In the end, Duncan's controversial art could no longer pay her bills in America. On May 9, 1915, she slipped away from her mounting debts and the "philistine darkness" of New York, bound for Europe with her Isadorables aboard the ship *Dante Alighieri.*

France would again prove a much more congenial base for Duncan's ambitions. Visual artists there, even before she danced specifically for *la gloire française,* had made her into something of a monument. In 1913 the new Théâtre des Champs-Elysées had opened in Paris, adorned by multiple images of the American dancer. Above its entrance the passionate sculptor Antoine Bourdelle (1861–1929) installed a bas-relief representing Duncan and Nijinsky paired in an imagined *pas de deux.* After seeing the pair dance at a soiree, Bourdelle had written in his diary, "It seemed to me, as I watched Madame Isadora Duncan sitting or reclining, that with each of her pauses she was offering me an antique marble throbbing with intensity."[77]

Inside the auditorium of the same theater, French Symbolist painter and writer Maurice Denis (1870–1943) used the fresco medium for his multiple images of Duncan as the nine Muses, dancing barefoot in her typical Greek-style tunics. The legendary Isadora, the French seemed to agree, had been apotheosized into art, though not at all immobilized in the process. For the price of a ticket, the flesh-and-blood dancer continued to make herself available to sold-out houses, but she preferred to think of her audience as a refined few—this despite her highly public protestations in New York about democratizing dance for the masses. "My dancing," she told one impresario, "is for the elite, for the artists, sculptors, painters, musicians, but not for the general public."[78]

## Dance at the Armory Show: Revolutionary Moves

In her bold fusion of "primitive" and modern dance forms, Duncan helped to pave the way for visual modernism—especially of the French variety—to invade and take root in America. Despite earlier incursions (such as Rodin's drawings of Duncan, which in 1908 rattled the foundations of figure drawing when shown in Alfred Stieglitz's Gallery 291) European modernism arrived en masse at New York's Armory Show of 1913. We have referred to this event in other contexts above, but it is necessary to take a broader look at it here, especially with regard to the range of its dance subjects, and for several important reasons: 1) dance revealed itself at the Armory Show as a versatile way of interrogating human form and movement; 2) dance subjects at the Armory Show positioned inventive new formal experiments alongside more traditional renderings of the figure; and 3) dance subjects foregrounded its potential to reveal aspects of human—perhaps even national—character, whether seen in individual or group dancers.

Because modernism originated in Europe, many critics were suspicious of its "un-American" character. Conservative critic Royal Cortissoz famously decried the Armory show's avant-garde art as an "invasion" of "aliens." Lacking what he called "aesthetic naturalization," the art would remain "foreign" and unassimilated. But the xenophobic reception given to modern art in the Armory Show was not universal; a few critics and many visual artists would pronounce it a turning point in their own professional lives. Some of the critics who defended it did so in terms that suggest its vitality and its nascent search, like Duncan's, for liberated art forms suitable to the new century. F. J. Gregg, writing during the show's New York venue, drew this distinction: "What is undoubtedly to be found in the Frenchmen is a quality in their work which, however it may irritate, or puzzle, or disturb, never produces dullness. . . . On the other hand, American art, or that part of it with which the ordinary man is perfectly satisfied, is deadly dull and suggests decay instead of growth."[79]

Was Gregg right? Certainly the Armory Show was the most vilified exhibition yet mounted in this country. And retrospective critical opinion has largely ratified his view. The Armory Show was indeed startling in its formal impudence, undercutting old aesthetic certainties and—perhaps worse—making much of the show's American work look decidedly old-fashioned. One can see this by placing the Armory Show's dance subjects on a stylistic continuum. Likely Picabia's Cubist *Dances at the Spring* (Armory Show cat. no. 415, discussed above) would occupy the most radical position. As one of the irritating or puzzling works Gregg noted, it came in for some of the same vitriolic criticism leveled at Duchamp's *Nude Descending a Staircase*. One critic declared that *Dances at the Spring* must be unfinished and offered to help Picabia to locate and bring forth the bodies of its dancers. On the radical end as well was Raymond Duchamp-Villon's sculpture *Danseurs* (1912, Armory Show cat. no. 612, unlocated) one of a series of experiments with solids and voids in the human form.[80]

At the opposite end, American Jerome Myers's *The Street Dance* (a realist composition of children dancing in a circle) might have been the most conservative of the Armory Show dance subjects. In marked contrast to Picabia's piece, Myers's painting was cited appreciatively by writers in the essay portion of the show's official catalog (volume 3). Like Myers, other American painters focused on dance as cultural narrative rather than as stylistic statement: George Bellows (who exhibited a total of five works at the Armory) showed one called *Dancer* (now unidentified), while Stuart Davis submitted a watercolor of a dance floor crowded with working-class types, *Dance* (1912, Armory Show cat. No. 814).[81]

But there was not a firm dichotomy between European and American works nor between works that emphasized form over content. There were French works, for example, that were memorable chiefly as conveyors of cultural history or ideology. The Armory Show's adoption of tried-and-true revolutionary ideals—its pine tree symbol, from a Revolutionary War battle flag, for example—reminded its audience of deliberate connections between American culture and political revolution. That revolutionary spirit was echoed in the New York show by an important French dance subject fraught with ideological and historic implications. Henri Rousseau's *The Celebration* or *The Centennial of the Revolution (Le Centenaire,* 1892) was shown in all three venues of the Armory Show. It reminded Americans of the shared cultural values affirmed by the French and American revolutions—values couched amiably by Rousseau in the rhythms of the dance. Rousseau painted a large group of male and female dancers, the women wearing liberty caps, circling around a tree. The scene is historically based, one of a whole body of secular festivals staged in Revolutionary-era France to reinforce communal values within a dramatically altered social order. What takes place in Rousseau's scene is a performance of the Carmagnole (popular during the Revolution) danced around the Tree of Liberty, a symbol in perfect accord with the Armory Show's own pine tree symbol.[82] Rousseau invokes other powerful symbols of the Revolution: at the far right is a group of three men accompanied by Liberty, or Marianne, the abstract deity of Gallic freedom. She too wears the Phrygian cap of liberty like Delacroix's majestic, bare-breasted heroine in his 1830 *Liberty Leading the People* (Louvre, Paris). Rousseau's stout republicanism forecasts the surge in French patriotism that would occur just a year after the Armory Show, when France entered the Great War. Was it because of long, historic friendship with France that American critics found nothing to object to in Rousseau's patriotic *Celebration* in dance form? More likely, it was that Rousseau's "naive," folkloric style needed no "aesthetic naturalization." While Rousseau appealed on one hand to the interest in folk art already demonstrated by European and American avant-gardes, other qualities (his lack of academic training, simplified forms and bold stylizations, a certain naiveté, and an imagined affiliation with the "primitive," then often synonymous with "folk") made him palatable to general American audiences as well.[83] And finally, Rousseau's painting was a link in a long chain of visual representations, images that—together with a constant traffic in ideas and performers—made for a nearly uninterrupted transatlantic cultural exchange.

# 10

# Dance, Visual Art, and America's Countercultures

## Revolutionizing Gender and Sexuality

The American painter Florine Stettheimer once reported seeing Duncan and the Russian sculptor Paul Troubetzkoy "dancing about together" at a private party in Paris. But Stettheimer, unlike so many of her artist compatriots, was not tempted to render that moment or any other Isadora idyll on canvas. She found Duncan's movements undisciplined, elusive, and—for her—unpaintable. Still, while she shied away from Duncan's powerful, unique physicality, Stettheimer found inventive ways to deal, through male subjects, with the new dance and the new sexuality, making frequent forays into pictorial androgyny. She was one of a new generation bent on demolishing old cultural rigidities, replacing them with new twentieth-century standards of sexual plasticity, a concept corresponding fortuitously to a new plasticity trumpeted in dance.[1] For example, Stettheimer often painted her male subjects—Duchamp's persona Rrose Sélavy, composer Virgil Thomson, and critic Carl Van Vechten—in female dancer's footgear. But when wild, exuberant dancing was called for (as in her *Natatorium Undine*, fig. 85, above), Stettheimer preferred the genteel anonymity of the tried-and-true bacchante.

If Stettheimer avoided Duncan as direct subject, she could not ignore her influence on modern dance. The painter's treatment of Nijinsky's androgyny in her canvas *Music* (fig. 83, above), clearly reveals the extent to which Duncan's movements and dress influenced the increasing feminization of the male dancer—especially by Diaghilev. As dance historian Lynn Garafola has noted, "In Nijinsky's case, the body was progressively feminized. Released from the decorum of conventional masculinity, it openly displayed its erotic attributes—a pliant, supple middle, soft, embracing arms, eyes lengthened and darkened with liner." Described thus, Nijinsky's torso and arms approach the celebrated Duncanesque movements. But in their deliberate eroticism, these new male heroes out-Duncan Isadora herself. Continues Garafola, "In the drawings of Robert Montenegro, Paul Iribe, and George Barbier especially, [Nijinsky's] pose is often languid, its curves dramatized by serpentine scarves and by gestures that circle inward on the body, as if announcing its availability."[2] That is seen as well in photographs of Nijinsky in *Le Spectre de la Rose* (see fig. 84).

Stettheimer has Nijinsky dancing that very role in *Music*. By emphasizing the imaginary, dreamlike nature of the scene, Stettheimer succeeded in neutralizing whatever offense might have accompanied his femininization.[3] This distancing—through the imaginary, antique, or exotic—safeguarded propriety and became a standard device for painters as well as choreographers experimenting with unorthodox treatments of sexuality. Costumes likewise sanitized the androgyny. Harem pants (adopted by Stettheimer and worn by her for decades), skirts, and tunics crossed gender boundaries with ease. With her own eccentric clothes, as well as her portrayal of gender-blurred bodies, Stettheimer used dance as a vehicle for creating an androgynous or bisexual visual vocabulary. She made dance communicate as one of the elements—along with speech and painting—of a new modernist discourse of the body.

The style and form of the redefined dancer's body, as just seen in Stettheimer's work, generated fascinating parallels in aesthetics. From a formal standpoint, the concept of plasticity played an important role in early twentieth-century recastings of movements in space. Plasticity is an old term, generally understood to be present in painting when figures are fully modeled and seem capable of moving freely in the pictorial space. In other words, they appear three-dimensional. Artists and critics in the era of Cézanne and the Cubists were especially concerned with plasticity as they reconfigured old notions of space and worked to valorize flatness as an alternative to illusionistic depth. Guillaume Apollinaire, for example, wrote a 1908 article on the "plastic virtues" of Picasso. For the next few decades the term was much in vogue, adapted by painters such as Mondrian, though often misunderstood (Georgia O'Keeffe remarked somewhat dismissively that she never really understood what it meant).[4]

In the early 1920s, even before Mondrian was developing his own Neoplasticism theories, a Russian named Alexei Sidorov published a book on *plastique*, or "free" dance, meaning "pure" movement in space. His was a codification of a free dance movement already underway in Russia. A number of *plastique* dance troupes emerged there in the 1910s, directly out of Isadora Duncan's dance. Like her, they aspired to a reunification of the body with the self. The concept of the *plastique* passed into distant quarters, even entering the dance vocabulary of the Denishawn school in Los Angeles, where the term *plastique* was often used to describe a dancer's movement in space. Concepts such as *plastique* do not translate perfectly from one discipline into another. Nonetheless, their dissemination reveals the desire of dancers and visual artists to communicate with each other through the developing dialects of modernism, soon to fuse into a language capable of expressing, if not unifying, the radical discourse of art, music, time, and modern consciousness itself.

Flowing as if through a permeable cultural membrane, modernist ideas from the visual arts continued to affect dancers well beyond the glory days of the Cubists and Futurists. Martha Graham, for example, paid close attention to a whole range of twentieth-century innovators, who repeatedly taught her lessons about finding underlying choreographic structures in the complex, fragmented spaces of modern painting. With them, she learned that symbol and representation could be used to communicate thoughts, feelings, even abstractions. As

George Beiswanger wrote, "With [Graham] as with Cézanne and Van Gogh, Picasso and Matisse—whose paintings she studied and whose writings she read—the surface of dance (the conventional idioms, the accepted evasions, the brittle shell) had to be 'broken up,' so that the underlying structure could be disclosed."[5]

## An Artist in Revolt against Compulsory Heterosexuality: Charles Demuth and Dance

In American art, the dominant culture has most often dictated acceptable subjects for artists. Yet, as the concept of the avant-garde grew in boldness and tenacity, twentieth-century artists increasingly tested the boundaries of acceptable behavior, and therefore, acceptable subject matter. The expression of subcultures, whether political, ethnic, or racial, found voice in dance and literature as well as in painting. Categories of behavior considered normal or abnormal were beginning to change under the influence of psychoanalysis, but clandestine sexual subcultures—especially the expression of homosexual themes and identities—were not yet publicly acceptable, and therefore not artistically representable. All of which makes the work of Charles Demuth, who frequently represented the homoerotic in his work, an especially subversive genre in his day. In most areas of his life Demuth kept his sexual orientation discreetly veiled behind a screen of public propriety, but in his art the preference emerges, adding a degree of complexity that enriches our perceptions of both the person and his art. But that is today's view; in Demuth's day the conventions of society demanded otherwise. As Jonathan Weinberg points out, even Marcel Duchamp, studied avant-gardist and sometime cross-dresser, argued against considering Demuth's art and sexuality together. "The little perverse tendency that he had was not important in Demuth's life," said Duchamp. "After all, everybody has a little perverse tendency in him. That quality in him had nothing to do with the quality of his work. It had nothing to do with his art."[6] However well-meaning, however protective Duchamp (and other friends) were of Demuth's privacy, they acted against the tide of cultural history, which today regards sexuality as one, but only one, of a range of important identity characteristics informing any artist—indeed, any person.

My interest here is to look at a few of the many images of same-sex love by Demuth—those, specifically, in which dance bodies forth sexuality. His choice of dance subjects is both vicarious and ironic: lame and diabetic, Demuth probably engaged in little dancing himself. But watching from the sidelines only sharpened his eye for analyzing both social constraints and transgressions. In 1929 Demuth exhibited *Dancing Sailors* (1917; fig. 138) at New York's new Museum of Modern Art. This watercolor, and a second, very similar one, each feature three dancing couples: two sailors dance with women while a third is paired with another sailor. What are the social implications of two men dancing together? In that era, before respectable young women could freely date servicemen, there was sometimes a shortage of women. In their absence men occasionally danced

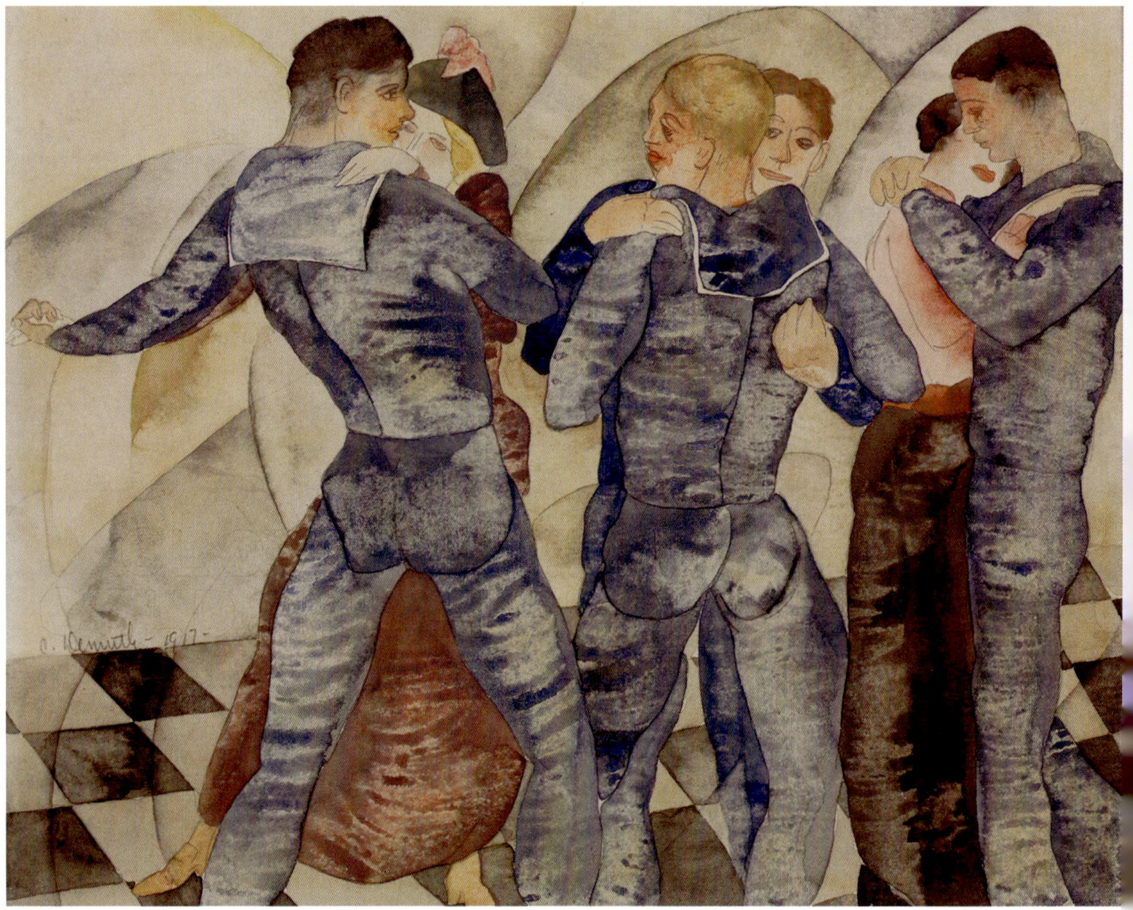

**Figure 138** Charles Demuth, *Dancing Sailors*, 1917, watercolor over graphite, 8 × 10 ¹/₁₀ inches. (Cleveland Museum of Art, Mr. and Mrs. William H. Marlatt Fund, 1980.9b)

with each other, usually in trendy fast dances. But this situation, as Weinberg points out, is different: there are women present, and—tellingly—all the couples are linked in similarly close embrace, clearly moving to slow music. A sexual interest is thus implicit in all three couples, yet except for a glance between two of the sailors, there is no evidence that anyone even notices the unconventional pairing of male sailors. What one must notice, however, are the bodies of the male dancers, viewed from behind, with their muscular physiques clearly visible beneath their tight sailor uniforms. These bodies Demuth portrays as unmistakable objects of sexual desire. By contrast, we see little of the women themselves or the long, loose clothes covering their bodies.

What's going on here? Some mild social unruliness, a bit of low-level cultural subversion? With sophisticated irony, Demuth's images point out ambivalent relationships within a repressed American culture. Dance, he shows us, is (like sex) a physical act, but one performed in public and governed by a set of social guidelines. Here those rules have been disregarded; Demuth sets up a mild but deliberate tension, clearly visible when one pauses at length over the artist's overt expression of male–male intimacy. But that too is part of what Demuth explores here: how social dance, with its intrinsic touching, allows couples—even a male couple—to test the limits of acceptable social behavior.[7] Dance has proved to be one of the most durable and inventive sites of resistance to the dominant culture. In time to the rhythmic pulsing of music, dancers—and we with them—are swept along past ordinary considerations of conventionality.

Like some modern painting, dance exposed the social dynamics of an era in ways both provocative and perilous. Making art expressive of countercultural ideals or practice led Demuth to popular dance halls and private parties where he could observe dancers at close range. As his friend Marsden Hartley wrote of Demuth, "Charles liked being in on these parties, those tiger-like stalkings after amusement down the courses of the night, he liked being swept into atmospheres and getting his own funny kick out of them, and they were big ideas and issues for Charles, bringing some of the best of his work out of him."[8] In his attraction to dance scenes and in the quality of work he produced from them, Demuth was not alone.

## Cabarets, Chorus Lines, and Dance Marathons: Images of America's Restless Vitality

Other artists who explored the seamier side of dance imagery included the American Adolf Dehn, whose Harlem-inspired prints of African American dancers we considered earlier. In both Europe and the United States, Dehn continued to expand his vocabulary of dance subjects, combining biting cultural criticism with his own louche inclinations. Following his student days in Minneapolis and New York, he spent most of the decade of the 1920s in Vienna, Berlin, and Paris. There he immersed himself in café and cabaret life, sketching dancers, prostitutes, musicians, and audiences with similar incisiveness. Sometimes it is difficult to distinguish between the former two occupations in Dehn's drawings from those years. He frequently contributed drawings to American publications, including *The Dial*, for which magazine he drew two *Dancers*. With their languid poses and seductive looks, one wonders if the title may be a euphemism deemed necessary for American audiences.[9] As Dehn's eye for satire sharpened, he became an irreverent observer of all kinds of social and physical types. He developed an animated drawing style well suited to convey the rhyming silhouettes of the fleshy, Teutonic forms on the dance floor. With a kind of linear athleticism, Dehn's prints throw certain contours into prominence, emphasizing the rhythmic movements of the dance. While living in Vienna Dehn met and married a Russian emigrée dancer, Mura Ziperovitch, who became his frequent model for dance subjects and who focused the artist's attention more closely on the world of the dance.[10]

Moving to Berlin in 1923, Dehn found a city rife with dissolution and ripe for satire of all kinds. Its stolid daytime respectability gave way by night to a morally ambiguous, decidedly cruder Berlin. George Grosz (1893–1959), part of Germany's Neue Sachlichkeit (New Objectivity) movement, was already

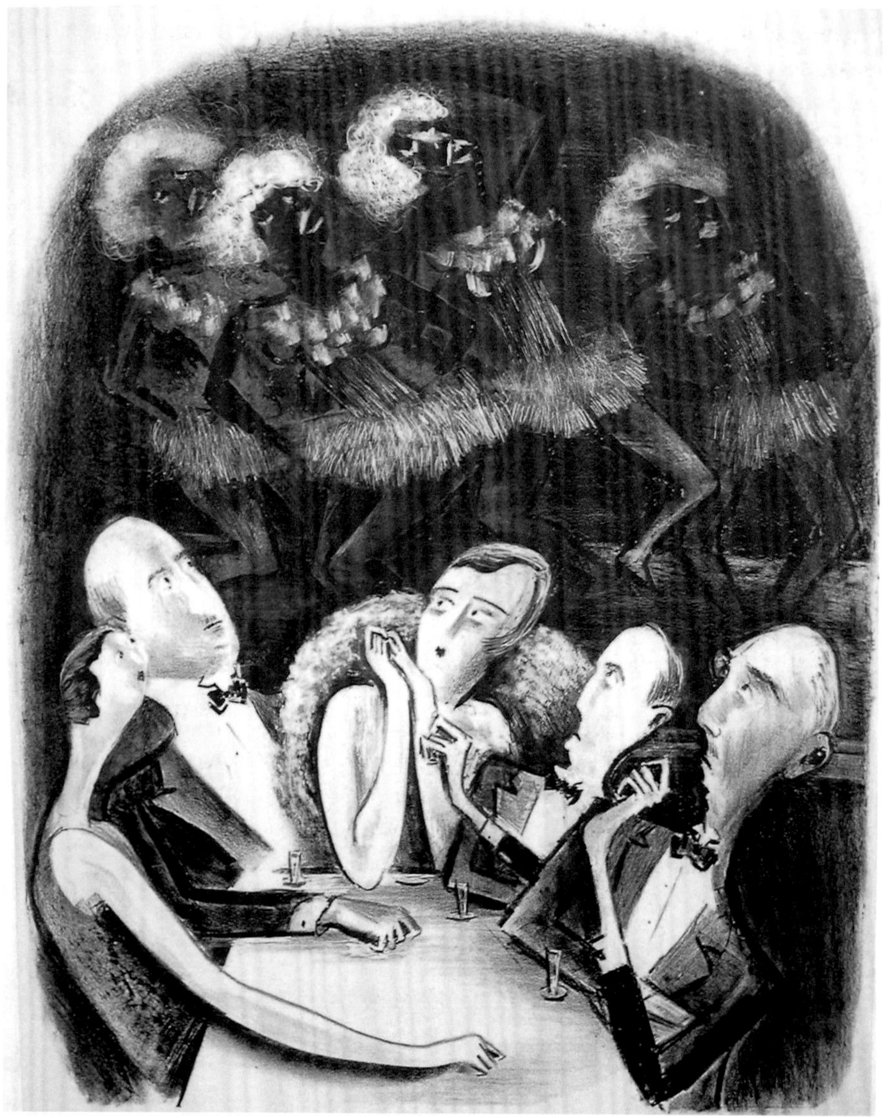

Figure 139 Adolf Dehn, *We Nordics*, 1931, lithograph, 13 ½ × 11 inches. (courtesy Dehn Quests)

spewing political vitriol in his own caricatures, such as *Tea Dance (Tanz Kaffee)* (c. 1925, National Gallery of Art, Washington, D.C.). Grosz took Dehn (who spoke fluent German) beneath the veneer of Berlin's hypocrisies. In a city where politics and race were highly volatile, Grosz and Dehn found that just getting the subjects down on paper made for expressive dynamite.[11] In *We Nordics* (1931; fig. 139) Dehn cast a cynical eye on a cabaret scene in which four African (or African American) dancers perform before a table of five effete Europeans, who affect shock at the spectacle before them. Honing his visual means to a purpose, Dehn plays up the contrast between the energy of the dancers, whose skin color, facial features, and hair are strongly emphasized, and the hyperrefined, enervated white spectators. Within a single lithograph, Dehn tapped into the tensions and hypocrisy embedded in attitudes of the emerging fascist elite: simultaneous fascination for and imagined superiority over the racial Other. It is clear where Dehn's cultural sympathies lie.

A taste for bawdy striptease or burlesque dancers often drew Dehn to vaudeville theaters. He understood its raw appeal—his own and other men's attraction to it—as a kind of *nostalgie de la boue*. Writing years later, Dehn analyzed the social implications of his burlesque subjects: "A burlesque number! For men only! For men who get tired of being noble, upright, and lonely. A couple hours of sublimation before going home to a dull or empty bed. . . . I tried to make the garish setting, the vulgar attempt to stimulate the audience, and the awkward pattern of the dancers a part of the design."[12]

Dehn's burlesque subjects, with their variously excited or morose male spectators, set up a fascinating contrast with a burlesque subject by the American printmaker Elizabeth Olds (1896–1991). Olds, who made many lithographs and drawings for the WPA/FAP Graphic Arts Division during the Depression, knew its rules: no nudes in government-underwritten works. Still, many artists—including women—were drawn to seminude burlesque dancers as subjects. By the time she produced her *Burlesque (Chorus Line)* (c. 1935–45; fig. 140),

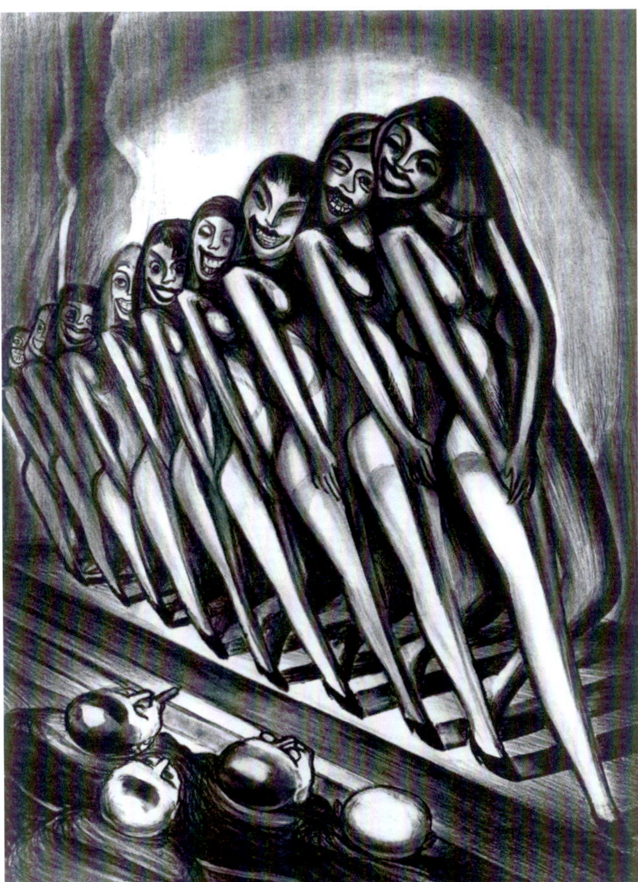

Figure 140 Elizabeth Olds, *Burlesque (Chorus Line)*, c. 1935–45, lithograph, 14 ½ × 10 ¾ inches. (Smithsonian American Art Museum, Transfer from Archives of American Art, Smithsonian Institution, 1984.31.40)

Olds had formed strong leftist political views. She had been influenced by José Clemente Orozco's murals at Dartmouth College, especially his linear stylizations and aggressive, active forms. As Helen Langa succinctly points out, Olds infused *Burlesque (Chorus Line)* with the formal ideals and countercultural politics she admired:

> By molding the dancers' bodies into a wall of angular energy and repeating their stiff-armed poses, exaggerating the artifice of their smiles and turning their linked bodies into a visual metaphor for "labor solidarity," [Olds] celebrated these women's strength. In characterizing their performance as labor, she undermined more exploitative tropes of representation that seemed to solicit a male viewer's voyeuristic gaze. And by emphasizing their multiracial identities, she may also have intended the print as an antiracist statement, inspired perhaps by Orozco's valorization of Mexican *indigenismo*.[13]

In the hands of Olds, a chorus line became an emblem of the restless vitality of American life, overlaid with multiple valences of social meaning. Dance proved itself once again a strong and able carrier of changing cultural ideas.

Another 1930s dance subject from the American demimonde is that of the taxi-dancer, or the dancer for hire. The anonymity of city life, especially for transplanted small-town men, meant that dance partners must often be paid for. Urban realist Reginald Marsh (1898–1954) knew this world well, and often painted its denizens, variously forthright or demure. In Marsh's *Ten Cents a Dance* (1933; fig. 141), a row of voluptuous taxi-dancers, like exotic night-blooming flowers, await selection under the gaze of a presumably male viewer. Here dance, or the mere anticipation of it, eases the strain of urban social isolation at a time of high unemployment and bleak poverty.

Dance marathons were curious and visually arresting social phenomena associated with the interwar period. Beginning as one of a raft of record-breaking fads that swept the United States in the 1920s, the dance marathon took on a new, darker tone during the Depression, when an odd mix of Americans—ranging from out-of-work bank clerks to would-be starlets—competed for cash prizes. Desperate couples struggled to remain on their feet hour after hour, dancing in a fatigued stumble, trying to stay awake longer than their competitors. In June 1928, a Madison Square Garden marathon, billed as the "Dance Derby of the Century" began with ninety-one couples, the hardiest of which danced for 481 hours. A few years later, in the depths of the Depression, the Wildwood marathon in New Jersey lasted an unimaginable eighty-one days. Expatriate Gertrude Stein, witnessing a Chicago dance marathon during an American lecture tour, described the scene in her hypnotic modernist prose: "Here there was nothing neither waking nor sleeping, they were all young ones and they were moving as their bodies were drooping. They had been six weeks without sleeping . . . when there were two of them one was more clinging than moving."[14] Photographers and a few other visual artists such as Reginald Marsh were present at such events, capturing couples caught up in a cheerless ritual of emptiness

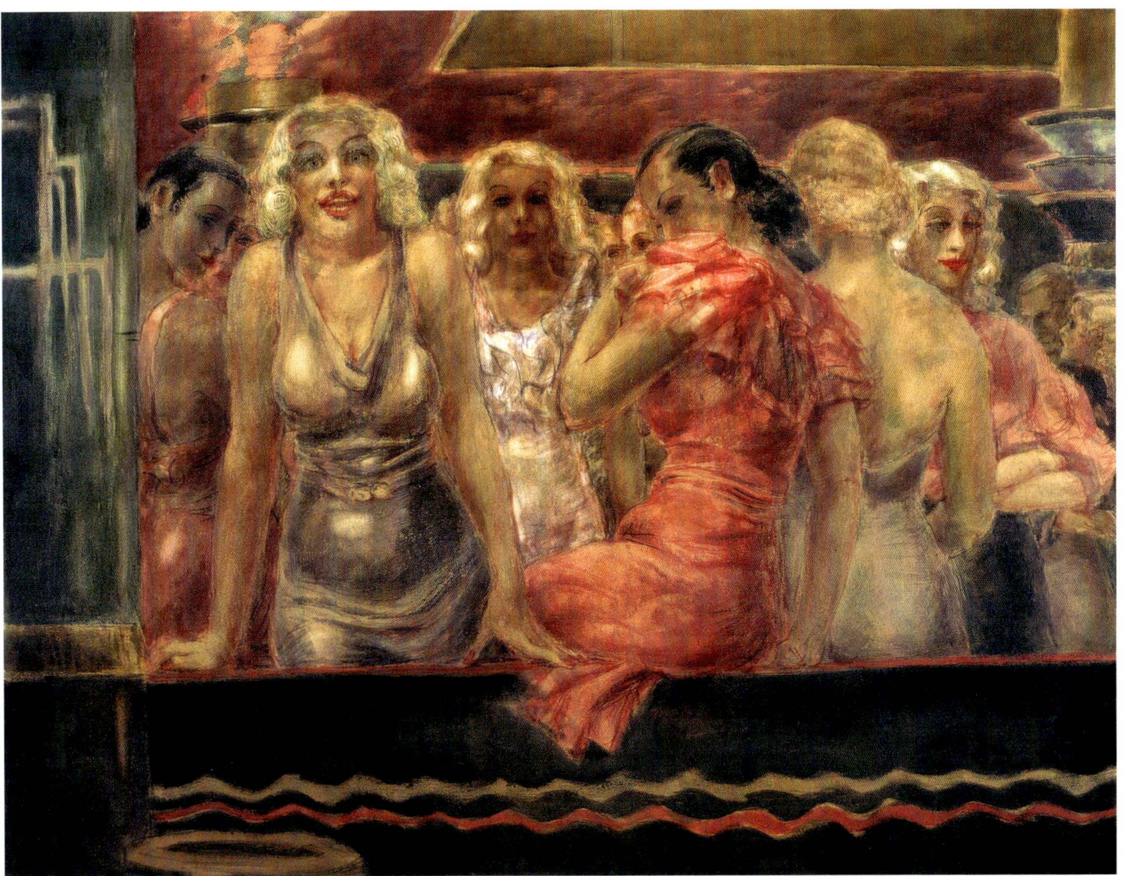

**Figure 141** Reginald Marsh, *Ten Cents a Dance*, 1933, egg tempera on panel, 36 × 48 inches. (Whitney Museum of American Art, New York, Felicia Meyer Marsh Bequest, 80.31.10; art © 2010 Estate of Reginald Marsh/Art Students League, New York/Artists Rights Society [ARS], New York; photo: Peter Accettola)

and despair, having abandoned, after many hours, any pretense of pleasure in the movements of the dance. As players in an eerie *danse macabre*, dance marathoners came to personalize the larger epic tragedy of the Great Depression, selling their energy in a dark mockery of the pleasures of dance. Like modern, antimonumental sculpture, the couples' hopes sag with the exhaustion and disillusionment of a whole era.

Philip Evergood (1901–75) used sharp disharmonies of color, distorted space, and elongated figure proportions to achieve a desired "nastiness" of effect in his strident *Dance Marathon* (1934; fig. 142).[15] Evergood acknowledged the influence of El Greco and the Italian Mannerists in his gawky, muscular dancers, who struggle as if caught within the spider-web pattern of the floorboards. Overhead an eerie skeleton's hand extends prize money, while a wall placard announces that it is day 49 of the torturous contest. Of his social realist subjects, *Dance Marathon*, while devoid of overt political slogans and raillery, remains one of Evergood's most poignant comments on the urban despair of the Depression

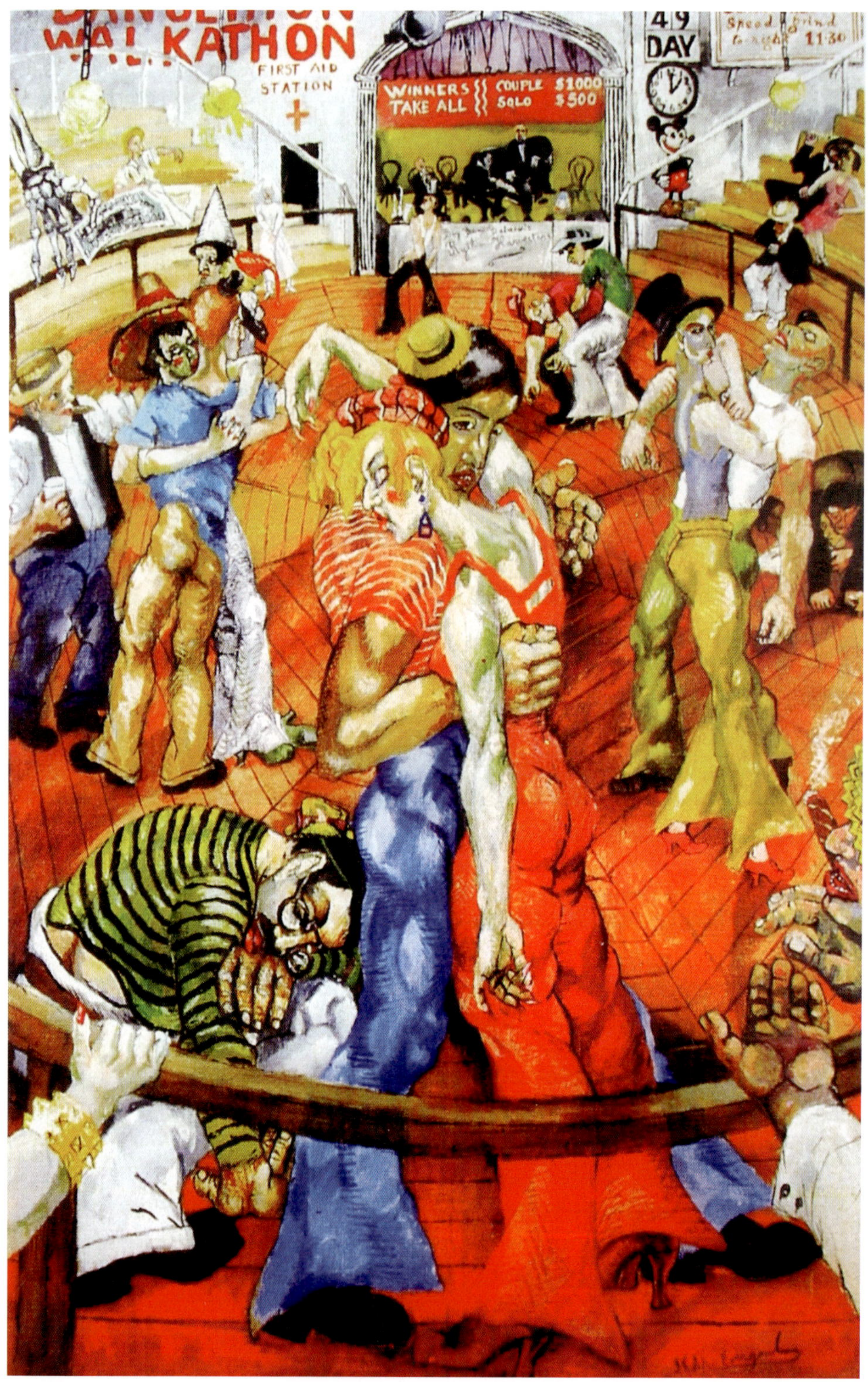



**Figure 142** Philip Evergood, *Dance Marathon*, 1934, oil on canvas, 60 1/16 × 40 1/16 inches. (Blanton Museum of Art, University of Texas at Austin, Gift of Mari and James A. Michener, 1991; photo: Rick Hall)

years, during which the artist threw his energies into radical political movements, walking picket lines and serving as president of the Artists Union. About the time he painted *Dance Marathon* Evergood joined the Public Works of Art Project, continuing with the WPA until 1937, a span in which his work, like that of other New York realists, maintained a stark opposition to the agrarian nostalgia generated by the regionalist painters of the Midwest.

As we have seen, dance has functioned in ways that have opened up, examined, and critiqued American culture. As a sometime carrier of cultural revolt, subversion, even scandal, it has been enlisted as a cultural weapon of considerable power. And that power has been enhanced by the expressions of visual artists. To the dominant culture, dance and dance images have sometimes created sites of resistance, expressive of counterculture values. At other moments, through its ability to engage public issues and opinion, dance has provided models for a liberated modern culture. As alive as the instant in which performed, dance's muscular immediacy animates the American present, then merges, through visual images, into a deathless continuum of shared memory.

# Conclusion

I f there is anything that is made clear by looking at a broad picture of the relationship between American art and dance, it is this: that dance has drawn on the nation's deepest resources of historical awareness and imaginative reflection. At important moments, it has embodied our culture's prevailing cultural assumptions or myths, while sometimes filtering them through the distorting lens of ideology. However manipulated, it is clear that dance and its visual art representations have each helped to define the character of the other. They are, in one fundamental sense, two different approaches to the problem of self-realization.

There was a belief, widespread in the early twentieth century, that the foundation of any nation's dance lies within the character of its people. In the United States, as we have seen, dance culture has been tied closely to its various regions, a notion that instantly recalls Alexis de Tocqueville's attempts to describe the character of American places. From his vantage point in the 1830s, the French visitor looked ahead to see America's solitudes disappearing. "One sees them," he wrote, "with a sort of melancholy pleasure; one is in some sort of a hurry to admire them."[1] What Tocqueville predicted about landscape has applied equally to American culture: it changes so rapidly that one must see it in a hurry. And dance, like the pulse of change itself, takes on heightened importance as a component of America's rushing cultural journey. Especially in the modern era, dance, with its inherent and unceasing references to motion, autonomy, and change, seems to confirm something of the essentially rootless or nomadic character of American life.

Still, velocity and change need not obscure America's search to define itself culturally. Links between national character (however quaint or murky the term) and cultural traditions can be studied if we slow down long enough to do so. Dance anthropologist Joann Kealiinohomoku argues that all forms of dance reflect their obvious origins in cultural traditions within which they developed.[2] This is as true for the United States (with its multiple cultural identities) as for a less mongrel people. As we have already seen, the varieties of American identity are reflected in many ways, not least in its diverse dance expressions.

As a subject for visual artists, dance has given new meaning to America's perennial myths, cherished identities, and most powerful dreams. Like every other nation, the United States has defined itself in part by its leisure pursuits. And social dance, in its endless variations, has been an important expression of

Americans at play. But alongside its potential for enjoyment, dance, like visual art, testifies to the abiding importance of spatial organization, physical pattern, and rhythmical motion in realizing aesthetic form. Dance's habitual patterns of movement acquire associated emotions that reflect culturally specific ideas about order and meaning.[3] Not infrequently, visual artists have been among the first to understand and record those ideas. As American dance has come to reflect an increasingly complex set of attitudes toward the moving body, visual artists have pressed dance into every part of their own realm, and drawn it out again with protean inventiveness. Everywhere, dance has helped to define the visual character of the modern world and to illuminate humanity's own complex interaction with that world. Even now, as globalization is eroding national styles (in dance as in all arts), American dance continually reinvents itself, while carrying fresh expressions around the world.

Empathy and distance are two sides of the same aesthetic coin. Often the aesthetic experience, in modern Western terms, has been characterized as a moment of "liminality," when individuals can step back—in a museum, for example—from everyday concerns and relations to look at their world with different thoughts and feelings. As the Swedish writer Goran Schildt has written, museums are settings in which we seek a state of "detached, timeless and exalted" contemplation that "grants us a kind of release from life's struggle and . . . [from] captivity in our own ego."[4] Observing ritual or dance can produce the same kind of liminal effect, enabling viewers to enter a quasi-ceremonial site where time and space differ from what lies outside. In this study, I have argued that—besides their other obvious affinities—dance and art participate symbiotically in generating that kind of experience. Whether transfixed by a painting or caught up in a dance performance, viewers themselves enact liberating aesthetic experiences, potentially deepening their own understanding of consciousness.

## Circling Back: A Postscript on Modernity, Postmodernity, and the Prodigality of Dance Imagery

Characterized by enormous aesthetic diversity, modernism broadly rejected empty historicism in style and ornamentation. Instead, modernism often emphasized physical process—in painting visible brushstrokes, and in sculpture chisel marks—in an effort to convey a quality of "honesty" also pursued in the other arts. Creative persons made an obsession of exploring the qualities of their medium, whether in dance, literature, painting, sculpture, or music. Visual artists' incorporation of dance and dancers into a wide range of visual representations created a rich and diverse record, in which are embedded all manner of nuanced responses to an era that first saw the concept of the mainstream enshrined, only to be relegated later in the century to the status of another outworn myth of modernism. Eventually, many historians came to agree with art critic Thomas McEvilley's view that "history no longer seems to have any shape, nor does it seem any longer to be going any place in particular."[5] That statement, in itself, invites reconsiderations of visual art and of its cultural siblings. Models of history have limited usefulness, each carrying its own benefits and dangers, not least of which is presuming to unveil formerly hidden structures. Without resorting to that kind of metaphysical posturing, can one merely observe that dance, like history, has lost its corresponding shape and direction? Without them, can dance take on new meaning as movement without a destination? And, finally, if an art form's primary social function is to redefine the communal self as the community changes, how successfully have visual artists responded to redefinition of dance, movement, and the body itself?

Critics still disagree on whether pluralism, the acceptance of a range of artistic intentions and styles, was intrinsic to modernism, or whether its birth coincided with a nebulous postmodern era. Regardless, artistic pluralism continues to reflect our culturally heterogeneous age, in which arbitrary chronological or stylistic termini lose secure meaning. In that spirit, it is appropriate to cast a departing eye on a few examples that fall beyond the endpoint of this study, if only to suggest dance's continuing metaphorical and formal relevance to visual art.

Both dance and visual art were seized, in the 1960s and 1970s, by questions about their very nature. Critics and choreographers began to wonder why—if dance's proper subject is movement—must it conform to music, or require a story or emotion? Critic Joan Acocella looks back at dancers who, during those decades, questioned their medium's formal bounds: "Their way of doing so was to de-theatricalize dance. That meant no music, much of the time. Often it also meant a suppression of structure."[6] Some dancers, such as those associated with two 1960s collectives in New York, Judson Dance Theatre and Grand Union, emphasized individual improvisation. Sometimes, their unpredictable individual performances, without selection, development, or climax, became strategies by which drama and group patterning could be undercut. Taking the long view, American dance had, in a sense, achieved a radical antithesis to the relentless, ritualistic patterning of the Shakers, for whom communal immersion and patterning totally subordinated the individual dancer. Separated by nearly two centuries, each kind of dance supplies an aspect of America's fluid cultural identity.

Such twentieth-century challenges within the American dance world paralleled questions asked concurrently by visual artists and art critics, most famously by Clement Greenberg, whose formalist arguments sought to exclude content from painting. In 1959 the painter Morris Louis (1912–62) painted *Saraband* (fig. 143), a work of lyrical, liquid color. Impressed by the staining technique developed by Helen Frankenthaler, and thinking to extend Greenberg's formalist arguments, Louis signed on to painting's "self-purification" process, in which figuration, narrative, and pictorial space recede.[7] Pure color, unburdened with thematic or emotional baggage, would remain. And paint, formerly assigned the task of transcribing the world's varied surfaces, was freed to express its own autonomy as a medium. Still, if *Saraband* purports to refuse a metaphorical role beyond art, it does so without firm conviction. By attaching such a title to a work in which luscious "veils" of warm color were allowed to flow at the whim of gravity, Louis created a new metaphor, perhaps unwittingly, for the unbridled flow of energy released in dance. A saraband is, after all, a sinuous dance popular

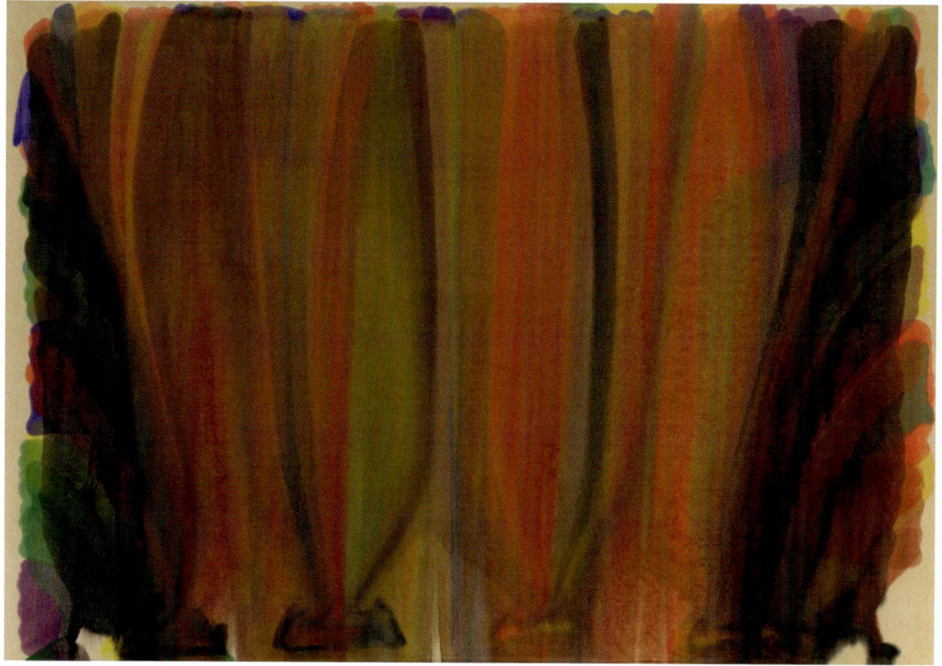

**Figure 143** Morris Louis, *Saraband*, 1959, acrylic resin on canvas, 8 feet 5 ⅛ inches × 12 feet 5 inches. (Solomon R. Guggenheim Museum, New York, 64.1685)

in European courts in the seventeenth and eighteenth centuries. Of either Persian or Arabic-Moorish origin, it was first considered wild and untamed, a "panto-mime of unparalleled suggestiveness." In Spain, stiff penalties of prison or exile were levied against those who dared to dance it. And Ben Jonson exclaimed, "How they are tickl'd with a light ayre! The bawdy Saraband."[8] As Spanish influence grew, the saraband passed into France where, in milder form, it became a favorite diversion at the court of Louis XIII. In an artist of lesser gravitas, one might suspect a Louis/Louis pun. The point is this: whatever his intent, Morris Louis has failed (happily, in my view) to eliminate all extra-artistic meaning from his work. The title's unmistakable reference to dance, combined with the strong lyrical allusion to sinuous, moving shapes, denies a vaunted purge of figural and thematic references.[9] *Saraband*'s post-painterly abstraction may indeed delight the eye, but it delights other faculties as well. In its persistent allusion to terpsi-chorean pleasures of the past, it refuses limitations as a "purified" visual experi-ence, drawing instead on the viewer's broader sensory intelligence.

In the next decade, the Minimalists banished (or re-banished) narrative, met-aphor, gesture, and personal feeling from art, striving through hard-edged geom-etry and industrial techniques and materials to approach complete impersonality in their artistic expression. But their goal of negating the messy complexity of the real world was supplanted in the late 1960s by artists who allowed narrative or metaphorical content to return to their work. Replacing timeless and sanitized geometry and hard industrial materials, they chose string, rubber, and other flex-ible materials to advance a variant of abstraction. In works such as *Rope Piece*

(1970, Whitney Museum of American Art, New York), Post-Minimalist sculptor Eva Hesse (1936–70) dipped lengths of rope into latex, then knotted and tangled them before suspending the resultant weblike form from wires attached to the ceiling. Something like Pollock's seemingly chaotic poured pieces, Hesse's *Rope Piece* achieved structure through variable forms that hang, drape, and change, casting shadows on the wall behind. Those shadows also call forth allusions to Man Ray's *The Rope Dancer Accompanies Herself with Her Shadows* (discussed in chapter 8) painted a half-century earlier. Out of Hesse's complex, clotted shapes—cast deliberately in formal disarray—emerge internal shapes, vertical in orientation, connected by gently outstretched arcs, which read as calligraphic abstractions of the human figure, drawn in space. Together they evoke the fluid, almost balletic quality of dance. Both Man Ray's and Hesse's pieces, like dance itself, challenge the idea of the art object as lasting and static. They wed what seems like rigor or system to a paradoxical spontaneity. And by undermining fixed form and scale, they create the possibility of changing iconographic interpretations, embodying both artists' sense of the essential absurdity of life.

In the wider arc of recent American painting, dance subjects have ranged from idealist figurative works to bold, straightforward abstraction. In his *Artist's Studio: The Dance* (1974, Museum of Modern Art, New York), Roy Lichtenstein (1923–97) combined elements of several of Matisse's paintings of the dance, including his 1912 *Nasturtiums with the Painting "Dance" II* (Metropolitan Museum of Art, New York), in which the French artist had already quoted from his own previous paintings of dance. Lichtenstein's trademark style of hard black outlines enclosing bright, crisp forms ensures that they can be seen at a distance, and so does Matisse's simplified, unfussy arrangement of dancing bodies, making this a doubly felicitous choice for one of Lichtenstein's many parodies of modernist icons. Asked about his appropriation of Matisse's *Dance*, Lichtenstein explained that he was trying to challenge accepted notions of painting and sensuality inherent in the subject of nude dancers. "Matisse loved to look at things and paint them—flowers, girls or whatever. . . . I've tried to take away anything [in Matisse's painting] that was beguiling,"[10] insisted Lichtenstein. With tongue in cheek and subversion on his mind, Lichtenstein made art about art about art. The quotations circle, just as Matisse's dancers do, endlessly.

Nancy Spero (1926–2009) also appreciated Matisse's dance paintings. In works such as her *Goddess II* (1985, collection of the artist), Spero borrowed some of his techniques for her own "attenuated moving figures," despite their very different approaches to decoration and political content in art. Mary Frank (b. 1933) studied dance in Martha Graham's classes in the late 1940s, then went on to make sculptures of bodies inspired by the dancers she saw there and by the organic shapes in the sculpture of Henry Moore. "[Graham] was ferocious and overwhelming," recalled Frank. "She talked about Greek ideas I wasn't interested in at the time, and she talked about sculpture. Particularly Henry Moore, the first sculptor I felt connected to."[11] Dance continued as a leitmotiv in Frank's work; she drew dancers in dimly lit rehearsal halls and befriended dancer Henrietta Bagley, whose wrapped dance movements inside lengths of stretchy cloth recalled the tubular forms Graham once created—a process of using the body as "material" subject to numinous transformations, and a vital part of the unremitting work (and play) of consciousness.

Joan Brown's (1938–90) many paintings of dance subjects in the 1970s explore the dynamics—and sometimes the ultimate futility—of human attempts to connect meaningfully with one another. In *The Last Dance* (1973, private collection), couples in a San Francisco ballroom are threatened by the macabre, apocalyptic presence of large rats, who approach and gnaw at them.

Performance artists in recent decades have used the theater, and sometimes dance, to explore alternative identities. Carolee Schneemann, Adrian Piper, and Laurie Anderson are among them, but it is Eleanor Antin (b. 1935), who turned her early training as an actress into fantasy dramas that explore aspects of the self. One of her best-known artistic personae was as *The Ballerina*, a part for which she prepared in the late 1970s by plunging deeply into ballet lessons prior to her "post-conceptual" performances.

American dancers, musicians, and choreographers in recent decades have collaborated with visual artists in stunning productions that continue to expand the dialogue between the two arts. Merce Cunningham (1919–2009), who began as a soloist with Martha Graham's company, was a fascinating transitional figure. As a choreographer, Cunningham's uncompromising abstraction was hailed as intrinsic to artistic modernism, as was his fascination with the creative process itself. His formal experiments extended from the use of chance to computer-generated steps, allowing indeterminacy to feed choreographic structure. The reception of such innovations depended on the critic's point of view. Detractors sometimes saw Cunningham's work as a descent into sterile formal exercises. Whatever the critical opinion, Cunningham was a creative force who integrated visual arts into his dances. In particular, he worked imaginatively with Robert Rauschenberg, Jasper Johns, Nam June Paik, Frank Stella, Robert Morris, Bruce Nauman, Morris Graves, and Andy Warhol, to name only the best known.[12] Even more recently, dancers such as Bill T. Jones have explored the integration of choreography with visual imagery produced by new media artists, who captured his voice and movements digitally, manipulating them to produce a virtual dance installation.[13] In such collaborations, it is as if the old dream of a *gesamtkunstwerk* has been reborn, bringing undreamed of solutions to an abiding challenge: how can the visual artist adjust the color, power, and shape of his or her visual means to suit or enhance the quality of the dance?

Dance reveals our desire for art spanning spectacle and a whole range of sensory gratifications. Through time and across fields, the dance between tradition and innovation is itself a deep part of human nature, and reveals, arguably, clues to a constantly evolving national consciousness.

Contemplative and mutually gifted in the organization of forms, visual artists and dancers have continued to sharpen our understandings of dance as part of the poetry and passion of life itself. Great dancers, like other extraordinary artists, make the world go round. And we, who can only gape at their creations, fasten on for the ride.

# Notes

## Preface

1. A few examples are John Collier and Ira Moskowitz, *American Indian Ceremonial Dances: Navajo, Pueblo, Apache, Zuñi* (New York: Bounty Books, 1972); Charlotte Heth, *Native American Dance: Ceremonies and Social Traditions* (Washington, D.C.: National Museum of the American Indian, Smithsonian Institution, 1992); James Mooney, *The Ghost-Dance Religion and the Sioux Outbreak of 1890* (Chicago: University of Chicago Press, 1965); Virginia More Roediger, *Ceremonial Costumes of the Pueblo Indians: Their Evolution, Fabrication, and Significance in the Prayer Drama* (Berkeley: University of California Press, 1991); and Sharyn R. Udall, "The Irresistible Other: Hopi Ritual Drama and Euro-American Audiences," in Udall, *Contested Terrain: Myth and Meanings in Southwest Art* (Albuquerque: University of New Mexico Press, 1996), 43–68. More generally, see Angela L. Miller et al., *American Encounters: Art, History, and Cultural Identity* (Upper Saddle River, N.J.: Pearson Education/Prentice Hall, 2008).

## Introduction

1. William Faulkner, interview with Jean Stein, *Paris Review* 12 (Spring 1956).
2. Taylor, quoted in Anna Kisselgoff, "Paul Taylor, Ballet's Beloved Enemy," *New York Times*, March 4, 2001, Art and Leisure, sec. 2, p. 11.
3. Angna Enters, *Artist's Life* (London: W. H. Allen, 1959), 30.
4. Joan Acocella, "The Flame: The Battle over Martha Graham's Dances," *New Yorker*, February 19 and 26, 2001, 194.
5. Pavlova, quoted in Mikka Gee, Judith Keller, and Anne Lyden, *Dance in Photography* (Los Angeles: J. Paul Getty Museum, 1999), n.p. My thanks to Amy Conger for this reference.
6. Graham, quoted in Barbara Morgan, *Martha Graham: Sixteen Dances in Photographs* (Dobbs Ferry, N.Y.: Morgan and Morgan, 1980), 11.
7. Mark Morris, interview on *The Newshour with Jim Lehrer*, PBS, March 23, 2001.

## Introduction to Part One

1. Matthew Arnold, *Civilization in the United States* (Boston: Cupples and Hurd, 1888), 170.
2. Graham, quoted in Walter Sorell, *The Dance through the Ages* (New York: Grosset and Dunlap, 1967), 195.
3. Carl Van Vechten, in *Parties* (New York: Knopf, 1930), reprinted in *Dance Index* 1, nos. 9, 10, 11 (September, October, November 1942): 186.

## Chapter 1. Expressing the Real or Imagined Heritage of a Nation

1. Thomas Hariot, quoted in *The New World: The First Pictures of America Made by John White and Jacques Le Moyne and Engraved by Theodore de Bry with Contemporary Narratives of the Huguenot Settlement in Florida, 1562–1565,*

*and the Virginia colony, 1585–1590,* ed. Stefan Lorant (New York: Duell, Sloan and Pearce, 1946), 247.

2. The French artist-cartographer Jacques Le Moyne (1533–88) accompanied an earlier expedition to Florida and South Carolina in 1564, making forty-two watercolors of Native American life, only one of which survives. Whether there were dance images among the group is unknown.

3. Not until 1784 was the first serious ballet production recorded in Philadelphia, a production called *La Forêt noire* starring French dancer Mme. Gardie and John Durang, America's only important dancer of the eighteenth century.

4. Lully (1632–87) was an influential figure in the court of Louis XIV, known for his dance and ballet music. He is credited with introducing new dances, such as the minuet, and for including fast-paced older forms such as the gigue, bourreé, and gavotte in his ballets. Lully was first to introduce women dancers on the French stage.

5. Allen Dodworth, *Dancing and Its Relation to Education and Social Life* (New York: Harpers, 1885). See also Ann Barzel, "European Dance Teachers in the United States," *Dance Index* 3, no. 3 (March 1944): 56–100.

6. John Cotton, quoted in Joseph E. Marks, *America Learns to Dance* (New York: Exposition Press, 1957), 15. As early as 1685 a dancing master named Francis Stepney had the audacity to set up a school of "mixt dancing" in Puritan New England, a venture quickly squelched, perhaps because instruction took place on Sunday. Stepney's affronts perhaps precipitated the famous tract of the next year, whose title tells all: "An Arrow against Profane and Promiscuous Dancing, drawne out of the Quiver of the Scriptures. By the Ministers of Christ at Boston in New England" (1686). The early church fathers—Chysostom, Ambrose, and Augustine, for example—had indeed given the Puritans ample ammunition against dance as an incitement to the flesh. On the other hand, though dance had its defenders throughout American history, the negativity of Puritan attitudes was not rigorously challenged until 1934, when Percy A. Scholes published *The Puritans and Music,* which gave a more balanced view of Puritan objections to dance, theater, and public entertainments of all kinds. More recently, dance sociologist Helen Thomas (*Dance, Modernity and Culture: Explorations in the Sociology of Dance* [London: Routledge, 1995], 31–35) has carefully weighed the causes and effects of Puritan attitudes toward dance, including the charge that the growth of professional art dance in the United States was thereby deterred.

7. E. D. Andrews, "The Dance in Shaker Ritual," in *Chronicles of the American Dance,* ed. Paul Magriel (New York: Da Capo, 1978), 12.

8. In the 1930s the modern dancer-choreographer Doris Humphrey presented *The Shakers,* in which she took a fresh look at Shaker ritual, employing their notion of "dancing one's sins away" in a theatrical performance that fused dance with song, narrative, and instrumental music. It was later filmed by Thomas Bouchard, with adaptations of Humphrey's choreography to suit cinematic requirements, and still images of the Humphrey-Charles Weidman production, photographed by Edward Steichen, appeared in *Vanity Fair* in 1933. *The Shakers* has been periodically revived by various companies.

9. Charlotte Cushman, quoted in Flo Morse, *The Shakers and the World's People* (Hanover: University Press of New England, 1980), vii.

10. The term "usable past" was invoked by critic Van Wyck Brooks, who urged Americans to open up the American past for new scrutiny, new interpretations:

"Discover, invent a usable past we certainly can, and that is what a vital criticism always does. . . . The past is an inexhaustible storehouse of apt attitudes and adaptable ideals; it opens of itself at the touch of desire; it yields up, now this treasure, now that, to anyone who comes to it armed with a capacity for personal choices" ("On Creating a Usable Past," *The Dial* 64 [April 11, 1918]: 337).

11. Quotes are from Washington Irving, *A History of New York from the Beginning of the World to the End of the Dutch Dynasty* (New York: Putnam, 1860), 405–6.

12. I am indebted here to Bryan Jay Wolfe's incisive interpretation of this painting in his *Romantic Re-Vision: Culture and Consciousness in Nineteenth-Century American Painting and Literature* (Chicago: University of Chicago Press, 1982), 131–40.

13. Irving, *A History of New York*, 311–12.

14. Quidor would remain interested in Irving's Knickerbocker tales, painting another dance scene two decades later in his *Peter Stuyvesant Watching Festivities on the Battery*, c. 1860 (Hunter Museum of American Art, Chattanooga, Tennessee).

15. Allen Dodworth, *Dancing*, quoted in Rosetta O'Neill, "The Dodworth Family and Ballroom Dancing in New York," in Magriel, *Chronicles of the American Dance*, 90.

16. Winifred E. Howe, *A History of the Metropolitan Museum of Art* (New York: Agilliss, 1913), n.p. It is not recorded how the Met dealt with the unusual floor in the grand hall: Dodworth had installed parquet inlaid with black walnut squares and lines to mark the correct angles for dancers' feet.

17. Robert W. Snyder and Rebecca Zurier, "Picturing the City," in Rebecca Zurier, Robert W. Snyder, and Virginia M. Mecklenburg, *Metropolitan Lives: The Ashcan Artists and Their New York* (Washington, D.C.: National Museum of American Art, 1995), 161.

18. David Bjelajac, *American Art: A Cultural History* (Upper Saddle River, N.J.: Prentice Hall, 2000), 290.

19. Rhea Childe Door, *What Eight Million Women Want* (Boston: Small, Maynard, 1910), quoted in Julie Malnig, "Two-Stepping to Glory: Social Dance and the Rhetoric of Social Mobility," in *Moving History/Dancing Cultures*, ed. Ann Dils and Ann Cooper Albright (Middletown, Conn.: Wesleyan University Press, 2001), 283.

20. From a 1904 study of Lower East Side social life by Columbia University graduate student Bella Mead, quoted in Bruce Weber, *Ashcan Kids: Children in the Art of Henri, Luks, Glackens, Bellows and Sloan* (New York: Berry-Hill Galleries, 1998), 14.

21. Eberle quoted in Christina Merriman, "New Bottles for New Wine," *Survey* 30 (May 3, 1913): 196–99.

22. Anonymous speaker, quoted in *Encyclopaedia Britannica*, 15th ed., s.v. "dance."

23. Mount, manuscript at Stony Brook, following an entry dated August 30, 1847, quoted in Barbara Novak, *American Painting of the Nineteenth Century* (New York: Harper and Row, 1979), 151. Mount's papers contain frequent references to his knowledge of Dutch art, including Ruysdael, Rembrandt, Hobbema, and Teniers.

24. Elizabeth Johns, *American Genre Painting: The Politics of Everyday Life* (New Haven, Conn.: Yale University Press, 1991), 25.

25. John Lewis Krimmel trained in Stuttgart and London, then immigrated to Philadelphia, where he taught drawing and made portraits before his death in 1822.

26. Mount, from *Christian Examiner* 15 (November 1833): 193 ff., quoted in Novak, *American Painting of the Nineteenth Century*, 145.

27. Mount, letter to brother Nelson from Catskill, October 1, 1843, quoted in Novak, *American Painting of the Nineteenth Century*, 306n3.

28. Dance as diversion for rural Americans engaged many painters at midcentury. Asher B. Durand, encountered above in his imagined recreation of a dance scene in Stuyvesant's New York, also turned his attention to rural American manners and amusements. His *Dance of the Haymakers* (1851, Detroit Institute of Arts), like Mount's, trades on rusticity and release—the old American ethic of earned leisure after hard physical labor.

29. Crockett, quoted in Foster Rhea Dulles, *A History of Recreation* (New York: Appleton-Century-Crofts, 1965), 37.

30. Emerson, quoted in John Wilmerding, *American Views: Essays on American Art* (Princeton, N.J.: Princeton University Press, 1991), 190.

31. Art historians have posited a variety of sources for Bingham's dancing figure extending back as far as the *Dancing Satyr* from the House of the Faun in Pompeii. E. Maurice Bloch, in his definitive *George Caleb Bingham: The Evolution of an Artist* (Berkeley: University of California Press, 1967), has documented Bingham's repeated quotation of classical sculptural sources in his painting. Such sources would have been available to the Missouri-based Bingham through instruction books and exhibitions he encountered during his occasional travels east. Thomas Hart Benton, whose twentieth-century Missouri career offers several parallels to Bingham's, painted figures whose muscularity and energy—more writhing and tense than Bingham's—also owe a considerable debt to Michelangelo.

32. Novak, *American Painting of the Nineteenth Century*, 165.

33. *Saint Louis Missouri Republican*, 27 November 1847, quoted in Johns, *American Genre Painting*, 86–87. Bingham's series depicting flatboatmen would grow to include at least twelve variations, in which subjects—besides dancing—play cards, watch cargo, or simply relax in port.

34. The tree was located in what is now the Calaveras Big Tree State Park.

35. I am thinking here of Cole's *The Oxbow* (1836, Metropolitan Museum of Art, New York) and Inness's *The Lackawanna Valley* (1855, National Gallery of Art, Washington, D.C.).

36. Thomas Hart Benton, "My American Epic in Paint," *Creative Arts* 3 (December 1928), xxxii.

37. Frances K. Pohl, *Framing America: A Social History of American Art* (New York: Thames and Hudson, 2002), 399.

38. Russell Lee, "Life on the American Frontier—1941 Version," *U.S. Camera* 4, no. 10 (October 1941), 41.

39. J. B. Colson, "The Art of the Human Document: Russell Lee in New Mexico," in J. B. Colson et al., *Far from Main Street: Three Photographers in Depression-Era New Mexico, Russell Lee, John Collier, Jr., and Jack Delano* (Santa Fe: Museum of New Mexico Press, 1994), 7.

40. See Augusta Fink, *I-Mary: A Biography of Mary Austin* (Tucson: University of Arizona Press, 1983), 245.

41. Andrew Lang, quoted in Jackson Lears, *No Place of Grace: Antimodernism and the Transformation of American Culture 1880–1920* (New York: Pantheon, 1981), 172–73.

42. Lears, *No Place of Grace*, 173.

43. Robert Coe, *Dance in America* (New York: E. P. Dutton, 1985), 142.

44. Elizabeth Hylbom, "Martha Graham's Technique Perfect," unidentified clipping in Broadmoor Art Academy Scrapbooks, Colorado Springs Fine Arts Center Library. Colorado painter and critic Archie Musick, for example, found Graham's dance inaccessible, wondering in print whether she was "artist or charlatan" (Musick, "The Transplanting of Culture," *Magazine of Art*, March 1937, 146).

45. Graham, quoted in Merle Armitage, *Martha Graham: The Early Years* (New York: Da Capo Press, 1978), 101.

46. Graham, quoted in Armitage, *Martha Graham*, 97. Graham's decision to simplify her productions was confirmed as well by an earlier experience with Georgia O'Keeffe, from whom she tried to borrow one of the painter's famous flower paintings to use as a backdrop in a new dance piece. "[O'Keeffe] refused," recalled Graham, "because she felt that it had nothing to do with the dance. And from that point on, I have tried to avoid a painting or a backdrop of any kind" (Graham, *Blood Memory* [New York: Doubleday, 1991], 133).

47. Noguchi, quoted in Robert Tracy, *Spaces of the Mind: Isamu Noghuchi's Dance Designs* (New York: Proscenium, 2001), 24.

48. Noguchi, *A Sculptor's World* (New York: Harper and Row, 1968), 47.

49. William Zorach, *Art Is My Life: The Autobiography of William Zorach* (Cleveland: World Publishing Company, 1967), 131.

50. John Martin, "To a Performer, Now High in Her Art, an Audience of Americans Pays Tribute," *New York Times*, February 8, 1931, www.nytimes.com/library/arts/02083.

51. Zorach, *Art Is My Life*, 131. My thanks to Sarah Burt for suggesting the Graham–Zorach connection.

52. Deborah Jowitt, "Dances with Sculpture," Tate Modern, London, November 1, 2006–January 21, 2007, http://www.tate.org.uk.

53. See Rosalind E. Krauss, *The Sculpture of David Smith: A Catalogue Raisonné* (New York: Garland, 1977), 164 for *Adagio* and 171 for *Boaz Dancing School*.

54. Nevelson, quoted in Carol Diehl, "The World of Mrs. N.," *Art in America*, January 2008, 109.

## Chapter 2. African American Dance and Art

1. This print is in the collection of the New York Historical Society. Its subtitle reads "View of the Stage on the fifty-seventh Night of Mr. T. D. Rice of Kentucky in His Original and Celebrated Extravaganza of JIM CROW on Which Occasion Every Department of the House Was Thronged to an Excess Unprecedented in the Records of Theatrical Attraction." It is further captioned "New York, 25th November 1833," although contemporary records indicate a more likely performance date of January 8, 1833. See Dale Cockrell, *"Jim Crow," Demons of Disorder: Early Blackface Minstrels and Their World* (Cambridge: Cambridge University Press, 1977).

2. Jim Crow was the minstrel character whose name became synonymous with a whole system of legal segregation that effectively separated the domains of whites and blacks and lasted until the 1960s.

3. Homer's engraving was published in the *Harper's Weekly* of December 21, 1861.

4. At the very beginning of his professional career Eakins had painted a dancing child in his *Street Scene, Seville* (1870), discussed in chapter 4.

5. Martin A. Berger, *Man Made: Thomas Eakins and the Construction of Gilded Age Manhood* (Berkeley: University of California Press, 2000), 32.

6. The Golliwog, emerging from folklore and the popular tales of Bertha Upton from the 1890s, was a jolly gnome, a fantastic froglike creature, a kind of Dutch knight-errant, whose adventures inspired Debussy.

7. A number of early films were made of the cakewalk, including *Bally-Hoo Cake Walk* (Biograph, 1903); *Cakewalk on the Beach of Coney Island* (Biograph, 1904); *Comedy Cake Walk* (Biograph, 1903); and *Cakewalk* (Pathé, before 1906). Several of these are in the collection of the Library of Congress. Yet another reincarnation of the minstrel show "walk around" would appear in Martha Graham's exploration of her country's cultural sensibility *American Document* (1938).

8. Bernstein, quoted in Gerard Jackson, *Theresa Bernstein: Expressions of Cape Ann & New York, 1914–1972* (Stamford, Conn.: Stamford Museum and Nature Center and Smith-Girard, 1989), n.p.

9. Harlem Renaissance is, as many scholars have noted, an inadequate term in its failure to account for African American cultural activities outside New York and before the 1920s. In the absence of a better term I retain it here.

10. William E. B. Du Bois, *The Negro* (1915; London: Oxford University Press, 1970), 5.

11. Douglas's style had developed from even more protean sources. His use of simplified shapes and exaggerated line evolved through two years of study with German painter Winold Reiss, who himself used Jugendstil graphics and German folk-art sources for his own brand of the "primitive."

12. Richard Jobson, *The Golden Trade* (Teighmouth: E. E. Speight and R. H. Walpole, 1904), 136.

13. Van Vechten, "The Lindy Hop," *Dance Index* 1, nos. 9, 10, 11 (September, October, November, 1942): 187.

14. William H. Johnson, quoted in Nora Holt, "Primitives on Exhibit," *New York Amsterdam News*, March 9, 1946, cited in Adelyn D. Breeskin, *William H. Johnson, 1901–1970* (Washington, D.C.: National Collection of American Art, 1972), 18.

15. Johnson, quoted in Richard J. Powell, "Re/Birth of a Nation," in *Rhapsodies in Black*, ed. Richard J. Powell (Berkeley: Hayward Gallery, Institute of International Visual Arts and University of California Press, 1997), 25.

16. Motley, statement written upon receiving the Harmon gold medal, 1929, quoted in Romare Bearden and Harry Henderson, *A History of African-American Artists* (New York: Pantheon, 1993), 152.

17. Emily Farnham, *Charles Demuth: Behind a Laughing Mask* (Norman: University of Oklahoma Press, 1971), 103. In a 1956 interview with Farnham, Marcel Duchamp reported that it was Demuth who first took him to Harlem, to the Little Savoy.

18. *The Masses* reader Carlotta Russell Lowell, quoted in Rebecca Zurier, *Art for the Masses (1911–1917): A Radical Magazine and Its Graphics* (New Haven, Conn.: Yale University Art Gallery, 1985), 156.

19. Van Gogh's *Bal à Arles* was illustrated in the Armory Show catalog as number 425. In 1920 it was again shown in New York in a major Van Gogh exhibit at the Montross Gallery. Although Van Gogh was much discussed, and had by then been recognized for some twenty years by French critics, American audiences were slow to appreciate him. At the Montross show's close none of Van Gogh's paintings had sold. But Davis would take up Van Gogh's palette and energetic brushstroke in his own Tioga landscape series, c. 1919. By contrast with Van Gogh, Picabia's *Dances at the Spring* (discussed in a later chapter) presented a stylistically radical interpretation of the dance, with its Cubist-type figures. Other dance subjects in the Armory Show catalog included a plaster *Danseurs* by sculptor Raymond Duchamp-Villon, an oil *Dancer* by George Bellows, and works by Jerome Myers, Robert W. Chanler, Bessie Potter Vonnoh, and Auguste Rodin.

20. Stuart Davis, "Autobiography" (New York: American Artists Group Monographs, 6, 1945), reprinted in Diane Kelder, ed., *Stuart Davis* (New York: Praeger, 1971), 23–24.

21. Davis, "On Abstract Art" (1935), reprinted in Barbara Rose, ed., *Readings in American Art since 1900* (New York: Praeger, 1968), 124.

22. Ibid.

23. Ione Robinson, letter to her parents dated September 20, 1928, quoted in Patricia Hills, ed. *Modern Art in the USA* (Upper Saddle River, N.J.: Prentice Hall, 2001), 86.

24. Ruellan, quoted in Joycelyn Pang Lumsdaine and Thomas O'Sullivan, *The Prints of Adolf Dehn: A Catalogue Raisonné* (Minnesota: Minnesota Historical Society Press, 1987), 24n77.

25. Gilbert Seldes, "Toujours Jazz," *The Dial* (August 1923), reprinted in *The Dial: Arts and Letters in the 1920s*, ed. Gaye L. Brown (Worcester, Mass.: Worcester Art Museum, 1981), 107.

26. Paul Colin, from his autobiography *La Croûte* (1957), quoted in Henry Louis Gates Jr. and Karen C. C. Dalton, introduction to *Josephine Baker and La Revue Nègre* (New York: Abrams, 1998), 9.

27. French dance critic André Levinson, quoted in Gates and Dalton, introduction, 7. For much more on the gender and racial politics that surround Josephine Baker's life and legend, see Brenda Dixon Gottschild, *The Black Dancing Body: A Geography from Coon to Cool* (New York: Palgrave Macmillan, 2003); Benetta Jules-Rosette, *Josephine Baker in Art and Life: The Icon and the Image* (Urbana: University of Illinois Press, 2007); and Olivia Lahs-Gonzales, ed. *Josephine Baker: Image and Icon* (Saint Louis: Reedy Press, 2006).

28. Geoffrey C. Ward and Ken Burns, *Jazz: A History of America's Music* (New York: Knopf, 2000), 156. Still extant today is a certain tension, or at least uncertainty, about the racial versus national identification of jazz. In the United States jazz had an early and abiding racial identification with African Americans, but gradually lost its identification as "black" or "white," becoming a nationalized form of cultural production. Abroad, especially in Paris, jazz was regarded as a quintessentially American cultural product, overlaid with African or "primitive" elements. Jazz dance is generally regarded as a creolized form, with rhythmic elements and body usage from sources in both African American and European American culture.

29. Baker became a naturalized French citizen in 1937 but retained ties to the United States and to her African American heritage there. She made several trips

to the United States in the 1960s to participate in civil rights demonstrations, and she returned in triumph to the New York stage in 1973.

30. Colin, quoted in Gates and Dalton, introduction, 9.

31. Wanda M. Corn, *The Great American Thing: Modern Art and National Identity, 1915–1935* (Berkeley: University of California Press, 1999), 116.

32. Norman Bryson, "Cultural Studies and Dance History," in *Meaning in Motion: New Cultural Studies of Dance*, ed. Jane C. Desmond (Durham, N.C.: Duke University Press, 1997), 75.

33. For Paul Colin's illustration of the caricatured Jane Marnac in *Pluie*, see Gates and Dalton, introduction, plate 3.

34. The interpretation of Matulka's personification of mechanical objects is bolstered by paintings he made in succeeding years, such as his *Gasoline Pumps* (c. 1934), which is illustrated in the catalog by Patterson Sims et al., *Jan Matulka 1890–1972* (Washington, D.C.: National Collection of Fine Arts and the Whitney Museum of American Art, 1980), cat. no. 59. It is also reminiscent of Paul Haviland's famous remark: "Man made the machine in his own image. . . . The phonograph is the image of his voice; the camera the image of his eye." Haviland, "We Are Living in the Age of the Machine," 291, no. 7–8 (September–October 1915): cover page.

35. Phyllis Rose, *Jazz Cleopatra: Josephine Baker in Her Time* (New York: Doubleday, 1989), 25; Anthea Kraut, "Primitivism and Diaspora: The Dance Performances of Josephine Baker, Zora Neale Hurston, and Katherine Dunham," *Theatre Journal* 55, no. 3 (October 2003): 440.

36. Less famous than Baker, perhaps because she pursued a career in modern dance, was Edna Guy, principal performer in the New Negro Art Theatre Dance Group, formed in 1931. Their pioneering work celebrated the black dance heritage in America, using African ritual and Negro spirituals as inspiration. Before the company's formation, John Sloan often hired Edna Guy, already a dancer, as a studio model for paintings. Unfortunately, he never portrayed her dancing. Instead, she provided rewarding figural and coloristic studies for him. Wrote Sloan: "Among all the racial strains we have in this country, the negro furnishes the most beautiful individuals. They are well termed 'colored people' and more artists might find them a rich field for color-sculptural study" (quoted in *The Art of John Sloan 1871–1951*, exhibition catalog [Brunswick, Maine: Walker Art Museum, Bowdoin College, 1962], n.p.). For Sloan's 1920s paintings of Guy, see nos. 790, 797, 800, 835, 836, 838 in Rowland Elzea, *John Sloan's Oil Paintings: A Catalogue Raisonné*, vol. 2 (Newark: University of Delaware Press and Associated University Presses, 1991).

37. Matthew Baigell, "American Art and National Identity: The 1920s," in *Critical Issues in American Art: A Book of Readings*, ed. Mary Ann Calo (Boulder, Colo.: Westview Press, 1998), 271–72.

## Introduction to Part Two

1. Israel Shenker, interview with Helen Gardner, *New York Times*, June 7, 1973, 56.

2. Wassily Kandinsky, *Concerning the Spiritual in Art* (New York: Dover, 1977), 50.

3. The exploration of human behavior was undertaken in many publications, notably Freud's *The Interpretation of Dreams*, which appeared in 1900.

4. Baigell, "American Art and National Identity: The 1920s," in Calo, *Critical Issues in American Art*, 271–72.

5. Doris Humphrey, quoted in Thomas E. Wartenberg, "Is Dance Elitist?" in *Philosophical Essays on Dance*, ed. Gordon Fancher and Gerald Myers (Durham, N.C.: American Dance Festival, 1981), 122–23.

## Chapter 3. Revisiting Arcadia

1. This description of paganism was devised by Malcolm Cowley, who in his durable study *Exile's Return* (New York: Viking, 1934) identified paganism as one of the animating features of the era of the early twentieth century in America.

2. Colette, *Oeuvres*, 3 vols. (Paris: Gallimard, 1984), 2:1284, quoted in Judith Thurman, *Secrets of the Flesh: A Life of Colette* (New York: Ballantine, 1999), 144.

3. Rodin, quoted in Sam Hunter, John Jacobus, and Daniel Wheeler, *Modern Art* (New York: Abrams, 2000), 63. Rodin's phrase is reminiscent of Baudelaire's famous assertion that everyday gesture and dress could express the heroic nature of modern life. In the search to free art from its bondage to literary illustration, high-flown allegory, and mythology and its religious successors, Baudelaire and Rodin pointed the way. We might argue whether the natural is inherently at odds with the conventions of Salon art, but the conceptual contrast is (and was) at least debatable.

4. Quoted in Marcel Raymond, *From Baudelaire to Surrealism* (New York: Wittenborn, Schultz, 1950), 58.

5. Quoted in ibid., 59.

6. Nathaniel Hawthorne, *The Marble Faun* (New York: New American Library, 1961), 69–70.

7. Quoted in Patricia C. F. Mandel, *Selection VII: American Paintings in the Museum's Collection, c. 1800–1930* (Providence: Rhode Island School of Design, 1977), 183n6.

8. Kendall, *Where She Danced* (New York: Alfred A. Knopf, 1979), 123.

9. Lawrence, *Lady Chatterley's Lover* (Garden City, N.Y.: International Collectors Library, n.d.), 222.

10. Later, James Joyce would honor that legacy of paganism and nature. In his *Ulysses*, which in T. S. Eliot's view destroyed the whole of the nineteenth century, Joyce's narrator weaves nature together with a pagan past, observing a deaf gardener "on the sombre lawn watching narrowly the dancing motes of grasshalms. To ourselves . . . new paganism . . . *omphalos*."

11. Curt Sachs, *World History of the Dance* (New York: W. W. Norton, 1937), 447.

12. Charles Eldredge, *American Imagination and Symbolist Painting* (New York University: Grey Art Gallery and Study Center, 1979), 18.

13. Mallarmé, quoted in Institute of Contemporary Art, *Art and Dance*, 13.

14. See discussion in Mandel, *Selection VII*, 211–12, citing Joseph Czestochowski.

15. The Pollaiuolo engraving passed from Pulitzer by bequest to the Metropolitan Museum of Art, New York, in 1917.

16. Kendall, *Where She Danced*, 87. Whitney took some dance lessons from Ruth St. Denis.

17. In the years immediately surrounding Zorach's *Dance*, a number of costume balls, popularly known as "Pagan Routs" or "Bals primitifs" were held in New

York's Greenwich Village. In this sense the word *pagan* signaled both a rejection of tradition and a declaration of modernity, especially popular with journalists who applied the term the New Paganism broadly, as in the Village's short-lived little magazine called *The Pagan*. In a similar vein, the Smithsonian American Art Museum has Marguerite Zorach's linoleum cut *The Dance* (1917), an image of women and children dancing exuberantly. Still another work of dancers by Marguerite Zorach is *Provincetown* (1921, Tom Veilleux Gallery, Portland, Maine).

18. Donna M. Cassidy, "John Marin's Dancing Nudes by the Seashore," *Smithsonian Studies in American Art* 4, no. 1 (Winter 1990), 82. Marin would have been familiar with Matisse's *Joy of Life* from at least 1909, when a reproduction of it was exhibited at Stieglitz's Gallery 291. He would likely also have seen Matisse's *Nasturtiums with the Painting "Dance" II* (1912), which was exhibited in the 1913 Armory Show, was acquired by prominent collector Scofield Thayer after 1923 and was reproduced in *The Dial* during that decade. Later, Marin pasted a photograph of Matisse's *The Dance* (1909) in his scrapbook, and throughout the 1930s and 1940s continued to collect reproductions of dancers and bathers by Matisse, Picasso, and Cézanne, affording him easy access to European prototypes. Matisse had a major U.S. exhibition at the Brooklyn Museum in 1928. Marin was also familiar with Matisse's mural *The Dance II (1931–33)*, at the Barnes Foundation near Philadelphia. Cassidy, 79.

19. Graham, from an early interview, quoted in Coe, *Dance in America*, 138.

## Chapter 4. Romantic Imports

1. Walter Sorell, *Dance through the Ages* (New York: Grosset and Dunlap, 1967), 80–81.

2. Lola de Valence was the Spanish ballerina Lola Melea who appeared at the Hippodrome in Paris with the Royal Ballet of Madrid in 1862. Manet also made an etching of her in 1863, an impression of which is in the Hunterian Art Gallery, University of Glasgow.

3. Two versions of Degas's *Spanish Dance* are listed as Bronze No. 20 (model date 1896–1911, Detroit Institute of Arts, 69.302), and Bronze No. 45 (model date 1882–95) *Dancer with Tambourine* is Bronze No. 12 (model date 1882–95). See Joseph S. Czestochowski and Anne Pingeot, eds., *Degas Sculptures: Catalogue Raisonné of the Bronzes* (Memphis: Torch Press and International Arts, 2002).

4. Philip Hone, *The Diary of Philip Hone*, quoted in *Dance Index* 6, no. 9 (1947): 222. Although the original never traveled to the United States, her famous dancer-choreographer brother Paul and her namesake niece did.

5. Quoted in Diane Waldman, *Joseph Cornell* (New York: George Braziller, 1977), 20.

6. Joseph Cornell, "Comment," *Dance Index* 6, no. 9 (1947): 203. Other Cornell works celebrating the ballet include several dedicated to the twentieth-century Russian dancer Tamara Toumanova, whom Cornell visited backstage. Dancer and artist exchanged small gifts; she provided sequins, beads, or feathers from her costumes, which the adoring but socially awkward Cornell then incorporated into worshipful collages and constructions like *A Swan Lake for Tamara Toumanova (Homage to the Romantic Ballet)* (1946, The Menil Collection, Houston). For more on these works, see Dickran Tashjian, *Joseph Cornell: Gifts of Desire* (Miami Beach, Fla.: Greenfield, 1992), 111 ff.

7.  See, for example, *Portrait of Ondine* (Smithsonian American Art Museum) and Cornell's cover design for *Dance Index* 3, nos. 9, 10, 11 (September, October, November 1944).

8. Cornell, quoted in Sandra Leonard Starr, *Joseph Cornell and the Ballet* (New York: Castelli, Feigen, Corcoran, 1983), 20.

9. For a fuller discussion on Cornell's Christian Science beliefs and their effect on his art, see ibid., 22–24.

10. Cornell and Duchamp shared a number of interests, including using box formats and assembling ready-made materials. Beginning in 1942 Cornell assisted Duchamp in assembling an edition of fabricated miniature reproductions of the Frenchman's earlier work (his *Boîte-en- valise*); thus, Cornell was thoroughly familiar with all Duchamp's work and may well have made knowing reference in his own work to the *Fresh Widow* construction. Cornell also compiled a thick dossier of Duchamp memorabilia. Their admiration was mutual; Duchamp called Cornell one of the most important and original twentieth-century American artists. *Joseph Cornell/Marcel Duchamp . . . In Resonance*, an exhibition exploring their many common interests, was mounted in 1999 by the Philadelphia Museum of Art.

11. Cornell's preoccupation, bordering on obsession, has resulted in a number of articles and catalogs based on his dance subjects See, for example, Starr, *Joseph Cornell and the Ballet.*

12.  Cornell was an avid collector of early dance films and owned prints of many, including one of Loïe Fuller in *Fire Dance* (see fig. 99). A catalog of dance films published by *Dance Index* (vol. 4 [1945]: 62 ff.) lists many films owned by Cornell.

13. Eakins, letter to his sister Caroline, Christmas 1869, quoted in Lloyd Goodrich, *Thomas Eakins: His Life and Work* (New York: Whitney Museum of American Art, 1933), 32.

14. Eakins, letter to his father, quoted in Darrel Sewell, *Thomas Eakins: Artist of Philadelphia* (Philadelphia: Philadelphia Museum of Art, 1982), 5.

15. Mary Cassatt to Emily Sartain, October 27, 1872, quoted in Nancy M. Mathews, ed. *Cassatt and Her Circle: Selected Letters* (New York: Abbeville, 1984), 109.

16. Cassatt's great friend Degas, fascinated by dance throughout his career, would himself produce small Spanish-themed bronze sculptures. See note 3, above.

17. Havelock Ellis, quoted in J. E. Crawford Flitch, *Modern Dancing and Dancers* (1912; Philadelphia: J. B. Lippincott, 1947), 196.

18. Trevor Fairbrother, *Sargent the Sensualist* (Seattle: Seattle Art Museum and Yale University Press, 2000), 99.

19.  Robert Hughes, *American Visions* (New York: Knopf, 1997), 251.

20.  James, quoted in Trevor Fairbrother, *John Singer Sargent* (New York: Abrams, 1994), 102.

21. Fairbrother, *John Singer Sargent*, 23.

22. Flitch, *Modern Dancing and Dancers*, 197.

23. H. I. Brock in the *New York Times*, quoted in Downes, *John Sargent: His Life and Work* (Boston: Little, Brown, 1925), 31. So impressed with Carmencita's talent was Sargent that he arranged a private performance for Isabella Stewart Gardner, who would become the owner of his *El Jaleo*. In a sketchbook Sargent later (1919) gave to Mrs. Gardner are twenty-one preparatory drawings for *El Jaleo* and four drawings, different in style and paper quality, which Warren Adelson and Elizabeth Oustinoff have suggested might be sketches of *La*

*Carmencita* (Adelson and Oustinoff, "Sargent's Spanish Dancer—a Discovery," *Antiques* 141, no. 3 [March 1992]: 471n14).

24. Sargent, quoted in Evan Charteris, *John Sargent* (New York: Scribner's Sons, 1927), 113.

25. Adolph Bolm, one of the Ballets Russes stars, toured Spain with Diaghilev in 1916, studying flamenco with José Otero. Bolm choreographed *The Birthday of the Infanta* for the Chicago Grand Opera in 1919. The Ballets Russes productions of *Las Meninas* (1916), *Le Tricorne* (1919, music by Manuel de Falla, scenery and costumes by Picasso), and *Cuadro Flamenco* (1921, with scenery and costumes by Picasso) similarly reflect the character of Spanish dance.

26. Matisse, for example, while in Seville in 1910 encountered a sixteen-year-old gypsy dancer named Dora, whom he called "a miracle of suppleness and rhythm . . . [who] revealed to me what the dance could be. . . . I compared her to the celebrated Is. Duncan, whose gestures cut across the flow of the music, where Dora by contrast prolonged the sound with her arabesques." Matisse, quoted in Hilary Spurling, *Matisse the Master* (New York: Knopf, 2005), 63.

27. Man Ray, quoted in Arturo Schwarz, *Man Ray: The Rigour of Imagination* (New York: Rizzoli, 1977), 39.

28. Henri de Toulouse-Lautrec (1864–1901) depicted Jane Avril on numerous occasions, including his famous poster of her performing the cancan at the Parisian nightclub the Divan Japonais (1893, color lithograph, Hunterian Art Gallery, University of Glasgow).

29. Editorial from *Harper's Weekly*, November 23, 1867, quoted in Lloyd Goodrich, *Winslow Homer's America, 1857–1880* (New York: Tudor, 1969), 85.

30. William Glackens, quoted in *William Glackens: The Formative Years* (New York: Kraushaar Galleries, 1991), 2.

31. Despite his efforts in Paris to refashion his career, Glackens would rely until 1919 on his work as magazine illustrator and newspaper artist to finance his painting.

32. John Marin (1870–1953), also resident in Paris in those years, made an etching of the subject: *Bal Bullier, Paris*, 1906, Museum of Fine Arts, Boston, Gift of L. Aaron Lebowich, 1950, 50.3261.

33. Cornell, letter to Marianne Moore, June 21, 1944, quoted in Tashjian, *Joseph Cornell*, 73.

34. Among those other Americans who knew Matisse from reproductions in *Camera Work* and admired him in the Armory Show was Man Ray, whose 1914 drawing *Figures Dancing in a Circle* (Los Angeles County Museum of Art) may owe something to Matisse's celebrated *Joy of Life*.

35. Matisse, quoted in James Johnson Sweeney, preface to Charlotte Trowbridge, *Dance Drawings of Martha Graham* (New York: The Dance Observer, 1945), n.p.

36. Isadora Duncan counted the dancers in Botticelli's *Primavera*, a reproduction of which hung in her childhood home, as an important early influence on her work.

37. Rodin's use of circling figures is essentially more serious, more allegorical, less allusive to a golden age than Matisse's. Many modern artists, including Rodin, saw the passions and pressures driving modern humanity flowing out of the same deeply rooted struggles apparent from earlier centuries, and often expressed in images of the dance. In Europe, the Church had for centuries been the great enemy of the dance, associating it with licentiousness and, perhaps more threatening still, with old pagan customs. Dance symbolized the

people's resistance to Christianity's efforts to root out old diabolical connotations. The round dance (the Reigen, rondo, or la Ronde), summoned fears of morbid, evil practices, mingled with themes of death, time, and the medieval Wheel of Fortune—all allegories of the inescapable cycles of human destiny outside orthodoxy. Naked women, demons and the Sabbat Noir were thematic and formal residues unforgotten by modern artists such as Rodin, who seems to have been aware of the allegorical power of dance imagery in formulating studies for such works as *The Burghers of Calais* and *The Gates of Hell*. Leading up to those summary groupings, Rodin scholar Albert Elsen found in some of the sculptor's figures much older themes of death from pre-Romantic sources: "I believe," wrote Elsen, "that [his print] *La Ronde* was inspired by Rodin's desire to create a modern Dance of Death and that. . . . Rodin's readings at the time in Baudelaire's *Les Fleurs du Mal* could also have inspired the concept of a fatal dance." For more on the sources and implementation of the *reigen* by Rodin, see Albert Elsen, "Rodin's 'La Ronde,'" *Burlington Magazine* 107, no. 747 (June 1965): 290–99.

38. In addition, a splendid Japanese Edo-period gold-leaf panel of a circle dance was shown at the Museum of Fine Arts, Boston, in 1911 on loan from, and in 1917 acquired by, the museum from Denman Ross, theorist and painter who lectured at Harvard on the theory of design. Ross was part of a circle of influential Bostonians (including Ernest Fenollosa and Arthur Wesley Dow) who actively promoted Japanese aesthetics in those years.

39. Other Europeans exploring such themes include the Swede Anders Zorn (1860–1920) in whose *Midsummer Dance* (1897, Nationalmuseum, Stockholm) whirling folk dancers celebrate the life-giving summer with outdoor dance, drink, and lovemaking. In a very different mood, Edvard Munch's *Dance of Life* (1899–1900, Nasjonalgalleriet, Oslo) casts a grim sexual narrative into a dance composition that shows Munch's essential pessimism about life and profound ambivalence about the power of women.

40. When Matisse's large red, blue, and green canvases of *Dance* and *Music* were shown in the 1910 Salon d'Automne, critics saw them as a challenge to the long-cherished separation between so-called "fine" and "decorative" art.

41. Goya, whose cartoons of the dance became tapestries, may qualify as a rare antecedent for Matisse; since both artists were thinking in terms of *decoration*. See John Hallmark Neff, "Matisse and Decoration: The Shchukin Panels," *Art in America* 63, no. 4 (July–August 1975): 40.

42. Gorky, quoted in Hughes, *American Visions*, 471.

43. The bacchic dance similarly inspired German American Hans Hofmann, who painted an abstract *Bacchanale* (1946, private collection).

44. R[obert] G[oodnough], "Review," *Art News* 49 (December 1950): 47, quoted in T. J. Clark, *Farewell to an Idea: Episodes from a History of Modernism* (New Haven, Conn.: Yale University Press, 1999), 308.

45. Other Pollock dance subjects are included and illustrated in *Jackson Pollock: A Catalogue Raisonné of Paintings, Drawings, and Other Works*, ed. Francis Valentine O'Connor and Eugene Victor Thaw (New Haven, Conn.: Yale University Press, 1978). They include *Dancing Head* (c. 1938–41, private collection); *The Night Dancer* (1944, private collection); *The Dancers* (1946, Tel Aviv Museum); *Shadows: Number 2, 1948* (1948, private collection); and *Untitled (Rhythmical Dance)* (1948, private collection).

46. Duncan, quoted in Coe, *Dance in America*, 125.

## Chapter 5. The Ballets Russes and the "Exotic" East

1. Cultural models were often drawn from Greek art, lauded by Joachim Winckelmann, leading eighteenth-century theoretician of Neoclassicism, who argued that only by imitating the Greek could modern artists again achieve greatness. At London's Royal Academy of the Arts, while under the spell of such thinking, American artist John Trumbull (1756–1843) saw a Hellenistic work known as *Invitation to the Dance*, from which he made a drawing called *The Dancing Faun* (1784–85, Arkansas Art Center, Little Rock). See Mark Antliff and Patricia Leighten, "Primitive," in *Critical Terms for Art History*, ed. Robert S. Nelson and Richard Shiff (Chicago: University of Chicago Press, 1996), 170.

2. T. S. Eliot, quoted in Frank Kermode, "Poet and Dancer before Diaghilev," in *Puzzles and Epiphanies* (London: Routledge and Kegan Paul, 1962), 3.

3. See *Mallarmé: Selected Prose Poems, Essays and Letters*, trans. Bradford Cook (Baltimore: Johns Hopkins University Press, 1956), 62.

4. Fokine created the ballet *Eunice* in 1907, featuring barefoot ballet dancers. In the spread of American ideas to Russia, Ruth St. Denis, another of modern dance's innovators, wanted to share the credit. To a Boston reviewer who suggested that Nijinsky, in his *L'Après-midi d'un Faune*, had invented the two-dimensional Egyptian-style movement she also used, St. Denis pointed out that her 1910 *Egypta* predated his *Faune* by two years. Further, she argued that she herself might well have provided the inspiration (Duncan's 1904–5 appearances notwithstanding) because her agent had taken photographs of her dances to Russia in 1908. See Suzanne Shelton, *Ruth St. Denis: A Biography of the Divine Dancer* (Austin: University of Texas Press, 1981), 132.

5. Sheldon Cheney, *A Primer of Modern Art* (New York: Boni and Liveright, 1924), 341, 343.

6. Diaghilev, quoted in Sorell, *The Dance through the Ages*, 163.

7. Hoffman quietly hired away a number of the Russian dancers from Diaghilev in Paris, then (with unauthorized use of Fokine's choreography and imitations of Baksts's decor) presented what she called *La Saison des Ballets Russes* in September 1911 at New York's Winter Garden.

8. Carl Van Vechten, "The Secret of the Russian Ballet," *Dance Index* 1, nos. 9, 10, 11 (September, October, November 1942): 164.

9. For more on the Philadelphia reaction to the Ballet Russes, see Sylvia Yount, "Rocking the Cradle of Liberty: Philadelphia's Adventures in Modernism," in Sylvia Yount and Elizabeth Johns, *To Be Modern: American Encounters with Cezanne and Company* (Philadelphia: Museum of American Art of the Pennsylvania Academy of the Fine Arts, 1996), 13–15.

10. Kendall, *Where She Danced*, 119.

11. Ibid., 118.

12. James Joyce, *Finnegans Wake* (1939), quoted in *Dance Index* 6, no. 4 (April, 1947): 94.

13. Rodin, quoted in Malvina Hoffman, *Yesterday Is Tomorrow* (New York: Crown, 1965), 118.

14. Burchfield, "Life and Career," autobiographical manuscript, 1955, quoted in John I. H. Baur, *Life and Work of Charles Burchfield: The Inlander* (Newark: University of Delaware Press, 1982), 27.

15. Joyce, quoted in *Dance Index* 6, no. 4 (April 1947): 94.

16. Frederick R. Karl, *Modern and Modernism: The Sovereignty of the Artist 1885–1925* (New York: Atheneum, 1988), 20–21. The leap to which Karl most likely

refers is Nijinsky's single, legendary leap performed in *Spectre of the Rose* (1911).

17. Unnamed critic, quoted in Lynn Garafola and Nancy Van Norman Baer, eds. *The Ballets Russes and Its World* (New Haven, Conn.: Yale University Press, 1999), 236. Not until Lincoln Kirstein championed Nijinsky's choreography starting in 1935 was the dancer given his due. Kirstein wrote, "Great as he was in the province of the performing dancer, Nijinsky was far greater as a practicing choreographer, in which function he either demonstrated or implied theories as profound as have ever been articulated about the classical theatrical dance" (309).

18. Stravinsky to fellow Russian exile Vladimir Ussachevsky, quoted in Richard Taruskin, "Orff's Musical and Moral Failings," *New York Times*, May 6, 2001, Arts and Leisure Sec. 2, p. 35.

19. Quoted in Joan Acocella, "The Lost Nijinsky," *New Yorker*, May 7, 2001, 94.

20. Stettheimer, quoted in Parker Tyler, *Florine Stettheimer: A Life in Art* (New York: Farrar, Straus, 1963), 128.

21. There is a persistent assertion in dance circles, perhaps apocryphal, that Nijinsky had wanted to dance *en pointe* in *The Firebird*, but was denied permission by Diaghilev.

22. Lynn Garafola, "The Travesty Dancer in Nineteenth-Century Ballet," in Dils and Albright, *Moving History/Dancing Cultures*, 213.

23. Tyler, *Florine Stettheimer*, 104. For more on Stettheimer's substantial theatrical endeavors, see Barbara Bloemink, *The Life and Art of Florine Stettheimer* (New Haven, Conn.: Yale University Press, 1995), esp. chap. 7.

24. Alfred David Lenz (1872–1926) made several bronze sculptures of Pavlova as the Dragonfly (*The Dragonfly*, 1916, Metropolitan Museum of Art, New York, 1920.17). The pale delicacy of Dresden porcelain also seemed to suit Pavlova's graceful demeanor. There is a porcelain sculpture (c. 1920) of Pavlova as *The Dragonfly* at New York's Museum of Modern Art, Department of Theatre Design. The emblem of the dragonfly or butterfly, made famous by Whistler and in Art Nouveau by Loïe Fuller, also proved a popular image for Pavlova, as well as for Florine Stettheimer. Stettheimer wrote poetry using the image, and Adolph Bolm asked the artist to create a butterfly for him.

25. Hoffman, *Yesterday Is Tomorrow*, 108.

26. Rodin, quoted in ibid., 118.

27. Hoffman, *Heads and Tales* (New York: Charles Scribner's Sons, 1936), 58.

28. Malvina Hoffman, *Sculpture Inside and Out* (New York: Bonanza, 1939), 154. From her sketches Hoffman modeled clay sketches in the round, followed by two-foot-high reliefs of the whole series. Some years later these were enlarged to four feet in height.

29. Arnold Genthe, *As I Remember* (New York: Reynal and Hitchcock, 1936), 178. There are, in fact, a few fragments of Pavlova on film taken at Universal Studios in Hollywood. She dances in *The Dying Swan* and *Oriental Fantasy* as well as several other pieces.

30. Hoffman, *Yesterday Is Tomorrow*, 230.

31. Max Weber, "The Fourth Dimension from a Plastic Point of View," *Camera Work* 31 (July 1910): 25.

32. Weber, "The Equilibrium of the Inanimate," lecture delivered at the Clarence H. White School of Photography (1916; reprinted in *Essays on Art: Max Weber* [Santa Fe: Gerald Peters Gallery, 2000], 71).

33. Josephine Nivison Hopper, quoted in Gail Levin, *Edward Hopper: An Intimate Biography* (Berkeley: University of California Press, 1995), 155.
34. Josephine Nivison to Robert Henri, letter of Oct. 15, 1921, quoted in ibid.
35. Louise Dahl-Wolfe, quoted in Margaretta K. Mitchell, *Recollections: Ten Women of Photography* (New York: Viking, 1979), 66.
36. Lynn Garafola, *Diaghilev's Ballets Russes* (New York: Da Capo Press, 1998), 33.
37. Natalie Curtis, married in 1917 to the painter Paul Burlin, ranged widely in her pursuit of indigenous American music and dance. The couple moved in modernist cultural circles, befriending Marcel Duchamp and Albert and Juliette Gleizes during the French artists' visits to New York in the mid-1910s. Curtis published several books, including *Negro Folksongs* (1918). She died in an accident in Paris on October 23, 1921.
38. *El Paso Herald*, March 25, 1922. For Nicholas Roerich the stamping nature of Pueblo dance, with incessant drums emphasizing the closeness of moccasined feet upon the earth, would also have recalled the rhythmic stamping of Stravinsky's *Le Sacre du Printemps*, a modern rite choreographed to resurrect ancient dance rhythms.
39. Bolm's protégé Lester Horton shared an interest in the dance of North American Indians, traveling into far-flung reservations and steeping himself in their ceremonials. Dances such as Horton's *Totem Incantation*, dealing with Native American puberty and marriage rites, came out of such early travels. Before his early death at age forty-seven in 1953, Horton took inspiration from several visual-arts sources: a *Guernica* piece was based on Picasso's images of traumatized individuals, and Paul Klee's visual caprices inspired Horton's *Another Touch of Klee* choreographed to a jazz score. One of Klee's caprices in an American collection is *A Balance-Capriccio* (1923, Museum of Modern Art, New York).
40. H. H. Arnason and Marla F. Prather, *History of Modern Art* (New York: Abrams and Prentice-Hall, 1998), 443.
41. Scholars debate the Nijinsky reference in this painting, which is one of the first in Kline's mature style. As neatly as this abstraction seems to allude to the dancer's turned-in body movements and unusual footwork, reprising by abstraction Nijinsky's uncanny energy-become-form, the documentation of this piece upon its entry into the collection of the Metropolitan Museum of Art (2006), indicates that the canvas may not refer at all to the dancer, having been titled arbitrarily as it was readied for Kline's first solo show at the Charles Egan gallery.
42. De Kooning, quoted in Denby, "Notes on the Accompanying Nijinsky Photographs," *Dance Index* 2, no. 3 (March 1943): 38.
43. Meynell quoted in D. Dodge Thompson, "John Singer Sargent's Javanese Dancers," *Antiques* 138 (July 1990): 129.
44. Ibid. A later artist whose work suggests a response to Muybridge was Joseph Cornell, whose 1933 collage in homage to dancer-choreographer Serge Lifar shows Lifar in two positions, one an afterimage of his forward motion (private collection).
45. See Flitch, *Modern Dancing and Dancers*, 194.
46. Charteris, *John Sargent*, 250–51.
47. Anon., "The New English Art Club," *Magazine of Art* 15 (1892): 123. One of Sargent's Javanese dancer drawings includes a full-body image and an arm detail of a dancer, seemingly swiftly drawn in order to capture the distinctive poses

and hand gestures (*Javanese Dancer, Arm and Hand Positions [from Sketchbook of Javanese Dancers]* 1889, Metropolitan Museum).

48. Sachs, *World History of the Dance,* 45–46.

49. Rodin's American student Malvina Hoffman responded with her *maître* to the angular gestures of the Cambodian dancers. Years later Hoffman described a visit to her studio by Helen Keller, who compensated for her absence of sight, speech, and hearing with an extraordinary capacity to learn through touch. Running her hands over the backward-turning fingers of Hoffman's sculpted Cambodian dancer, Keller recognized the subject instantly by this characteristic, unmistakable gesture. See Hoffman, *Sculpture Inside and Out,* 73.

50. The lure of Egyptian themes had already permeated France before the arrival of the Ballets Russes; Colette, following her divorce in 1906, had become a music hall performer, causing a sensation in her Rêve d'Egypte in 1907.

51. Beardsley's pen drawing *Salome with the Head of John the Baptist* (1893) is in the collection of the Princeton University Library. Corinth's *Salomé* (1899; Museum der Bildenden Künste, Leipzig) was exhibited to huge success in the 1900 Berlin Secession exhibition. As late as 1912, while living in Paris, the American painter Florine Stettheimer was aghast that the dealer Knoedler paid 500,000 francs for Henri Regnault's *Salomé* (1870), outbidding the Louvre. Tyler, *Florine Stettheimer,* 35. Regnault's *Salomé* eventually entered the collection of the Metropolitan Museum of Art. By 1896 it was cited in a series of articles by American artist Will H. Low as anticipating a shift toward the decorative in American art. Low, "A Century of Painting," *McClure's Magazine* 7 (September 1896).

52. Aubrey Beardsley (1872–98) illustrated Wilde's play with a series of line block prints. *The Stomach Dance* (1894, Hunterian Art Gallery, University of Glasgow) shows Salome performing the Dance of the Seven Veils.

53. See, for example, Rhonda Garelick, *Electric Salome: Loïe Fuller's Performance of Modernism* (Princeton, N.J.: Princeton University Press, 2007).

54. T. J. Clark, *The Painting of Modern Life: Paris in the Art of Manet and His Followers* (Princeton, N.J.: Princeton University Press, 1984), 211–12.

55. Norman Bryson, "Cultural Studies and Dance History," in Desmond, *Meaning in Motion,* 69.

56. Charles Rearick, *Pleasures of the Belle Epoque: Entertainment and Festivity in Turn-of-the-Century France* (New Haven, Conn.: Yale University Press, 1985), 83–84.

57. Julie Townsend has discussed Fuller's audiences in much more complex and nuanced terms, While some critics and spectators saw her as a "chaste ethereal spirit," others saw her performances as "erotically invested." Only in posthumous reconsiderations did candid views of Fuller's own sexuality emerge; like most public figures of her day, she kept her lesbian orientation private. See Townsend, "Alchemic Visions and Technological Advances: Sexual Morphology in Loie Fuller's Dance," in *Dancing Desires: Choreographing Sexualities on and off the Stage,* ed. Jane C. Desmond (Madison: University of Wisconsin Press, 2001), 83.

58. *Le Figaro,* 25 January 1893, quoted in Richard Nelson Current and Marcia Ewing Current, *Loïe Fuller: Goddess of Light* (Boston: Northeastern University Press, 1997), 52.

59. There are, in fact, multiple dance models she could have chosen from biblical sources: Jephthah's daughter, the daughters of Shiloh, as well as David and all Israel when they danced before the Lord.

60. Unnamed critic, quoted in Current and Current, *Loïe Fuller*, 83.

61. Another vehicle for Fuller's portrayal of Salomé, described as a "tragic pantomime in two acts," was produced in 1907 at the Théâtre des Arts, Paris. The score from that production, composed by Florent Schmitt, was later used for the 1913 Ballets Russes production of *La Tragédie de Salomé* at the Théâtre des Champs-Elysées.

62. Canadian-born Tanguay (1878–1947) began her stage career at age eight in the United States, shocking audiences with risqué songs and dances such as "I Don't Care." Thanks to roles such as her Salomé, Tanguay became vaudeville's highest-paid performer before losing her fortune in the stock market crash of 1929.

63. Allan posed for several famous photographers, including Clarence White and Edward Weston, then exhibited their images of her in New York. Writing to Weston in 1915, Allan said, "Your photographs are causing a sensation here in New York. I am very proud to show them. . . . Enclosed my check for my prints." In what looks like her Salomé costume, Allan posed again for Weston the next year in an outdoor setting, probably near the photographer's California studio. *Maud Allan with a Century Plant, Euphoric* shows the dancer with outstretched arms and ecstatic upturned gaze. Complex cultural assumptions collide in Allan's Salomé. At a time when something vaguely shameful—or at least ugly—was associated with the bare female foot, Allan enlisted the religious art of the Renaissance to redeem her daring act of dancing barefoot on the London stage. Traveling in Italy, she pointed to the barefoot Madonnas of Titian and Veronese as justification for removing her own shoes. While unshod like Titian's or Veronese's biblical women, Allan's Salomé differed importantly from them in that she *danced*. And in dancing she exerted a potentially assertive brand of female sexuality, raising all manner of late-Victorian anxieties about women in general, and in particular about female power, otherness and the colonized East. Exotic, seductive, emasculating, Allan's Salomé dance represents the quintessence of the oriental Other, invoking the cultural phenomenon Edward Said described as Orientalism, a polarizing discourse that long legitimized the domination of Eastern peoples by those in the West. See Edward Said, *Orientalism* (New York: Vintage, 1979). As Amy Koritz writes, "The dark continents of Western femininity and Orientalism meet in Allan's depiction of Salome." Amy Koritz, "Dancing the Orient for England: Maud Allan's *The Vision of Salome*" in Jane C. Desmond, ed. *Meaning in Motion: New Cultural Studies of Dance* (Durham: Duke Univ. Press, 1997), 138.

64. Levin, *Edward Hopper*, 182.

65. This work, listed as no. 603 in the Armory Show catalog, was last traced to a private collection in Paris, 1963. A photograph of it appears on the University of Virginia "crossroads" website on the Armory Show.

66. Noguchi, quoted in Tracy, *Spaces of the Mind*, 37.

67. Henri diary, November 7, 1902, quoted in Bennard B. Perlman, *Robert Henri: His Life and Art* (New York: Dover, 1991), 57.

68. Henri's friend Arthur B. Davies shared an interest in Jesseca Penn during the same period (1902), but the two painters approached the dancer's portrait differently. Unlike Henri, who posed her in anticipation of movement, Davies

asked Penn to begin by dancing for him, then pausing to hold certain positions until he could capture them in pastels. "[Penn] was particularly ecstatic in her appreciation of Davies," recalled a friend. Dudley Crafts Watson, quoted in Bennard B. Perlman, *The Lives, Loves and Art of Arthur B. Davies* (Albany: State University of New York Press, 1998), 128.

69. Robert Henri, *The Art Spirit* (Philadelphia: J. B. Lippincott, 1923), 17.

70. Ibid., 55.

71. Ibid., 17.

72. Henri composition-class talk, March 3, 1911, Beinecke Rare Book and Manuscript Library, Yale University.

73. Decidedly of Duncan, a 1916 drawing by Henri (now unlocated) captures the bulk of the dancer's torso, swathed in diaphanous drapery, arms raised in her typical lifting gesture.

74. Henri, quoted in "Isadora Duncan and the Libertarian Spirit," *The Modern School*, April 1915, 37.

75. Henri, quoted in William Innes Homer, *Robert Henri and His Circle* (Ithaca, N.Y.: Cornell University Press, 1969), 159.

76. Henri's oil portrait *Betalo Rubino, Dramatic Dancer* (1915), is in the collection of the Saint Louis Art Museum, Forest Park, Saint Louis, Missouri.

77. Henri, letter to Frank Crowninshield, May 6, 1919, quoted in Homer, *Robert Henri and His Circle*, 196. Roshanara was, in fact, a British dancer who specialized in the dances of India. She performed with Loïe Fuller, Pavlova, and Adolph Bolm's Ballet Intime.

78. Flitch, *Modern Dancing and Dancers*, 192–93. A less edifying version of St. Denis's *Cobra* at the Hudson Theatre is described by the dancer's biographer Suzanne Shelton, who identifies the source as a Coney Island routine, where St. Denis saw a snake charmer. She dashed home to improvise snake eyes from ordinary hat pins soldered onto finger rings. "With green stones glittering on each index and small finger, Ruthie pantomimed the coiling and hissing of two serpents, her arms gliding and darting in sinister foreplay . . . Several ladies swooned" (Shelton, *Ruth St. Denis*, 57).

79. The dashing and socially prominent Kessler, besides being a painter, became a devoted supporter of St. Denis. In Berlin Kessler commissioned Belgian designer Henry van de Velde to decorate his apartment (perhaps shown in the photograph) in the fashionable Art Nouveau or Jugendstil. Kessler introduced St. Denis to several other Berlin artists, including Ludwig von Hoffman and Hans Schlesinger, who sketched or painted her and joined Kessler in the circle of her ardent artist-admirers. Besides his attention to St. Denis, Kessler was also a friend and patron of theater designer Gordon Craig and, through Craig, became a friend to his lover, Isadora Duncan. Later he would befriend Josephine Baker on her tour of European capitals. In 1926, at Kessler's home in Berlin, Baker was much taken with a large Maillol sculpture called *Crouching Woman*, around which she danced playfully. To Kessler, the scene was "one genius speaking to another" (Kessler, quoted in Jean Claude Baker and Chris Chase, *Josephine: The Hungry Heart* [New York: Cooper Square Press, 1993], 128. The photograph is in the Denishawn Collection, No. 548, New York Public Library.

80. About the same time (c. 1916) sculptor Allan Clark (1896–1950) undertook a similar pose of Ted Shawn.

81. Cyrus Dallin to Edward Weston, quoted in Amy Conger, "Edward Weston's Early Photography" (PhD diss., University of New Mexico, 1982), 176.

## Introduction to Part Three

1. Stein, quoted in Coe, *Dance in America*, 189.
2. Pablo Picasso, quoted in Alfred Barr, *Picasso: Fifty Years of His Art* (New York, Museum of Modern Art, 1946), 270–71.
3. T. S. Eliot, "Burnt Norton," in *Four Quartets* (New York: Harcourt, Brace and World, 1943), 15–16.
4. W. B. Yeats, *Essays and Introductions* (New York: Macmillan, 1961), 287.

## Chapter 6. Loïe Fuller, Art Nouveau, and the Technological Present

1. Buffalo Bill Cody, war veteran and frontier scout, assembled a troupe which performed "fancy rifle shooting," dances by Native Americans, and plays, including one called *Twenty Days, or Buffalo Bill's Pledge*, in which Fuller appeared as a deserted waif in 1882. She had not yet begun her dancing career.
2. *New York Post*, February 16, 1892, 7.
3. William Butler Yeats, quoted in Lincoln Kirstein, *Dance: A Short History of Classic Theatrical Dancing* (Princeton, N.J.: Princeton Book Company, 1987), 268.
4. The approximate date of Whistler's drawings can be verified by a letter from Isabella Stewart Gardner asking Whistler to show her "the whirling tracings of Loie Fuller that you pencilled" (quoted in Margaret F. MacDonald, *James McNeill Whistler, Drawings Pastels, and Watercolours: A Catalogue Raisonné* [New Haven, Conn.: Yale University Press, 1995), no. 1346.
5. Only rarely had Whistler previously attempted to suggest dance movement. In an exceptional sketch for his painting of the "Gold Girl," Connie Gilchrist (fig. 127, discussed in chapter 9) Whistler had drawn repeated outlines on the fast-moving legs of the rope-skipping dancer (catalogue raisonné no. 710, *Sketch of Harmony in Yellow and Gold: The Gold Girl—Connie Gilchrist*, c. 1870s, British Museum).
6. That seems to be the case with his *Dancer No. 1* (c. 1900, Cleveland Museum of Art, Whistler Catalogue Raisonné, no. 1624), a drawing once thought to be of Loïe Fuller (perhaps because of the draperies she holds), but now identified as another favorite model. In this drawing and a series of similar Whistler works the dancer rises lightly on one foot, a momentary pose which the artist recorded quickly, then could rework in ink or pastel using his skilled visual memory. See MacDonald, *James McNeill Whistler*, nos. 1624–29.
7. Clare de Morinni, "Loïe Fuller, The Fairy of Light," in Magriel, *Chronicles of the American Dance*, 209. One of the dances Whistler saw Fuller perform at the Folies Bergère was *Le Papillon*, perhaps an extra attraction for an artist who had already adopted the butterfly as his own signature.
8. Mallarmé, quoted in Coe, *Dance in America*, 124.
9. *Paris Lantern*, April 26, 1895. In Alexander's *Repose*, his sitter belongs to a tradition of purposely decorative female subjects within the Aesthetic Movement, whose artists tended to submerge their model's identity into their compositions, decreasing narrative content while blurring boundaries among portraits, genre, and formal studies. Critic Sadakichi Hartmann said that Alexander's subjects "are not women, they are merely his means of expression" (Hartmann, quoted in Bailey Van Hook, "Decorative Images of American Women: The Aristocratic Aesthetic of the Late Nineteenth Century," *Smithsonian Studies in American Art* 4, no. 1 [Winter, 1990], 56). In her book on Alexander, scholar Sarah J. Moore suggests that Alexander's sitter in *Repose*,

despite the *Paris Lantern*'s suggestion that it was Fuller, may well have been his wife. A later Alexander painting that may also allude to Loïe Fuller is *The Butterfly* (c. 1906, private collection), whose female subject is likened to a decorative butterfly. Metaphorically, that painting calls up inevitable associations both to Fuller's famous butterfly dance as well as to the pervasive motif of the butterfly in Whistlerian terms. My thanks to Sarah Burt and to Sarah J. Moore for their insights and references.

10. A slightly later painting by Childe Hassam, *Tanagra (The Builders, New York)* (1918, Smithsonian American Art Museum, Washington, D.C.) clearly pictures the idea of these separate spheres. Within a decorative, dreamy interior a woman reflects on an ancient Greek statuette of a dancer, while behind her, through a window, the viewer sees male laborers working outside.

11. De Morinni, "Loie Fuller: The Fairy of Light," 210. The lithograph is documented in the Toulouse-Lautrec catalogue raisonné: Lee D. Wittrock *Toulouse-Lautrec: The Complete Prints* (New York: Sotheby Parke Bernet Publications, 1986),17 1/1.

12. From "The Journal of Julius Rolshoven," unpublished memoir written in the mid-1920s, Fine Arts Library, University of New Mexico, Albuquerque, 143–44. My thanks to Virginia Couse Leavitt for this reference.

13. For more on Maryhill and the Rodin works acquired for it by Loïe Fuller and Samuel Hill, see *Rodin: The Maryhill Collection*, exh. cat. (Malibu: J. Paul Getty Museum and Connor Museum, Pullman, Wash., 1975).

14. Fuller, quoted in Garelick, *Electric Salome*, 39. Edison, whose pioneering use of new motion picture technology led him to film many moving subjects, asked Fuller if he could record her dancing on film. Wary of motion pictures, like Isadora Duncan, Fuller declined.

15. Fuller, quoted in Current and Current, *Loïe Fuller*, 97.

16. Covielle, "Danse, musique, lumière chez la Loïe Fuller," *L'Eclair*, May 5, 1914.

17. For more on Fuller's synaesthesia, see Richard Hobbs, ed., *Impressions of French Modernity: Art and Literature in France 1850–1900* (New York: Manchester University Press, 1998), esp. chap. 8.

18. As dance historian Julie Townsend concludes, "Fuller's technological effects, the effacement of her body and the impersonality of her performance prefigures modernist concerns with the decentered or impersonal subject, mechanization, and antinarrative strategies" (Townsend, "Alchemic Visions and Technological Advances," in Desmond, *Dancing Desires*, 78–79).

19. Unnamed critic, quoted in Current and Current, *Loïe Fuller*, 176.

20. Vauxcelles, unidentified clipping dated May 10, 1914, Bibliothèque de L'Arsenal, Paris, quoted in Current and Current, *Loïe Fuller*, 210.

21. Isadora Duncan, *My Life* (New York: Boni and Liveright, 1927), 95.

22. Current and Current, *Loïe Fuller*, 303.

23. *Boston Herald*, April 22, 1896.

24. Hugh Morton, "Loïe Fuller and Her Strange Art," *Metropolitan Magazine* (1896?), 277–83, clipping in Theatre Collection, New York Public Library.

25. Fuller, quoted in Current and Current, *Loïe Fuller*, 204.

26. A curious legacy of Fuller's light-enhanced movement reappeared in performances of a troupe of "sacred dancers" brought to New York in 1924 by the Russian-born mystic Georges I. Gurdjieff. Purportedly descended from ancient Asian dances, and intended to convey both an aesthetic component and a form of esoteric knowledge, these performances featured dancers wearing wide sashes

in the seven colors of the spectrum. They began lined up in spectral order: red, orange, yellow, green, blue, indigo, and violet. When the dance began, the colors moved and shifted, giving viewers, as one observer reported, the illusion of "watching white light pressed very slowly through a prism and breaking into its spectral color" (Louise Welch, *Orage with Gurdjieff in America* [Boston: Routledge and Kegan Paul, 1982], chap. 1). Gurdjieff, then doyen of a community of mystics at the Château du Prieuré near Paris, could not have been unaware of the prismatic effects Loïe Fuller had long achieved with light, especially since in that year (1924) she was given a retrospective at the Louvre.

## Chapter 7. Social Dance

1. This painting entered the collection of the Museum of Fine Arts, Boston, in 1937.

2. Ann Douglas, *Terrible Honesty: Mongrel Manhattan in the 1920s* (New York: Farrar, Straus and Giroux, 1995), 69–70.

3. Another of Balanchine's early efforts in the United States was to choreograph a number called "5 A.M." for Josephine Baker, who had briefly returned from France for a season in 1935–36 with New York's Ziegfeld Follies.

4. Kirstein, program notes for *Alma Mater*, quoted in *The Key Reporter* 68, no. 1 (Fall 2002): 13. The music for the ballet was by Kay Swift.

5. The so-called "animal dances" became enormously popular in the United States and in Europe. In France, the Grizzly Bear, known as "la danse de l'ours," was described in the publication *La Vie parisienne* (1913): "Facing one another, they swayed their bodies to the left and the right, the man with affected heaviness, the woman more lightly, both of them laughing, talking, snapping their fingers. Then they slowly crouched all the way down to the ground continuing to look at and provoke one another mouth to mouth. . . . To finish, the man bruskly grabbed the woman by the waist, turned her upside down, then threw her, legs up, head down, onto her haunches" (cited in Jody Blake, *Le Tumulte Noir: Modernist Art and Popular Entertainment in Jazz-Age Paris, 1900–1930* [University Park: Pennsylvania State University Press, 1999], 43). Futurist Gino Severini's lively oil *The Bear Dance at the Moulin Rouge* (1913, Musée National d'Art Moderne, Centre National d'Art et de Culture Georges Pompidou, Paris) hints at the athleticism required in the Grizzly Bear.

6. Genthe, *As I Remember*, 176. Everywhere they went, Pavlova and Mordkin became dancing demigods in the minds of Americans, artistic in physical appearance as well as in performance. A unnamed critic in San Francisco wrote, for example, that Mordkin "is physically fit to be a sculptor's model, and thought and emotion as well as manly beauty mark his face" (Winthrop Palmer, *Theatrical Dancing in America* [New Brunswick, N.J.: A. S. Barnes, 1978], 175).

7. Pavlova, for example, introduced three ballroom dances—the Pavlovana, the Gavotte Renaissance, and the Czarina Waltz.

8. Flitch, *Modern Dancing and Dancers*, 198.

9. Apollinaire, from his novel *La Femme Assise*, quoted in Lincoln Kirstein, "Elie Nadelman: Sculptor of the Dance," *Dance Index* 7, no. 6 (1948): 135.

10. Such ballroom performances fanned out across the country and helped to disseminate the new dances to small-town America. In 1914 Ted Shawn, soon thereafter the partner of Ruth St. Denis, worked his way East by performing ballroom dances at stops along the Santa Fe Railroad. See Shelton, *Ruth St. Denis*, 120.

11. Nadelman, "Notes for a Catalogue," *Camera Work* 32 (October 1910): 41. As a collector of folk art, Nadelman owned mechanical toys of dancers, which may also have served as inspiration for some of his sculptures.

12. Genthe, *As I Remember*, 183.

13. Beatrice Wood, *Beatrice Wood: Mama of Dada* [film], Wild Wolf Productions, 1993.

14. Wood, letter to William Innes Homer, October 8, 1974, quoted in Homer, ed., *Avant-Garde Painting and Sculpture in America 1910–1925* (Wilmington: Delaware Art Museum, 1975), 150.

15. Henri-Pierre Roché, *Victor*, vol. 4 of Jean Clair, ed. *Marcel Duchamp* (Paris: Musée National d'Art Moderne, Centre Georges Pompidou, 1977), 55, quoted in Francis M. Nauman, *New York Dada 1915–23* (New York: Abrams, 1994), 186.

16. For more on the Greenwich Village balls, see Steven Watson, *Strange Bedfellows: The First American Avant-Garde* (New York: Abbeville Press, 1991), 228–30.

17. Lewis Mumford, "Machinery and the Modern Style," *New Republic*, August 3, 1921.

18. Robert Crunden, *Body and Soul: The Making of American Modernism* (New York: Basic Books, 2000), 101.

19. John Dos Passos, *Manhattan Transfer* (Boston: Harper and Brothers, 1925), 228.

20. Ibid., 144. It is useful to recognize that Dos Passos, besides his use of social dance themes, was a fan of the Ballets Russes as well, starting with their performances in Boston in February 1916.

21. Even earlier, Francis Luis Mora (1874–1940) had painted the same subject in his *Ball at the Art Students League* (1910, private collection). Mora, a muralist and illustrator, had also studied at the league.

22. George Bellows, quoted in Lauris Mason and Joan Ludman, *The Lithographs of George Bellows: A Catalogue Raisonné* (Millwood, N.Y.: KTO Press, 1977), 92.

## Chapter 8. American Vernacular

1. Marin, statement for "291" exhibition, January 1913, published in *Camera Work* 42–43 (April–July 1913): 18.

2. Duchamp, quoted in Caroline Cros, *Marcel Duchamp* (London: Reaktion Books, 2006), 27.

3. J. Edgar Chamberlain, "Review of John Marin Exhibition," *Camera Work* 42–43 (April–July 1913); 23.

4. Ibid.

5. So central to the image of the mechanistic modern were Manhattan's skyscrapers that visual artists mapped machine images onto many dance or dancelike subjects. Wanda Corn has reproduced a cartoon review of George Antheil's *Ballet Mécanique*, performed at Carnegie Hall in 1927 (Corn, *The Great American Thing*, fig. 94). Although composed as a symphonic rather than a dance performance, the cartoon construction workers in *El Rivetor* give the mechanistic sounds a new dimension—that of imagined movement. Dance, and its infinitely variable visual possibilities, could enhance the mechanistic idea dramatically. In fantasies of the machine/body, the machine as the human body's Other reveals its comedic side in this cartoon, as well as in such works as Chaplin's *Modern*

*Times*. Perhaps in response to Antheil's *Ballet Mécanique*, Russian dancer-choreographer Adolph Bolm staged an enthusiastically received *Mechanical Ballet* in 1931. Performed in the Hollywood Bowl, Bolm's lavish production included pistons, dynamos, and gears among its cast.

6. Sheldon Cheney, quoted in Hughes, *American Visions*, p. 405.

7. Sculptor Malvina Hoffman, for example, won an Honorable Mention for her airy caprice *Pavlova Dancing the Gavotte* (1915).

8. Umberto Boccioni, "The Italian Futurist Painters and Sculptors" in *Catalogue Deluxe of the Department of Fine Arts, Panama-Pacific International Exposition*, ed. John E. D. Trask and J. Nilsen Laurvik (San Francisco: Paul Elder, 1915), 1:124–25.

9. *San Francisco Call*, June 2, 1915.

10. Italian critic Maurizio Fagiolo dell'Arco, quoted in Garafola, *Diaghilev's Ballets Russes*, 80. Balla's set was, in fact, a blow-up of one of his own paintings, made three-dimensional. At a keyboard of light controls behind the scene, Balla created forty-nine different settings during the brief five minutes of the light ballet, performed entirely without dancers.

11. Futurist painting and sculpture were important components of the Museum of Modern Art's 1936 exhibition *Cubism and Abstract Art* as well as its 1949 show *Twentieth-Century Italian Art*.

12. Van Vechten, "The Secret of the Russian Ballet," 164.

13. F. T. Marinetti, "Manifesto of Futurist Dance," *Italian Futurista* (July 1917), reprinted in *Dance Observer* 2, no. 7 (October 1935).

14. In his dance manifesto Marinetti also imagined a wartime Dance of the Shrapnel and a Dance of the Aviatrix; in the latter, a female dancer could "simulate with jerks and weavings of her body the successive efforts of a plane trying to take off" (cited in RoseLee Goldberg, *Performance: Live Art 1909 to the Present* [New York: Abrams, 1979], 18). See also Antonella Majoochi, "La danza futurista," *Futurismo-Oggi* 20, nos. 5–7 (May–July 1988): 17–22.

15. F. T. Marinetti, *Futurist Painting: Technical Manefesto, 11 April 1910*. Originally published in the catalog of the Futurists' 1913 London exhibition, it was collected, in slightly altered form, with other Futurist manifestoes published in Italy in 1914.

16. Severini, in the introduction to the catalog of his London exhibition, 1913, quoted in Joshua C. Taylor, *Futurism* (New York: Museum of Modern Art, 1961), 66.

17. Taylor, *Futurism*, 69.

18. Christian Brinton, *Impressions of the Art at the Panama-Pacific Exposition* (New York: John Lane, 1916), 20. According to its catalog, American painter Everett Shinn exhibited a now-unlocated painting titled *Yellow Dancer* at the Panama-Pacific Exposition.

19. Stella, quoted in Hughes, *American Visions*, 376.

20. Bryson, "Cultural Studies and Dance History," in Desmond, *Meaning in Motion*, 72.

21. Graham, quoted in Merle Armitage, *Martha Graham* (New York: Dance Horizons, 1966), 105. Graham's humanist sources were rooted in cultural anthropology, myth, and depth psychology, and were often land based. Even so, she described the American land as "divine machinery." Graham, quoted in Mark Franko, *Dancing Modernism/Performing Politics* (Bloomington: Indiana University Press, 1995), 54.

22. Picabia, quoted in "French Artists Spur on an American Art," *New York Tribune*, October 24, 1915, sect. 4, p. 2.

23. According to Willard Bohn, Napierkowska was eventually deported for the lewdness of her dancing (Bohn, "The Abstract Vision of Marius de Zayas," *Art Bulletin* 62, no. 3 [September 1980]: 676).

24. For more on the Picabia–Duncan relationship, see Peter Kurth, *Isadora: A Sensational Life* (Boston: Little, Brown, 2001), 367–69.

25. *New York Evening Post* critic, 1915, quoted in Perlman, *The Lives, Loves and Art of Arthur B. Davies*, 270.

26. Man Ray had already produced a work called *Isadora Duncan Nue* (1912, unlocated) and had drawn his *Figures Dancing in a Circle* (1914, Los Angeles County Museum of Art) and used his evolving "disarticulated" figure style in his oil *Dance Interpretation* (1915) and, further modified, in his drawing *Ballet-Silhouette* (1916), the latter two serving as cover illustrations for the catalogs of his first and second exhibitions at New York's Daniel Gallery. Reproduced in Man Ray, *Self-Portrait* (Boston: Little, Brown, 1963), 57, 65.

27. Ray, *Self Portrait*, 65–66.

28. I am indebted for the narrative of the making of this painting to Francis M. Naumann's *New York Dada 1915–23* (New York: Abrams, 1994). Again, there is a curious reminder here of the rope-skipping dancer Connie Gilchrist, whose performances in 1879 had inspired Whistler to undertake radical new chromatic studies.

29. Ray, quoted in Arturo Schwarz, "An Interview with Man Ray: 'This is not for America,'" *Arts Magazine* 51 (May 1977): 118.

30. Man Ray, *Self-Portrait*, 65.

31. Jean Arp, 1915 exhibition preface, quoted in Arp, "Abstract Art, Concrete Art" (c. 1942), reprinted in Herschel B. Chipp, *Theories of Modern Art* (Berkeley: University of California Press, 1968), 390.

32. Ray, *Self-Portrait*, 80.

33. Ibid., 272–73, cited in Blake, *Le Tumulte Noir*, 130.

34. Calder, quoted in James Johnson Sweeney, *Calder* (New York: Museum of Modern Art, 1945), 28.

35. Graham, *Blood Memory*, 166.

36. Calder and Sweeney quoted in Jean Lipman, *Alexander Calder and His Magical Mobiles* (New York: Hudson Hills Press, 1981), 19, 44. Calder's interest in dance, both formally and metaphorically, may have been enhanced by his father's attention to dance subjects. Alexander Stirling Calder (1870–1945), also a sculptor, used dance images in works such as *The Dance of Life Begins Early*, a bronze of 1938 (Smithsonian American Art Museum, Washington, D.C.) and a well-known bronze medal called *Life as a Dance* (c. 1938, Fogg Art Museum, Harvard University, Cambridge, Mass.).

37. Mrs. Theo van Doesburg, quoted in Institute of Contemporary Art, Boston, *Art and Dance*, 35. A more psychologically grounded view is advanced by Peter Gay in *Modernism: The Lure of Heresy* (New York: W. W. Norton, 2008), 138–39. Gay avers that Mondrian's reluctance to come into physical contact with a partner made the Charleston—danced without touching—the artist's favorite. Mondrian's fear of intimacy, argues Gay, was linked to the artist's withdrawal from nature and his conviction that the technological triumphs cities represented made them infinitely preferable to nature itself.

38. Mondrian, "Liberation from Oppression in Art and Life," in *Plastic Art and Pure Plastic Art and Other Essays* (New York: Wittenborn, 1945), 47.

39. Mondrian produced a pair of these *Fox Trot* paintings; the earlier one is *Fox Trot B* (1929). Both belonged to the collection of the Société Anonyme assembled by Katherine Dreier and later given to the Yale University Art Gallery. Decades after Mondrian's black and white *Fox Trot A*, Andy Warhol painted a tongue-in-cheek parody of it. Warhol's (also in black and white) is *Dance Diagram (2) Fox Trot: "The Double Twinkle-Man"* (1962, Andy Warhol Museum, Pittsburgh). It is one of a series of dance diagram paintings Warhol exhibited flat on the floor, as if to instruct potential dancers. They featured numbered footprints and arrows to indicate the sequence of steps. Like Mondrian's *Fox Trot*, its direction and movement are based on intersecting horizontal and vertical lines.

40. Piet Mondrian, *The New Art—The New Life: The Collected Writings of Piet Mondrian*, ed. and trans. Harry Holtzman and Martin S. James (Boston: G. K. Hall, 1986), 148–49.

41. Mondrian, "Liberation from Oppression in Art and Life," 47.

## Chapter 9. Class, Vice, and the Revolt against Puritanism

1. Olga Maynard, *The American Ballet* (Philadelphia: Macrae Smith, 1959), 24.

2. Duncan, *My Life*, 19.

3. Marie was dismissed from the company in 1882 for unspecified reasons, after which she disappears from history, although it is likely that she fell into prostitution, like her sister Antoinette. A younger sister Charlotte escaped this all-too-common fate of the ballet *rats* to become a successful dancer, choreographer, and teacher. See Martine Kahane, "Little Dancer, Aged Fourteen—The Model," in Czestochowski and Pingeot, *Degas Sculptures*, 101–8.

4. "The Palace Theatre," *Morning Advertiser*, March 7, 1908, 2.

5. Thomas, *Dance, Modernity and Culture*, 69.

6. John Martin, *American Dancing* (New York: Dance Horizons, 1967), 132.

7. Max Weber scholar Percy North reports that the painter saw Duncan dance at Carnegie Hall in 1909. In her farewell performance there on December 2 Duncan not only danced barefoot and in gauzy costume, but was also visibly pregnant.

8. John Corbin in *Hampton*, July 1911, quoted in Current and Current, *Loïe Fuller*, 205.

9. Max Eastman, quoted in Robert Gottlieb, "Free Spirit," review of Peter Kurth, *Isadora: A Sensational Life*, *The New York Times Book Review*, December 30, 2001, 13. Photographer Arnold Genthe agreed with Eastman's claim for Duncan, extending her liberating results: "As a creative genius she was both artist and liberator," wrote Genthe, "releasing by her courage and heavenly grace, not the dance alone, but womankind, from the fetters of puritanism" (Genthe, *As I Remember*, 179).

10. Coe, *Dance in America*, 125.

11. For information on Murphy's *Within the Quota* I am indebted to Corn, *The Great American Thing;* see 102–4 therein for more on Murphy's ballet as an example of transatlantic themes in the 1920s.

12. Choreographer Alwin Nikolais stated the connection to Wood's painting, noted in Julia L. Foulkes, *Modern Bodies: Dance and American Modernism from Martha Graham to Alvin Ailey* (Chapel Hill: University of North Carolina Press, 2002), 148–49.

13. Goodrich, from a speech given January 29, 1965, Abraham Walkowitz File, Whitney Museum of American Art Papers, Archives of American Art, Smithsonian Institution, roll N692, frame 255.

14. Anonymous Saint Louis reviewer, quoted in Kendall, *Where She Danced*, 119.

15. The changes in American culture seen as a "commercialization of life" are discussed in Larzer Ziff, *The American 1890s: Life and Times of a Lost Generation* (New York: Viking, 1966), 14.

16. Allen, quoted in Kendall, *Where She Danced*, 127.

17. Ibid., 123.

18. Floyd Dell, *Women as World Builders: Studies in Modern Feminism* (New York: Hyperion, 1976), 44–45. Eastman, quoted in Kurth, *Isadora*, 327.

19. See, for example, Jane C. Desmond, introduction to *Meaning in Motion: New Cultural Studies of Dance*.

20. Duncan to Gordon Craig, 1905, quoted in Kurth, *Isadora*, 185.

21. Duncan, quoted in Coe, *Dance in America*, 125.

22. Nietzsche, from *Thus Spake Zarathustra* in *The Portable Nietzsche*, comp. and trans. Walter Kaufmann (New York: Viking, 1968), 153.

23. Nietzsche, quoted in Morgan, *Martha Graham*, 146.

24. Duncan, *Ecrits sur la Danse* (1927), quoted in Mark Franko, *Dancing Modernism/Performing Politics* (Bloomington: Indiana University Press, 1995), 18.

25. Edward Steichen, *A Life in Photography* (Garden City, N.Y.: Doubleday, 1963), following plate 83.

26. "What is great in man is that he is a bridge and not an end" wrote Nietzsche. In her 1927 essay "I See America Dancing," in *The Art of the Dance*, ed. Sheldon Cheney (New York: Theatre Arts, 1928), Duncan credited Nietzsche with creating the spirit of dance: "Nietzsche was the first dancing philosopher," she declared.

27. Janet Flanner, "Isadora," *New Yorker*, January 1, 1927.

28. Duncan, *My Life*, 156, 158.

29. Joann Kealiinohomoku, "An Anthropologist Looks at Ballet as a Form of Ethnic Dance," in Dils and Albright, *Moving History/Dancing Cultures*, 40.

30. Duncan, "I See America Dancing," in *The Art of the Dance*, 48–49.

31. Duncan, quoted in Kendall, *Where She Danced*, 60.

32. Later, in the ballets of the 1920s, female dancers took on modern proportions: slim, boyish, and fashionable. Female curves were out; flattened breasts were in. The costumes of these "new women," often flappers, more closely reflected street wear. When the Russian Ballet danced in Chicago in 1921, the Marshall Field Department Store produced a whole line of women's streetwear based on designer Nicholas Roerich's costume designs for *The Snow Maiden*.

33. Alain Corbin, quoted in Michelle Perrot, ed., *A History of Private Life: From the Fires of Revolution to the Great War* (Cambridge, Mass.: Belknap Press of Harvard University Press, 1990), 667.

34. Colette, *Paysages et portraits* (Paris: Flammarion, 1958), 150–54.

35. Kendall, *Where She Danced*, 85.

36. Duncan, speaking to Augustin Daly, the first American theatrical manager of his time, quoted in Kirstein, *Dance*, 265. For more on Duncan and Whitman, see Ruth L. Bohan, "'I Sing the Body Electric': Isadora Duncan, Walt Whitman, and the Dance," in *The Cambridge Companion to Walt Whitman*, ed. Ezra Greenspan (Cambridge: Cambridge University Press, 1995), 166–93.

37. Duncan, "I See America Dancing," in *The Art of the Dance*, 48–49.

38. Allan Ross Macdougall, "Isadora Duncan and the Artists," in *Nijinsky, Pavlova, Duncan: Three Lives in Dance*, ed. Paul Magriel (New York: Da Capo, 1977), 61.

39. Duncan, "The Dancer and Nature," c. 1905, in *The Art of the Dance*.

40. Duncan, *The Art of the Dance*, 88.

41. Duncan, *My Life*, 174.

42. Maria-Theresa, "The Truth about the Duncan Creed," *The Dance Magazine*, June 1926, 13.

43. Duncan, *The Art of the Dance*, 74–76. A number of visual artists depicted Duncan's dancing protégés, including the American painter F. Luis Mora (1874–1940), whose lively pastel (*Isadora Duncan*, n.d. Hood Museum of Art, Dartmouth College, Hanover, N.H.) portrays the children in a gauzy, fast-moving swirl surrounding Isadora, directing their movements from her central position.

44. Modern views of children and artistic practice, whether in the fields of dance or the visual arts, were far from settled in those years, giving rise to lively debate. Children's art, for example, had active proponents on both sides of the Atlantic, including Wassily Kandinsky, theorist of the avant-garde. As early as 1912 Kandinsky was praising children's art, declaring, "There is an unconscious and enormous force in the child which manifests itself here and which puts the work of the child on an equally high (and often much higher!) level as the work of the adult." In his publication *Der Blaue Reiter* Kandinsky reproduced several drawings by children. This publication, which came early to the attention of gallery owner Alfred Stieglitz in New York was perhaps one of the stimuli that prompted Stieglitz's interest in the art of children. Stieglitz reprinted excerpts of Kandinsky in his publication *Camera Work* and exhibited the work of children in his Gallery 291 in 1912, 1914, and 1916. Stieglitz-circle regular Sadakichi Hartmann reviewed the first of those shows for *Camera Work*, arguing along the same lines as Duncan. Like her, Hartmann hailed a child's honesty and closeness to nature: "Children draw when they feel the impulse," wrote Hartmann. "The idea is vague as mist on a light summer morning. The motif develops while the children are at work. The directness of the performance triumphs over all technical obstructions."

45. As early as 1868, Ruskin had advocated a revival of traditional fairy tales to Anglo-American children's literature. Such antirational lore, common in the outlook of primitives and children, shared a mutual basis in animism and wish fulfillment. Writing in 1908, an author of medieval romances suggested, "The present day is exhibiting a curiously vivid interest in fairy tales. . . . Perhaps our very materialism is responsible for this new hunger after fantasy." Escapism flourished within both popular and more erudite art. W. B. Yeats collected and immortalized Irish lore in *The Celtic Twilight* (1893), while J. M. Barrie's *Peter Pan* found enthusiastic adult audiences in both America and England.

46. Robert Henri, quoted in Perlman, *Robert Henri*, 118.

47. Kandinsky, *Concerning the Spiritual in Art*, 50.

48. Kandinsky, *Concerning the Spiritual in Art*, 50.

49. Duncan quoted this statement of Rodin's in her program notes (Dance Collection, New York Public Library for the Performing Arts).

50. Rodin, quoted in Denys Sutton, *Triumphant Satyr: The World of Auguste Rodin* (London: Country Life, 1966), 103.

51. According to Duncan, Rodin's overwhelming presence in her studio, paired with her proper American upbringing, prevented her from a full initiation into the delights of the flesh: "How often I have regretted," she later wrote, "this childish miscomprehension which lost to me the divine chance of giving my virginity to the Great God Pan, the mighty Rodin. Surely Art and all Life would have been richer thereby!" It was a mistake she atoned for repeatedly with other lovers. See Duncan, *My Life*, 90–91.

52. Abraham Lerner and Bartlett Cowdrey, Abraham Walkowitz oral history interview, Smithsonian Institution, December 8 and 22, 1958.

53. Duncan, quoted in Abraham Walkowitz, *Isadora Duncan in Her Dances* (Girard, Ks.: Haldeman-Julius, 1945), frontispiece.

54. Marie Theresa, "Isadora the Artist," in ibid., 7.

55. Since the nineteenth century, the ideal of what was known as the "Grecian Bend" had also been incorporated into American social dance. Allen Dodworth, discussed in chapter 1 as the arbiter of grace in American social dance of his era, advocated a slight forward inclination of the body akin to the "beautiful curved line" of ancient Grecian statuary. This attitude should be maintained by graceful social dancers, argued Dodworth, at all times. Dodworth, *Dancing and Its Relation to Education and Social Life*, quoted in O'Neill, "The Dodworth Family," in Magriel, *Chronicles of the American Dance*, 95.

56. Duncan, *My Life*, 316.

57. Quoted in Jean Selz, *Modern Sculpture* (New York: Braziller, 1963), 72.

58. Van Vechten, quoted in Kurth, *Isadora*, 344. "The New Isadora," in Paul Magriel, *Isadora Duncan* (New York: Henry Holt, 1948), 30–31.

59. Van Vechten to Stein, misdated April 5, 1917, in Carl Van Vechten, *Letters of Carl Van Vechten*, ed. Bruce Kellner (New Haven, Conn.: Yale University Press, 1987), 23–24.

60. Quoted in Gottlieb, "Free Spirit," 12. Eventually Duncan, whose own leftist politics extended beyond France (or America) to the cause of world revolution, took her rousing version of the French anthem on the road, performing throughout Europe and North and South America.

61. San Francisco artist Harry Cassie Best (1863–1936) painted Duncan in 1895, the year before she left California to seek her fame in New York (portrait now unlocated). And Bay Area painter and illustrator Ray Boynton (1883–1951) saw her as a dancing nymph in *Bacchante-Isadora Duncan* (1917, Oakland Museum, Oakland, Calif.).

62. Arnold Genthe, *Isadora Duncan: Twenty-Four Studies* (New York: Mitchell Kennerley, 1929).

63. Genthe, "Isadora, Prophet of the Dance," in Walkowitz, *Isadora Duncan in her Dances*, 9.

64. Duncan, *My Life*, 327.

65. Sandburg, "Isadora Duncan," in *Carl Sandburg: Breathing Tokens*, ed. Margaret Sandburg (New York: Harcourt Brace Jovanovich, 1978), 60.

66. Worth noting, though perhaps only coincidental to Russell's color choice for *Synchromy in Orange*, is the appellation "tango" given to a certain orangish hue during those years in Paris. See Blake, *Le Tumulte Noir*, 48. In 1925, long after Russell had returned to the United States, the poet Blaise Cendrars wrote to him suggesting that he develop a synchromist ballet for the Ballets Suédois in Paris. Russell and Cendrars had met in France in 1917, and the poet's verse *Ma Danse* had been published alongside one of Russell's drawings in a French

periodical. Russell expressed enthusiasm at Cendrars's suggested synchromist ballet, and the prospective outcome—colored shapes in an abstract kinetic spectacle—might have been revolutionary. Sadly, before anything came of it, the Ballets Suédois disbanded. See Gail Levin, "The Ballets Suédois and American Culture," in Nancy Van Norman Baer, *Paris Modern: The Swedish Ballet 1920–1925* (San Francisco: Fine Arts Museums of San Francisco, 1995), 125–26.

67. Sloan, diary entry from February 15, 1911, *John Sloan's New York Scene: From the Diaries, Notes and Correspondence 1906–1913*, ed. Bruce St. John (New York: Harper and Row, 1965), n.p.

68. Sloan, quoted in Dartmouth College exhibition catalog *John Sloan Paintings and Prints* (Hanover, N.H.: Dartmouth College, 1946), 51.

69. See Peter Morse, *John Sloan's Prints: A Catalogue Raisonné of the Etchings, Lithographs, and Posters* (New Haven, Conn.: Yale University Press, 1969), 376.

70. Floyd Dell, *Homecoming: An Autobiography* (New York: Farrar and Rhinehart, 1933), 274–75.

71. Flanner, "Isadora."

72. Mabel Dodge to Gertrude Stein, n.d. (contextually, January 1915), in Patricia R. Everett, *A History of Having a Great Many Times Not Continued to Be Friends* (Albuquerque: University of New Mexico Press, 1996), 240.

73. Duncan, quoted in Kurth, *Isadora*, 334.

74. Genthe, *As I Remember*, 179.

75. Quoted in Irma Duncan and Allan Ross Macdougall, *Isadora Duncan's Russian Days and Her Last Years in France* (New York: Covici-Friede, 1929), 168.

76. Coe, *Dance in America*, 125.

77. Bourdelle, quoted in Sorell, *The Dance through the Ages*, 178.

78. Duncan, *My Life*, 70.

79. F. J. Gregg, "The Attitude of the Americans," *Arts and Decoration*, March 1913, reprinted in Rose, *Readings in American Art since 1900*, 76.

80. Duchamp-Villon's *Danseurs* was purchased from the Armory Show by Arthur B. Davies.

81. Davis's painting is illustrated in the "Gallery K" portion of the University of Virginia's Armory Show website, http://xroads.virginia.edu.

82. Dance historian Judith Chazin Bennahum points out that such festivals were staged, in part, to replace the old rituals of Revolution-banned Christianity: "[The Liberty Tree revelers] danced ritualistically in a latter-day paganism, with . . . the props of a new religion invented by the young radicals." Bennahum, *Dance in the Shadow of the Guillotine* (Carbondale: Southern Illinois University Press, 1998), 129.

83. Within the next decade Americans would begin to look more closely at their own folk paintings for ways to augment their historical identity. The Whitney Studio Club held an exhibition of American folk art in 1924. In 1931 dealer Edith Halpert started an American Folk Art Gallery in New York, and in 1932 the Museum of Modern Art exhibited *American Folk Art: The Art of the Common Man in America 1750–1950*.

## Chapter 10. Dance, Visual Art, and America's Countercultures

1. A little later, Martha Graham would express her own revolt against dance's classical tradition in gendered terms. Ballet she considered artificial and effeminate; instead, she favored dance whose "urge is *masculine* and *creative* rather than *imitative*." Eventually, she reworked the feminine, blending it with what

dance historian Mark Franko calls "a double consciousness through which Graham articulates her own experience in male terms, but also reintroduces the feminine" (Franko, *Dancing Modernism/Performing Politics*, 56).

2. Lynn Garafola, "Reconfiguring the Sexes," in Garafola and Baer, *The Ballets Russes and Its World*, 263.

3. Joseph Cornell, the indefatigable balletomane and devoté of the consummately romantic rose, also interpreted *Le Spectre de la Rose* in a work of 1941.

4. Piet Mondrian incorporated the term *plasticism* into his own theory of art, which reduced painting's means to line, space, and color, arranged in the most elemental compositions. For Mondrian, Neoplasticism became more than a style; it was a statement of faith in an art of universal harmonies.

5. Beiswanger, quoted in Morgan, *Martha Graham*, 145.

6. Duchamp, quoted in Jonathan Weinberg, *Speaking for Vice: Homosexuality in the Art of Charles Demuth, Marsden Hartley, and the First American Avant-Garde* (New Haven, Conn.: Yale University Press, 1993), xiii.

7. Demuth also explored the subject of physical contact between men in a group of slightly earlier watercolors of Turkish baths; see Weinberg, *Speaking for Vice*, figs. 35, 38, and 39.

8. Marsden Hartley, "Farewell, Charles," (1935), in *On Art*, ed. Gail R. Scott (New York: Horizon Press, 1982), 97.

9. One of Dehn's close associates in Vienna was the poet e. e. cummings (1894–1962), another of the city's transient illuminati and frequenter of its nightlife. Besides his poetry, Cummings also contributed an ink and graphite drawing called *Dancers* to the *Dial*.

10. Urban realist Guy Pène du Bois (1884–1958) painted *Mura Dehn in Dance Costume* a few years later (1932, private collection).

11. Grosz's mordant comments on German society would force him to flee his homeland for New York, where he settled in 1933.

12. Adolf Dehn, "O Woman! O Frailty!" *The Magazine of the Year*, February 1948, 133.

13. Helen Langa, "Elizabeth Olds: Gender Difference and Indifference," *Woman's Art Journal* 22, no. 2 (Fall 2001/Winter 2002): 7.

14. Stein, from *Everybody's Autobiography*, quoted in Janet Malcolm, "Gertrude Stein's War," *New Yorker*, June 2, 2003, 77.

15. Evergood, in John I. H. Baur, *Philip Evergood* (New York: Harry N. Abrams, 1972).

## Conclusion

1. Tocqueville, quoted in Hughes, *American Visions*, 147.

2. Joann Kealiinohomoku, "An Anthropologist Looks at Ballet as a Form of Ethnic Dance," in Dils and Albright, *Moving History/Dancing Cultures*, 33.

3. Deidre Sklar, "Five Premises for a Culturally Sensitive Approach to Dance," in Dils and Albright, *Moving History/Dancing Cultures*, 30–31.

4. Goran Schildt, "The Idea of the Museum," in *The Idea of the Museum: Philosophical, Artistic, and Political Questions*, ed. L. Aagaard-Mogensen (Lewiston, N.Y.: E. Mellen Press, 1988), 89.

5. Thomas McEvilley, *Art and Otherness: Crisis in Cultural Identity* (Kingston, NY: McPherson, 1992), 133.

6. Joan Acocella, "Think Pieces," *New Yorker*, May 24, 2010, 78.

7. Frankenthaler (1928–2011) herself thought in terms of the fluid gestures of dance, for she recorded that she was drawn to Jackson Pollock's "dancelike use of arms and legs" in his famous drip paintings made on the floor (Marilyn Stokstad, *Art History*, 2nd ed. [New York: Harry N. Abrams, 2002], 1137).

8. Jonson, quoted in Sorell, *The Dance through the Ages*, 74.

9. Almost inevitably, some of the same criticism has been leveled against modern choreographers such as Paul Taylor, accused of subverting abstraction (and thereby betraying modernism) by inserting specific content into some pieces. Such discussions raise the old question of whether abstract form, whether in painting or in dance, can ever be completely nonreferential. If it is true that modern dance, like modernist painting, has been progressively liberated from narrative function toward an exploration of purified form, one must conclude that in both endeavors—dance and painting—the liberation has been only relative.

10. Jean-Claude Lebensztejn, "Eight Statements: Roy Lichtenstein," *Art in America* 63, no. 4 (July–August 1975): 68.

11. Mary Frank, quoted in Eleanor Munro, *Originals: American Women Artists* (New York: Simon and Schuster, 1979), 298.

12. Between 1954 and 1964, for example, Cunningham worked at least twenty times with Rauschenberg, who provided sets for dances often scored by John Cage.

13. *After Ghostcatching* (2010) was a tenth-anniversary reworking of a virtual dance for stereoscopic display presented at the Site Santa Fe Eighth International Biennial in 2010. Jones collaborated with the Openended Group (Mark Downie, Shelley Eshkar, and Paul Kaiser), who provided visual and sound design, using three-dimensional moving drawing and projection to integrate art, dance, and technology.

# Bibliography


**Archival Sources**

Joseph Cornell Papers, Archives of American Art, Smithsonian Institution.

Isadora Duncan and Loïe Fuller Archives, San Francisco Performing Arts Library and Museum.

Elizabeth McCausland Papers, Archives of American Art, Smithsonian Institution.

Julius Rolshoven Journal, University of New Mexico Fine Arts Library, Albuquerque.

Abraham Walkowitz File, Whitney Museum of American Art Papers, Archives of American Art, Smithsonian Institution.

Abraham Walkowitz Interview, conducted by Abram Lerner and May Bartlett Cowdrey, December 8 and 22, 1958; Archives of American Art, Smithsonian Institution.

Robert Henri Papers, Beinecke Rare Book and Manuscript Library, Yale University.

National Archives and Records Administration, Records of the Treasury Relief Art Project.

**Theses and Ditssertations**

Conger, Amy. "Edward Weston's Early Photography." PhD diss., University of New Mexico, 1982.

Groff, Diane Price. "Arnold Rönnebeck: An Avant-Garde Spirit in the West." Master's thesis, University of Denver, 1991.

Lundahl, Vera. "Compositional Form in Modern Dance and Modern Art." PhD diss. Texas Woman's University, 1983.

McAfee, Cheryl Jaye. "The Ecstasy of Dance in Art: Isadora Duncan as Muse." Master's thesis, Arizona State University, 1997.

**Books and Catalogs**

Amberg, George. *Art in Modern Ballet.* New York: Pantheon, 1946.

Anon. *The Official Guide Book of the Panama California Exposition, San Diego, 1915.*

Armitage, Merle. *Dance Memoranda* Edited by Edwin Corle. New York: Duell, Sloan and Pearce, 1947.

———. *Martha Graham.* New York: Dance Horizons, 1966.

———, ed. *Martha Graham: The Early Years.* 1937. Reprint, New York: Da Capo Press, 1978.

Arnason, H. H., and Marla F. Prather. *History of Modern Art.* 4th ed. New York: Abrams and Prentice-Hall, 1998.

Arnold, Matthew. *Civilization in the United States*. Boston: Cupples and Hurd, 1888.

Arthur, Susan E. *Elizabeth Olds: Retrospective Exhibition*. Austin, Tex.: The RGK Foundation, 1986.

*The Armory Show International Exhibition of Modern Art 1913*. Vol. 3, Contemporary and Retrospective Documents. Arno Series of Contemporary Art. New York: Arno Press, 1972.

Baer, Nancy Van Norman. *Paris Modern: The Swedish Ballet 1920–1925*. San Francisco: Fine Arts Museums of San Francisco, 1995.

Baigell, Matthew. *Thomas Hart Benton*. New York: Abrams, 1974.

Baker, Jean-Claude, and Chris Chase. *Josephine: The Hungry Heart*. New York: Cooper Square Press, 1993.

Baldwin, Neil. *Man Ray American Artist*. New York: Da Capo Press, 2000.

Banes, Sally. *Dancing Women: Female Bodies on Stage*. London: Routledge, 1998.

Barr, Alfred. *Picasso: Fifty Years of His Art*. New York: Museum of Modern Art, 1946.

Baur, John I. H. *Life and Work of Charles Burchfield: The Inlander*. Newark: University of Delaware Press, 1982.

———. *Philip Evergood*. New York: Harry N. Abrams, 1972.

Bearden, Romare, and Harry Henderson. *A History of African-American Artists*. New York: Pantheon, 1993.

Berg, Shelly. *Le Sacre du Printemps: Seven Productions from Nijinsky to Martha Graham*. Ann Arbor, Mich.: UMI Research Press, 1988.

Berger, Martin A. *Man Made: Thomas Eakins and the Construction of Gilded Age Manhood*. Berkeley: University of California Press, 2000.

Bjelajac, David. *American Art: A Cultural History*. Upper Saddle River, N.J.: Prentice-Hall, 2000.

Blake, Jody. *Le Tumulte Noir: Modernist Art and Popular Entertainment in Jazz-Age Paris, 1900–1930*. University Park: Pennsylvania State University Press, 1999.

Bloemink, Barbara J. *The Life and Art of Florine Stettheimer*. New Haven, Conn.: Yale University Press, 1995.

Breeskin, Adelyn D. *William H. Johnson, 1901–1970*. Washington, D.C.: National Collection of American Art, 1972.

Brinton, Christian. *Impressions of the Art at the Panama-Pacific Exposition*. New York: John Lane, 1916.

Brown, Gay. *The Dial: Arts and Letters in the 1920s*. Worcester, Mass.: Worcester Art Museum, 1981.

Brown, Milton. *The Story of the Armory Show*. New York: Abbeville, 1988.

*Calder*. Amsterdam: Stedelijk Museum, 1967. Exhibition catalog.

Caldwell, Helen. *Michio Ito: The Dancer and His Dances*. Berkeley: University of California Press, 1977.

Calo, Mary Ann, ed. *Critical Issues in American Art: A Book of Readings*. Boulder, Colo.: Westview Press, 1998.

Cassidy, Donna. *Painting the Musical City: Jazz and Cultural Identity in American Art, 1910–1940.* Washington, D.C.: Smithsonian Institution Press, 1997.

*Cecilia Beaux: Portrait of an Artist.* Philadelphia: Pennsylvania Academy of the Fine Arts., 1974. Exhibition catalog.

Chandler, Arthur. *The Aesthetics of Piet Mondrian.* New York: MSS Information Corporation, 1972.

Charteris, Evan. *John Sargent.* New York: Scribner, 1927.

Cheney, Sheldon. *A Primer of Modern Art.* 11th ed. 1924. Reprint, New York: Tudor, 1945.

Chipp, Herschel B. *Theories of Modern Art.* Berkeley: University of California Press, 1968.

Cikovsky, Nicolai, Jr., and Franklin Kelly. *Winslow Homer.* Washington, D.C.: National Gallery of Art, 1995.

Clark, Carol, Nancy Mowll Mathews, and Gwendolyn Owens. *Maurice Brazil Prendergast; Charles Prendergast: A Catalogue Raisonné.* Munich: Prestel-Verlag, 1990.

Clark, Garth. *Gilded Vessel: The Lustrous Art and Life of Beatrice Wood.* Madison, Wisc.: Guild Publishing, 2001.

Clark, T. J. *Farewell to an Idea: Episodes from a History of Modernism.* New Haven, Conn.: Yale University Press, 1999.

———. *The Painting of Modern Life: Paris in the Art of Manet and His Followers.* Princeton, N.J.: Princeton University Press, 1984.

Cockrell, Dale. *"Jim Crow," Demons of Disorder: Early Blackface Minstrels and Their World.* Cambridge: Cambridge University Press, 1977.

Coe, Robert. *Dance in America.* New York: E. P. Dutton, 1985.

Colette. *Paysages et portraits.* Paris: Flammarion, 1958.

Colson, J. B., et al. *Far from Main Street: Three Photographers in Depression-Era New Mexico, Russell Lee, John Collier, Jr., Jack Delano.* Santa Fe: Museum of New Mexico Press, 1994.

Conningham, Frederic A. *Currier & Ives Prints: An Illustrated Check List.* New York: Crown, 1983.

Cooper, Harry, and Ron Spronk. *Mondrian: The Transatlantic Paintings.* New Haven, Conn.: Yale University Press, 2001.

Corn, Wanda M. *The Great American Thing: Modern Art and National Identity, 1915–1935.* Berkeley: University of California Press, 1999.

Craven, Thomas, ed. *A Treasury of American Prints: A Selection of One Hundred Etchings and Lithographs by the Foremost Living American Artists.* New York: Simon and Schuster, 1939.

Cronin, Vincent. *Paris on the Eve 1900–1914.* New York. St. Martins, 1990.

Cros, Caroline. *Marcel Duchamp.* London: Reaktion Books, 2006.

Crunden, Robert M. *Body and Soul: The Making of American Modernism.* New York: Basic Books, 2000.

Current, Richard Nelson, and Marcia Ewing Current. *Loïe Fuller: Goddess of Light.* Boston: Northeastern University Press, 1997.

Curry, David Park. *James McNeill Whistler at the Freer Gallery of Art.* Washington, D.C.: Freer Gallery of Art, 1984.

Czestochowski, Joseph. *The Drawings and Paintings of Ira Moskowitz.* New York: Landmark, 1990.

Czestochowski, Joseph S., and Anne Pingeot, eds. *Degas Sculptures: Catalogue Raisonné of the Bronzes.* Memphis: Torch Press and International Arts, 2002.

Daly, Ann. *Done into Dance: Isadora Duncan in America.* Middletown, Conn.: Wesleyan University Press, 2002.

*The Dance in Art* Edited by Wallace S. Baldinger. Eugene: University of Oregon Museum of Art, 1963.

Danzker, Jo-Anne Birnie. *Loie Fuller: Getanzter Jugendstil.* Munich: Museum Villa Stuck, 1995.

Dell, Floyd. *Homecoming: An Autobiography.* New York: Farrar and Rhinehart, 1933.

————. *Women as World Builders: Studies in Modern Feminism.* New York: Hyperion, 1976.

DeMille, Agnes. *The Book of the Dance.* New York: Golden, 1963.

Denby, Edwin. *Dance Writings and Poetry.* Edited by Robert Cornfield. New Haven, Conn.: Yale University Press, 1998.

Desmond, Jane, ed. *Dancing Desires: Choreographing Sexualities on and off the Stage.* Madison: University of Wisconsin Press, 2001.

————, ed. *Meaning in Motion: New Cultural Studies in Dance.* Durham, N.C.: Duke University Press, 1997.

*Diaghilev and Russian Stage Designers.* Washington, D.C.: International Exhibitions Foundation, 1972–74.

Dickens, Charles. *American Notes.* 1842. Reprint, New York: Modern Library, 1996.

Dils, Ann, and Ann Cooper Albright, eds. *Moving History/Dancing Cultures: A Dance History Reader.* Middletown, Conn.: Wesleyan Univ. Press, 2001.

Dixon Gottschild, Brenda. *The Black Dancing Body: A Geography from Coon to Cool.* New York: Palgrave Macmillan, 2003.

Dodworth, Allen. *Dancing and Its Relation to Education and Social Life.* New York: Harpers, 1885.

Dos Passos, John. *Manhattan Transfer.* Boston: Harper and Brothers, 1925.

Douglas, Ann. *Terrible Honesty: Mongrel Manhattan in the 1920s.* New York: Farrar, Straus and Giroux, 1995.

Downes, William. *John Sargent: His Life and Work.* Boston: Little, Brown, 1925.

Du Bois, William E. B. *The Negro.* 1915. Reprint, London: Oxford University Press, 1970.

Dulles, Foster Rhea. *A History of Recreation.* New York: Appleton-Century-Crofts, 1965.

Duncan, Irma, and Allan Ross Macdougall. *Isadora Duncan's Russian Days and Her Last Years in France.* New York: Covici-Friede, 1929.

Duncan, Isadora. *The Art of the Dance.* Edited by Sheldon Cheney. New York: Theatre Arts, Inc., 1928.

———. *My Life.* New York: Boni and Liveright, 1927.

Eldredge, Charles. *American Imagination and Symbolist Painting.* New York University: Grey Art Gallery, 1979.

Eliot, T. S. *Four Quartets.* New York: Harcourt, Brace and World, 1943.

Elsen, Albert E. *Rodin.* New York: Museum of Modern Art, 1963.

Elzea, Rowland. *John Sloan's Oil Paintings: A Catalogue Raisonné.* 2 vols. Newark: University of Delaware Press and Associated University Presses, 1991.

Enters, Angna. *Artist's Life.* London: W. H. Allen, 1959.

———. *First Person Plural.* New York: Stackpole Sons, 1937.

Everett, Patricia R. *A History of Having a Great Many Times Not Continued to Be Friends.* Albuquerque: University of New Mexico Press, 1996.

Fairbrother, Trevor. *John Singer Sargent.* New York: Abrams, 1994.

———. *John Singer Sargent the Sensualist.* Seattle: Seattle Art Museum and Yale University Press, 2000.

Fancher, Gordon, and Gerald Myers, eds. *Philosophical Essays on Dance.* Durham, N.C.: American Dance Festival, 1981.

Farnham, Emily. *Charles Demuth: Behind a Laughing Mask.* Norman: University of Oklahoma Press, 1971.

Flitch, J. E. Crawford. *Modern Dancing and Dancers.* 1912. Reprint, Philadelphia: J. B. Lippincott, 1947.

Foulkes, Julia. *Modern Bodies: Dance and American Modernism from Martha Graham to Alvin Ailey.* Chapel Hill: University of North Carolina Press, 2002.

Franko, Mark. *Dancing Modernism/Performing Politics.* Bloomington: Indiana University Press, 1995.

———. *The Work of Dance: Labor, Movement, and Identity in the 1930s.* Middletown, Conn.: Wesleyan University Press, 2002.

Fuller, Loie, intro. Anatole France. *Fifteen Years of a Dancer's Life.* Boston: Small, Maynard, 1913.

Garafola, Lynn. *Diaghilev's Ballets Russes.* 1989. Reprint, New York: Da Capo Press, 1998.

Garafola, Lynn, and Nancy Van Norman Baer, eds. *The Ballets Russes and Its World.* New Haven, Conn.: Yale University Press, 1999.

Garelick, Rhonda K. *Electric Salome: Loïe Fuller's Performance of Modernism.* Princeton, N.J.: Princeton University Press, 2007.

Gay, Peter. *Modernism: The Lure of Heresy.* New York: W. W. Norton and Company, 2008.

Gates, Henry Louis, Jr., and Karen C. C. Dalton. Introduction to *Josephine Baker and La Revue Nègre: Paul Colin's Lithographs of Le Tumulte Noir in Paris, 1927.* New York: Abrams, 1998.

Gee, Mikka, Judith Keller, and Anne Lyden. *Dance in Photography.* Los Angeles: J. Paul Getty Museum, 1999.

Gelman, Barbara, ed. and intro. *The Wood Engravings of Winslow Homer.* New York: Bounty Books, 1969.

Genthe, Arnold. *As I Remember: The Autobiography of Arnold Genthe.* New York: Reynal and Hitchcock, 1936.

———. *The Book of the Dance.* New York: Mitchell Kennerley, 1916.

Glackens, Ira. *William Glackens and the Ashcan Group.* New York: Crown, 1957.

Golding, John. *Paths to the Absolute: Mondrian, Malevich, Kandinsky, Pollock, Newman, Rothko and Still.* Princeton, N.J.: Princeton University Press, 2000.

Goodrich, Lloyd, *Thomas Eakins: His Life and Work.* New York: Whitney Museum of American Art, 1933.

———. *Winslow Homer's America, 1857–1880.* New York: Tudor, 1969.

Goodwin, Sarah Webster. *Kitsch and Culture: The Dance of Death in Nineteenth-Century Literature and Graphic Arts.* New York: Garland Publishing, Inc. 1988.

Graham, Martha. *Blood Memory.* New York: Doubleday, 1991.

Guadagnini, Walter. *Matisse.* Edison, N.J.: Chartwell, 1993.

Hall, Edward T. *The Dance of Life: The Other Dimension of Time.* New York: Random House, 1983.

Harris, Margaret Haile. *Loïe Fuller, Magician of Light.* Richmond, Va.: Richmond Museum, 1979.

Harrison, Jane. *Ancient Art and Ritual.* New York: Henry Holt, 1913.

Haskins, James. *Black Dance in America: A History through Its People.* New York: Thomas Y. Crowell, 1990.

Hawthorne, Nathaniel. *The Marble Faun.* 1860. Reprint, New York: New American Library, 1961.

Hendricks, Gordon. *Eadweard Muybridge: The Father of the Motion Picture.* New York: Viking, 1975.

———. *The Life and Work of Winslow Homer.* New York: Abrams, 1979.

Heller, Adele, and Lois Rudnick, eds. *1915, the Cultural Moment.* New Brunswick, N.J.: Rutgers University Press, 1991.

Henri, Robert. *The Art Spirit.* Philadelphia: J. B. Lippincott, 1923.

Hills, Patricia, ed. *Modern Art in the USA.* Upper Saddle River, N.J.: Prentice Hall, 2001.

———. *Painting Harlem Modern: The Art of Jacob Lawrence.* Berkeley: University of California Press, 2009.

———. *Syncopated Rhythms: 20th-Century African American Art from the George and Joyce Wein Collection.* Boston: Boston University Art Gallery, 2005.

Hobbs, Richard, ed. *Impressions of French Modernity: Art and Literature in France 1850–1900.* New York: Manchester University Press, 1998.

Hoffman, Katherine. *Georgia O'Keeffe: A Celebration of Music and Dance.* New York: George Braziller, 1997.

Hoffman, Malvina. *Heads and Tales.* New York: Charles Scribner's Sons, 1936.

———. *Sculpture Inside and Out.* New York: Bonanza Books, 1939.

———. *Yesterday Is Tomorrow: A Personal History*. New York: Crown, 1965.

Hoffman, Marilyn Friedman. *Marguerite and William Zorach: The Cubist Years 1915–1918*. Manchester, N.H.: Currier Gallery of Art, 1987.

Homer, William Innes, ed. *Avant-Garde Painting and Sculpture in America 1910–1925*. Wilmington: Delaware Art Museum and University of Delaware, 1975.

———. *Robert Henri and His Circle*. Ithaca, N.Y.: Cornell University Press, 1969.

Horgan, Paul. *Henriette Wyeth: The Artifice of Blue Light*. Santa Fe: Museum of New Mexico Press, 1994.

Howe, Winifred E. *A History of the Metropolitan Museum of Art*. New York: Agilliss, 1913.

Hughes, Robert. *American Visions*. New York: Knopf, 1997.

Hunter, Sam, John Jacobus, and Daniel Wheeler. *Modern Art*. 3rd rev. ed. New York: Abrams, 2000.

Ingles, Elisabeth. *Bakst: The Art of Theatre and Dance*. London: Parkstone Press, 2000.

Institute of Contemporary Art, Boston. *Art and Dance: Images of the Modern Dialogue 1890–1980*. Boston: Institute of Contemporary Art and Toledo Museum of Art, 1982.

Irving, Washington [as Dietrich Knickerbocker]. *A History of New York from the Beginning of the World to the End of the Dutch Dynasty*. New York: Putnam, 1860.

Jackson, Gerard. *Theresa Bernstein: Expressions of Cape Ann & New York, 1914–1972*. Stamford, Conn.: Stamford Museum and Nature Center and Smith-Girard, 1989. Exhibition catalog.

Jenkins, Nicholas, ed. *By With To and From: A Lincoln Kirstein Reader*. New York: Farrar, Straus and Giroux, 1991.

Jobson, Richard. *The Golden Trade*. Teighmouth: E. E. Speight and R. H. Walpole, 1904.

Johns, Elizabeth. *American Genre Painting: The Politics of Everyday Life*. New Haven, Conn.: Yale University Press, 1991.

*John Sloan Paintings and Prints*. Hanover, N.H.: Dartmouth College, 1946. Exhibition catalog.

Jules-Rosette, Benetta. *Josephine Baker in Art and Life: The Icon and the Image*. Urbana: University of Illinois Press, 2007.

Kandinsky, Wassily. *Concerning the Spiritual in Art*. Translated by M. T. H. Sadler. 1914. Reprint, New York: Dover, 1977.

Karl, Frederick R. *Modern and Modernism: The Sovereignty of the Artist 1885–1925*. New York: Atheneum, 1988.

Kelder, Diane, ed. *Stuart Davis*. New York: Praeger, 1971.

Kendall, Elizabeth. *Where She Danced*. New York: Alfred A. Knopf, 1979.

Kermode, Frank. *Puzzles and Epiphanies*. London: Routledge and Kegan Paul, 1962.

Kirschke, Amy Helene. *Aaron Douglas: Art, Race and the Harlem Renaissance*. Jackson: University Press of Mississippi, 1995.

Kirstein, Lincoln. *Dance: A Short History of Classic Theatrical Dancing.* 1935. Reprint, Princeton, N.J.: Princeton Book Company, 1987.

———. *Elie Nadelman.* New York: Eakins Press, 1973.

Kraus, Richard, and Sarah Chapman. *History of the Dance in Art and Education.* 2nd ed. Englewood Cliffs, N.J.: Prentice-Hall, Inc., 1981.

Krauss, Rosalind E. *The Sculpture of David Smith: A Catalogue Raisonné.* New York: Garland, 1977.

———. *Terminal Iron Works: The Sculpture of David Smith.* 1971. Reprint, Cambridge, Mass.: MIT Press, 1979.

Kurth, Peter. *Isadora: A Sensational Life.* Boston: Little, Brown, 2001.

Lahs-Gonzales, Olivia, ed. *Josephine Baker: Image and Icon.* Saint Louis: Reedy Press, 2006.

Lawrence, D. H. *Lady Chatterley's Lover.* 1928. Reprint, Garden City, N.Y.: International Collectors Library, n.d.

Lears, Jackson. *No Place of Grace: Antimodernism and the Transformation of American Culture 1880–1920.* New York: Pantheon, 1981.

Levin, Gail. *Edward Hopper: An Intimate Biography.* Berkeley: University of California Press, 1995.

Levin, Gail, and Judith Tick. *Aaron Copland's America: A Cultural Perspective.* New York: Watson-Guptill, 2000.

Lipman, Jean. *Alexander Calder and His Magical Mobiles.* New York: Hudson Hills Press, 1981.

Lorant, Stefan, ed. *The New World: The First Pictures of America Made by John White and Jacques Le Moyne and Engraved by Theodore de Bry with Contemporary Narratives of the Huguenot Settlement in Florida, 1562–1565, and the Virginia colony, 1585–1590.* New York: Duell, Sloan and Pearce, 1946.

Loughery, John. *John Sloan: Painter and Rebel.* New York: Henry Holt, 1995.

Lumsdaine, Joycelyn Pang, Thomas O'Sullivan. *The Prints of Adolf Dehn: A Catalogue Raisonné.* Saint Paul: Minnesota Historical Society Press, 1987.

MacDonald, Margaret F. *James McNeill Whistler, Drawings, Pastels, and Watercolours: A Catalogue Raisonné.* New Haven, Conn.: Yale University Press, 1995.

Magriel, Paul, ed. *Chronicles of the American Dance.* New York: Henry Holt, 1948.

———, ed. *Isadora Duncan.* New York: Henry Holt, 1948.

———, ed. *Nijinsky, Pavlova, Duncan: Three Lives in Dance.* New York: Da Capo, 1977.

Mandel, Patricia C. F. *Selection VII: American Paintings in the Museum's Collection, c. 1800–1930.* Providence: Rhode Island School of Design, 1977.

Manning, Susan. *Modern Dance, Negro Dance: Race in Motion.* Minneapolis: University of Minnesota Press, 2006.

Marks, Joseph E. *America Learns to Dance.* New York: Exposition Press, 1957.

Marter, Joan. *Alexander Calder.* Cambridge: Cambridge University Press, 1991.

Martin, John. *American Dancing*. New York: Dance Horizons, 1967.

Mason, Lauris, with Joan Ludman. *The Lithographs of George Bellows: A Catalogue Raisonné*. Millwood, N.Y.: KTO Press, 1977.

Mathews, Nancy M., ed. *Cassatt and Her Circle: Selected Letters*. New York: Abbeville, 1984.

Maynard, Olga. *The American Ballet*. Philadelphia: Macrae Smith, 1959.

McCarren, Felicia. *Dance Pathologies: Performance, Poetics, Medicine*. Stanford: Stanford University Press, 1998.

McDonagh, Don. *Martha Graham*. New York: Praeger, 1973.

McDonnell, Patricia. *On the Edge of Your Seat: Popular Theater and Film in Early Twentieth-Century American Art*. New Haven, Conn.: Yale University Press and Frederick R. Weisman Art Museum, University of Minnesota, 2002.

McEvilley, Thomas. *Art and Otherness: Crisis in Cultural Identity*. Kingston, N.Y.: McPherson, 1992.

McGrath, Robert L. *Paul Sample: Painter of the American Scene*. Hanover, N.H.: Dartmouth College, Hood Museum of Art, 1988. Exhibition catalog.

Meech, Julia, and Gabriel Weisberg. *Japonisme Comes to America: The Japanese Impact on the Graphic Arts 1876–1925*. New York: Abrams, 1990.

Mitchell, Margaretta K. *Recollections: Ten Women of Photography*. New York: Viking, 1979.

Mondrian, Piet. *The New Art—The New Life: The Collected Writings of Piet Mondrian*. Edited and translated by Harry Holtzman and Martin S. James. Boston: Documents of Twentieth Century Art, 1986.

Morgan, Barbara. *Martha Graham: Sixteen Dances in Photographs*. 1941. Reprint, Dobbs Ferry, N.Y.: Morgan and Morgan, 1980.

Morse, Flo. *The Shakers and the World's People*. Hanover: University Press of New England, 1980.

Morse, Peter. *John Sloan's Prints: A Catalogue Raisonné of the Etchings, Lithographs, and Posters*. New Haven, Conn.: Yale University Press, 1969.

Munro, Eleanor. *Originals: American Women Artists*. New York: Simon and Schuster, 1979.

Myers, Jane, and Linda Ayres. *George Bellows: The Artist and His Lithographs 1916–1924*. Fort Worth, Tex.: Amon Carter Museum, 1988.

Naumann, Francis M. *Conversion to Modernism: The Early Work of Man Ray*. New Brunswick, N.J.: Rutgers University Press, 2003.

———. *New York Dada 1915–23*. New York: Abrams, 1994.

Naumann, Francis M., with Beth Venn. *Making Mischief: Dada Invades New York*. New York: Whitney Museum of American Art, 1996.

Nectoux, Jean-Michel, ed. *Afternoon of a Faun: Mallarmé, Debussy, Nijinsky*. New York: Vendome Press, 1987.

Newhall, Nancy, ed. *The Daybooks of Edward Weston*. Vol. 2, *California*. New York: Horizon, 1961.

Nietzsche, Friedrich. *Thus Spake Zarathustra*. In *The Portable Nietzsche*. Compiled and translated by Walter Kaufmann. New York: Viking, 1968.

Noguchi, Isamu. *A Sculptor's World.* New York: Harper and Row, 1968.

Norton, Leslie. *Leonide Massine and the 20th Century Ballet.* Jefferson, N.C.: McFarland and Company, 2004.

Novak, Barbara. *American Painting of the Nineteenth Century.* New York: Harper and Row, 1979.

Nygren, Edward J., and Frances Fralin. *Eadweard Muybridge: Extraordinary Motion.* Washington, D.C.: Corcoran Gallery, 1986.

O'Connor, Francis Valentine, and Eugene Victor Thaw, eds. *Jackson Pollock: A Catalogue Raisonné of Paintings, Drawings, and Other Works.* New Haven, Conn.: Yale University Press, 1978.

Padgette, Paul. Introduction to Carl Van Vechten, *The Dance Photography of Carl Van Vechten.* New York: Macmillan, 1981.

Palmer, Winthrop. *Theatrical Dancing in America.* 2nd ed. New Brunswick, N.J.: A. S. Barnes, 1978.

Perlman, Bennard B. *The Lives, Loves and Art of Arthur B. Davies.* Albany: State University of New York Press, 1998.

———. *Robert Henri: His Life and Art.* New York: Dover, 1991.

Perrot, Michelle, ed., *A History of Private Life: From the Fires of Revolution to the Great War.* Translated by Arthur Goldhammer. Cambridge, Mass.: Belknap Press of Harvard University Press, 1990.

Pohl, Frances K. *Framing America: A Social History of American Art.* New York: Thames and Hudson, 2002.

Pollock, Griselda. *Mary Cassatt: Painter of Modern Women.* London: Thames and Hudson, 1998.

Powell, Richard J., et al. *Rhapsodies in Black: Art of the Harlem Renaissance.* Berkeley: University of California Press and the Hayward Gallery, 1997.

Pyne, Kathleen. *Art and the Higher Life: Painting and Evolutionary Thought in Late Nineteenth-Century America.* Austin: University of Texas Press, 1996.

Ray, Man. *Self-Portrait.* Boston: Little, Brown, 1963.

Raymond, Marcel. *From Baudelaire to Surrealism.* New York: Wittenborn, Schultz, 1950.

Rearick, Charles. *Pleasures of the Belle Epoque: Entertainment and Festivity in Turn-of-the-Century France.* New Haven, Conn.: Yale University Press, 1985.

Rembert, Virginia Pitts. *Piet Mondrian in the USA.* Dulles, Va.: Parkstone Press, 2002.

Reynolds, Nancy, and Malcolm McCormick. *No Fixed Points: Dance in the Twentieth Century.* New Haven, Conn.: Yale University Press, 2003.

Rose, Barbara, ed. *Readings in American Art since 1900.* New York: Praeger, 1968.

Rose, Phyllis. *Jazz Cleopatra: Josephine Baker in Her Time.* New York: Doubleday, 1989.

Rosenfeld, Paul. *By Way of Art: Criticisms of Music, Literature, Painting, Sculpture, and the Dance.* Essay Index Reprint Series. 1928. Reprint, Freeport, N.Y.: Books for Libraries Press, Inc., 1967.

Rudnick, Lois. *Utopian Vistas: The Mabel Dodge Luhan House and the American Counterculture*. Albuquerque: University of New Mexico Press, 1996.

Rust, Frances. *Dance in Society*. London: Routledge and Kegan Paul, 1969.

Sachs, Curt. *World History of the Dance*. Translated by Bessie Schönberg. New York: W. W. Norton, 1937.

Sawelson-Gorse, Naomi, ed. *Women in Dada*. Cambridge, Mass.: MIT Press, 1998.

Schendler, Sylvan. *Eakins*. New York: Little, Brown, 1967.

Schwarz, Arturo. *Man Ray: The Rigour of Imagination*. New York: Rizzoli, 1977.

Scott, Gail R., ed. *On Art*. New York: Horizon Press, 1982.

Selz, Jean. *Modern Sculpture*. Translated by Annette Michelson. New York: Braziller, 1963.

Sewell, Darrel. *Thomas Eakins: Artist of Philadelphia*. Philadelphia: Philadelphia Museum of Art, 1982.

Shattuck, Roger. *The Banquet Years: The Origins of the Avant Garde in France 1885 to World War I*. New York: Vintage, 1955, rev. ed. 1968.

Shelton, Suzanne. *Ruth St. Denis: A Biography of the Divine Dancer*. Austin: University of Texas Press, 1981.

Sims, Patterson, et al. *Jan Matulka 1890–1972*. Washington, D.C.: Whitney Museum of American Art and Smithsonian Institution, 1980. Exhibition catalog.

Sloan, John. *The Gist of Art*. New York: American Artists Group, 1939; rev. ed. 1944.

———. *John Sloan's New York Scene: From the Diaries, Notes and Correspondence 1906–1913*. Edited by Bruce St. John. New York: Harper and Row, 1965.

Sorell, Walter. *The Dance through the Ages*. New York: Grosset and Dunlap, 1967.

Sorini, Emiliano. *Gropper–Catalogue Raisonné of the Etchings*. San Francisco: Alan Wofsy Fine Arts, 1998.

Starr, Sandra Leonard. *Joseph Cornell and the Ballet*. New York: Castelli, Feigen, Corcoran, 1983.

Steichen, Edward. *A Life in Photography*. Garden City, N.Y.: Doubleday, 1963.

Steichen, Joanna, ed. *Steichen's Legacy: Photographs, 1895–1973*. New York: Alfred A. Knopf, 2000.

Stevens, Mark, and Annalyn Swan. *de Kooning: An American Master*. New York: Alfred A. Knopf, 2004.

Stieglitz, Alfred. *Camera Work: The Complete Illustrations 1903–1917*. Cologne: Taschen, 1997.

Stokstad, Marilyn. *Art History*. 2nd ed. New York: Harry N. Abrams, 2002.

Stovall, Tyler. *Paris Noir: African-Americans in the City of Light*. New York: Houghton-Mifflin, 1996.

Stratton, Suzanne L. *Spain, Espagne, Spanien: Foreign Artists Discover Spain 1800–1900*. New York: The Equitable Gallery and The Spanish Institute, 1993.

Sutton, Denys. *Triumphant Satyr: The World of Auguste Rodin*. London: Country Life, 1966.

Sweeney, James Johnson. *Calder*. New York: Museum of Modern Art, 1945. Exhibition catalog.

Tarbell, Roberta. *Peggy Bacon*. Washington, D.C.: National Collection of Fine Arts, 1975. Exhibition catalog.

———. *William and Marguerite Zorach: The Maine Years*. Rockland, Maine: Farnsworth Library and Art Museum, 1979.

Tashjian, Dickran. *Joseph Cornell: Gifts of Desire*. Miami Beach: Greenfield, 1992.

———. *William Carlos Williams and the American Scene, 1920–1940*. New York: Whitney Museum of American Art, 1978.

Taylor, Joshua C. *Futurism*. New York: Museum of Modern Art, 1961.

Thomas, Helen. *Dance, Modernity and Culture: Explorations in the Sociology of Dance*. London: Routledge, 1995.

———, ed. *Dance, Gender and Culture*. London: Macmillan, 1993.

Thompson, Robert Farris. *African Art in Motion: Icon and Act in the Collection of Katherine Coryton White*. Berkeley: University of California Press and National Gallery of Art, 1974.

Thorp, Nigel, ed. *Whistler on Art: Selected Letters and Writings*. Washington, D.C.: Smithsonian Institution Press, 1994.

Thurman, Judith. *Secrets of the Flesh: A Life of Colette*. New York: Ballantine, 1999.

Todd, Frank Morton. *The Story of the Exposition*. 5 vols. New York: G. P. Putnam's Sons, 1921.

Tracy, Robert. *Spaces of the Mind: Isamu Noguchi's Dance Designs*. New York: Proscenium, 2001.

Trowbridge, Charlotte. *Dance Drawings of Martha Graham*. New York: The Dance Observer, 1945.

Tyler, Parker. *Florine Stettheimer: A Life in Art*. New York: Farrar, Straus, 1963.

Van Vechten, Carl. *The Dance Photography of Carl Van Vechten*. New York: Schirmer, 1981.

———. *Letters of Carl Van Vechten*. Edited by Bruce Kellner. New Haven, Conn.: Yale University Press, 1987.

Volk, Mary Crawford. *El Jaleo*. Washington, D.C.: National Gallery of Art, 1992.

Waldman, Diane. *Joseph Cornell*. New York: George Braziller, 1977.

Walker, John. *James Abbott McNeill Whistler*. New York: Abrams, 1987.

Walkowitz, Abraham. *Isadora Duncan in Her Dances*. Girard, Kans.: Haldeman-Julius, 1945.

Wallace, Carol McD, Don McDonagh, Jean L. Druesedow, Laurence Libin, and Constance Old. *Dance: A Very Social History*. New York: Metropolitan Museum of Art, 1986.

Ward, Geoffrey C., and Ken Burns. *Jazz: A History of America's Music*. New York: Knopf, 2000.

Weber, Bruce. *Ashcan Kids: Children in the Art of Henri, Luks, Glackens, Bellows and Sloan*. New York: Berry-Hill Galleries, 1998.

Weber, Max. *Max Weber: Essays on Art*. Santa Fe: Gerald Peters Gallery, 2000.

Weinberg, Jonathan. *Speaking for Vice: Homosexuality in the Art of Charles Demuth, Marsden Hartley, and the First American Avant-Garde*. New Haven, Conn.: Yale University Press, 1993.

*William Glackens: The Formative Years*. New York: Kraushaar Galleries, 1991. Exhibition catalog.

Wilmerding, John. *American Views: Essays on American Art*. Princeton, N.J.: Princeton University Press, 1991.

Witkin, Lee D. *Kyra Markham, American Fantasist, 1891–1967*. New York: The Witkin Gallery, Inc. 1981.

Wittrock, Wolfgang. *Toulouse-Lautrec: The Complete Prints*. New York: Sotheby Parke Bernet Publications, 1986.

Wolf, Bryan Jay. *Romantic Re-Vision: Culture and Consciousness in Nineteenth-Century American Painting and Literature*. Chicago: University of Chicago Press, 1982.

Wood, Beatrice. *I Shock Myself: The Autobiography of Beatrice Wood*. San Francisco: Chronicle, 1985.

Yeats, W. B. *Essays and Introductions*. New York: Macmillan, 1961.

Yount, Sylvia, and Elizabeth Johns. *To Be Modern: American Encounters with Cézanne and Company*. Philadelphia: Museum of American Art of the Pennsylvania Academy of the Fine Arts, 1996.

Ziff, Larzer. *The American 1890s: Life and Times of a Lost Generation*. New York: Viking, 1966.

Zigrosser, Carl. *The Complete Etchings of John Marin*. Philadelphia: Philadelphia Museum of Art, 1969.

Zorach, William. *Art Is My Life*. Cleveland: World Publishing Company, 1967.

Zurier, Rebecca. *Art for the Masses (1911–1917): A Radical Magazine and Its Graphics*. New Haven, Conn.: Yale University Art Gallery, 1985. Exhibition catalog.

Zurier, Rebecca, Robert W. Snyder, and Virginia M. Mecklenburg. *Metropolitan Lives: The Ashcan Artists and Their New York*. Washington, D.C.: National Museum of American Art, 1995.

## Articles

Acocella, Joan. "The Flame: The Battle over Martha Graham's Dances." *New Yorker*, February 19 and 26, 2001, 180–95.

———. "The Lost Nijinsky." *New Yorker*, May 7, 2001, 94–97.

———. "Think Pieces." *New Yorker*, May 24, 2010, 77–79.

Adelson, Warren, and Elizabeth Oustinoff. "Sargent's Spanish Dancer—a Discovery." *Antiques* 141, no. 3 (March 1992): 460–71.

Ades, Dawn. "Cornell and Duchamp." *Burlington Magazine* 141, no. 1152 (March 1999): 195–98.

Anderson, Jack. "At Some Point, You Can't Argue with Eminence." *New York Times,* March 4, 2001, Arts and Leisure Sec. 2, p. 11.

Anon. "Evolution of La Loïe's Dance." *New York World Herald*, August 27, 1893.

———. "The New English Art Club." *Magazine of Art* 15 (1892): 123.

Antliff, Mark, and Patricia Leighten. "Primitive." In *Critical Terms for Art History*. Edited by Robert S. Nelson and Richard Shiff. Chicago: University of Chicago Press, 1996.

Armstrong, Carol M. "Edgar Degas and the Representation of the Female Body." In *The Female Body in Western Culture: Contemporary Perspectives*. Edited by Susan Rubin Suleiman, 223–242. Cambridge, Mass.: Harvard University Press, 1986.

Barzel, Ann. "European Dance Teachers in the United States." *Dance Index* 3, no. 3 (March 1944): 56–100.

Benton, Thomas Hart. "My American Epic in Paint." *Creative Arts* 3 (December 1928): xxxi–xxxvi.

Borshuk, Michael. "An Intelligence of the Body: Disruptive Parody through Dance in the Early Performances of Josephine Baker." In *Embodying Liberation: The Black Body in American Dance*. Edited by Dorothea Fischer-Horning and Alison D. Goeller, 41–57. Hamburg: Lit Verlag Munster, 2001.

Brooks, Van Wyck. "On Creating a Usable Past." *The Dial* 64 (April 11, 1918): 337–41.

Cassidy, Donna M. "John Marin's Dancing Nudes by the Seashore: Images of the New Eve." *Smithsonian Studies in American Art* 4, no. 1 (Winter 1990): 71–91.

Chamberlain, J. Edgar. "Review of John Marin Exhibition." *Camera Work* 42–43 (April–July 1913): 23.

Cornell, Joseph. "Comment." *Dance Index* 6, no. 9 (1947): 203.

Covielle. "Danse, musique, lumière chez la Loïe Fuller." *L'Eclair*, May 5, 1914.

Dehn, Adolf. "O Woman! O Frailty!" *Magazine of the Year,* February 1948, 133–34.

Deresiewicz, William. "The Salome Factor: How the Sexualization of Concert Dance Helped End a Golden Age." *The American Scholar* 74, no. 2 (Spring 2005): 112–16.

De Souza, Pauline. "Black Awakening: Gender and Representation in the Harlem Renaissance." In *Women Artists and Modernism*. Edited by Katy Deepwell, 55–69. Manchester: Manchester University Press, 1998.

Diehl, Carol. "The World of Mrs. N." *Art in America*, January 2008, 106–11.

Dunning, Jennifer. "Still Paying Heed to Graham's Cry." *New York Times,* September 16, 2001, Arts and Leisure, 18.

Elsen, Albert. "Rodin's 'La Ronde.'" *Burlington Magazine* 107, no. 747 (June 1965): 290–99.

Faulkner, William. Interview with Jean Stein. *Paris Review* 12 (Spring 1956).

Flanner, Janet. "Isadora." *New Yorker,* January 1, 1927.

"French Artists Spur on an American Art." *New York Tribune,* October 24, 1915, sect. 4, p. 2.

Garelick, Rhonda. "Electric Salomé: Loie Fuller at the Exposition Universelle of 1900." In *Imperialism and Theater: Essays on World Theater, Drama and Performance.* Edited by J. Ellen Gainor. New York: Routledge, 1995.

Goldscheider, Cécile. "Rodin et la danse." *Art de France* 3 (1963): 321–35.

Gottlieb, Robert. "Free Spirit." Review of Peter Kurth, *Isadora: A Sensational Life. New York Times Book Review,* December 30, 2001, 11–13.

Hand, John O. "Futurism in America." *Art Journal* 41 (Winter 1981): 337–42.

Heller, Nancy G. "What's There, What's Not: A Performer's View of Sargent's *El Jaleo.*" *American Art* 14, no. 1 (Spring 2000): 8–23.

Haviland, Paul. "We Are Living in the Age of the Machine." *291,* no. 7–8 (September–October 1915): cover page.

Inglis, William. "Is Modern Dancing Indecent?" *Harper's Weekly,* May 17, 1913, 11–12.

"Isadora Duncan and the Libertarian Spirit." *The Modern School,* April 1915, 37–38.

Keller, Marie T. "Clara Tice, 'Queen of Greenwich Village.'" In *Women in Dada.* Edited by Naomi Sawelson-Gorse, 414–41. Cambridge, Mass.: MIT Press, 1998.

Kirstein, Lincoln. "Elie Nadelman: Sculptor of the Dance." *Dance Index* 7, no. 6 (1948): 131–51.

Kisselgoff, Anna. "Paul Taylor, Ballet's Beloved Enemy." *New York Times,* March 4, 2001, Arts and Leisure sec. 2, pp. 1, 11.

Kraut, Anthea. "Between Primitivism and Diaspora: The Dance Performances of Josephine Baker, Zora Neale Hurston, and Katharine Dunham." *Theatre Journal* 55, no. 3 (October 2003): 433–50.

Langa, Helen. "Elizabeth Olds: Gender Difference and Indifference." *Woman's Art Journal* 22, no. 2 (Fall 2001/Winter 2002): 5–10.

Lebensztejn, Jean-Claude. "Eight Statements." *Art in America* 63, no. 4 (July–August 1975): 65–75.

Lee, Russell. "Life on the American Frontier—1941 Version." *U.S. Camera* 4, no. 10 (October, 1941): 41 et passim.

Low, Will H. "A Century of Painting." *McClure's Magazine* 7 (September 1896): 65–72.

Majocchi, Antonella. "La danza futurista." *Futurismo-Oggi* 20, nos. 5–7 (May–July 1988): 17–22.

Malcolm, Janet. "Gertrude Stein's War." *New Yorker,* June 2, 2003, 74–83.

Maria-Theresa. "The Truth about the Duncan Creed." *The Dance Magazine,* June 1926: 12–15.

Marinetti, F. T. "Manifesto of Futurist Dance." *Italian Futurista* (July 1917). Reprinted in *Dance Observer* 2, no. 7 (October 1935).

Martin, John. "To a Performer, Now High in Her Art, an Audience of Americans Pays Tribute." *New York Times,* February 8, 1931, http://www.nytimes.com/library/arts/02083.

Merriman, Christina. "New Bottles for New Wine." *Survey* 30 (May 3, 1913): 196–99.

Mondrian, Piet. "Liberation from Oppression in Art and Life." In *Plastic Art and Pure Plastic Art and Other Essays,* 37–48. New York: Wittenborn, 1945.

Mumford, Lewis. "Machinery and the Modern Style." *New Republic,* August 3, 1921.

Nadelman, Elie. "Notes for a Catalogue." *Camera Work* 32 (October 1910): 41.

Neff, John Hallmark. "Matisse and Decoration: The Shchukin Panels." *Art in America* 63, no. 4 (July–August 1975): 39–48.

Platt, Susan. "Elizabeth McCausland: Art, Politics and Sexuality." In *Women Artists and Modernism.* Edited by Katy Deepwell, 83–96. Manchester: Manchester University Press, 1998.

Polcari, Stephen. "Martha Graham and Abstract Expressionism." *Smithsonian Studies in American Art* 4, no. 1 (Winter 1990): 3–28.

Ratcliff, Carter. "In Detail: Matisse's *Dance.*" *Portfolio* 3, no. 4 (July–August 1981): 38–45.

Rudhyar, Dane. "The Indian Dances for Power." *Dance Observer* 1, no. 6 (August–September 1934): 64.

Sandburg, Carl. "Isadora Duncan." In *Carl Sandburg: Breathing Tokens.* Edited by Margaret Sandburg. New York: Harcourt Brace Jovanovich, 1978.

Schildt, Goran. "The Idea of the Museum." In *The Idea of the Museum: Philosophical, Artistic, and Political Questions.* Edited by L. Aagaard-Mogensen, 81–90. Lewiston, N.Y.: E. Mellen, 1988.

Schwarz, Arturo. "An Interview with Man Ray: 'This is not for America.'" *Arts Magazine* 51 (May 1977): 116–21.

Shenker, Israel. Interview with Helen Gardner. *New York Times,* June 7, 1973, 56.

Sommer, Sally R. "The Stage Apprenticeship of Loie Fuller." *Dancescope* (n.d.): 23–34.

Sontag, Susan. "Dancer and the Dance" and "Lincoln Kirstein." In *Where the Stress Falls,* 187–193, 194–96. New York: Farrar, Straus and Giroux, 2001.

Taruskin, Richard. "Orff's Musical and Moral Failings." *New York Times,* May 6, 2001, Arts and Leisure Sec. 2, p. 35.

Thompson, D. Dodge. "John Singer Sargent's Javanese Dancers." *Antiques* 138 (July 1990): 125–33.

Townsend, Julie. "Alchemic Visions and Technological Advances: Sexual Morphology in Loie Fuller's Dance." In *Dancing Desires: Choreographic Sexualities on and off the Stage.* Edited by Jane C. Desmond, 73–96. Madison: University of Wisconsin Press, 2001.

Van Vechten, Carl. "The Lindy Hop." 1930. Reprinted in *Dance Index* 1, nos. 9, 10, 11 (September, October, November, 1942): 187.

———. "The Secret of the Russian Ballet." 1915. Reprinted in *Dance Index* 1, nos. 9, 10, 11 (September, October, November 1942): 164.

Weber, Max. "The Fourth Dimension from a Plastic Point of View." *Camera Work* 31 (July 1910): 25.

### Films and Videos

Beatrice Wood. *Mama of Dada*. Wild Wolf Productions, 1993.

Martha Graham. *An American Original*. Kultur Films, 1988.

———. *The Dancer Revealed*. Kultur Films/WNET-TV, 1994.

*Annabella* (one-minute film, hand colored, of a skirt dancer). Produced by Thomas A. Edison. n.d.

*Man Ray*. American Masters Series, PBS/WNET, 1997.

*Picasso and Braque Go to the Movies*. Arthouse Films, 2008.

# Index

Note: Page numbers in *italics* refer to figures. Alternate titles of works of art appear in brackets following the titles used in the text.

New Orleans, 62, *63*, 63–64

New York: architecture as dance and, 199–201, *200*, *201*, 293n5; avant-gardists support for Duncan in, 247–48; Bal des Beaux Arts of 1932 and, 200–201; Ballets Russes tours and, 190; dance halls and, 22; dancing as marker of social class and, 23, 30–31, 35–36; Duncan's avant-gardists support in, 247–48; Futurism exhibitions and, 203, 294n11; Hippodrome and, 112, 190; imagined immigrant experience in dance scenes and, 6, 20, *20*–23, *22*, 272n10; immigrant experience as upwardly mobile and, 24, *24*; immigrant experience documentation by visual artists and, 26, *26*–27, 63, 144; immigrant experience in photographs, 24–25, *25*

Nietzsche, Friedrich, 232–33, 297n26

*Nightlife* (Motley), 71, *73*

Nijinsky, Vaslav: Abstract Expressionism as influenced by, 153, *153*, *154*, *155*, *156*; abstraction of figures and, 137–38; androgynous iconography and, *141*, 141–42, 253–54, 285n21; *L'Après-midi d'un Faune* (Debussy), 138, *139*, 140, 151–52, 284n4; *Cleopatra* (ballet), 144, 151; energy of dance and, 150–51; faun image as influence on visual arts and, 138, *139*; *Large Clown [Nijinsky as Petrouchka]*, 153, *154*; modernism in dance innovations and, 284n4; modernism influences of, 138, *139*, 140, 285n17; modernist primitivism and, 140; *Music* (Stettheimer), *141*, 141–42; *Nijinsky* (Kline), 153, *155*, 156, 286n41; *Nijinsky as the Harlequin Petrouchka* (Elliott and Fry), 153, *153*; *Nijinsky Dancing [L'Après-midi d'un Faune]* (Tice), 138, *139*; plasticism and, 156; *Le Spectre de la Rose*, 140, *141*, 141, 253, 284n16, 301n3; travesty paradigm and, 141, *141*; *Vaslav Nijinsky in Le Spectre de la Rose* (Hoppe), 141, *141*; visual arts influences of, 138, *139*, 150–51. *See also* Ballets Russes (Russian Ballets)

*Nijinsky as the Harlequin Petrouchka* (Elliott and Fry), 153, *153*

*Nijinsky Dancing [L'Après-midi d'un Faune]* (Tice), 138, *139*

Nivison Hopper, Jo, 150–51

Noguchi, Isamu, 4, 46–48, 51–52, 164–65, *165*

North, Percy, 296n7

nostalgia for innocence of frontier, 41–42. *See also* memories

*Nude Descending a Staircase* (Duchamp), 199, 251

*Nude Women Dancing* (Muybridge), 158, *159*

nudity and dance images: archaic circle dance and, 105, 129–30, 280n18, 282n34; burlesque and, 259, 259–60; Dionysian Bacchanal and, 242, *243*; liberation of the senses and, 105–6, *106*, 280n18; modernism influences and, 138, *139*; paganism and, 100–101, *101*; plasticism and, *171*, 171–72, 289n80; portraiture and, 165, *166*, 167, 288n38. *See also* dance and dancers

*La Nuit [Ballet of the Night]*, 16

O'Keeffe, Georgia, 254, 275n46

Olds, Elizabeth, *Burlesque [Chorus Line]*, 259, 259–60

Olowe of Ise (Yoruba peoples, Nigeria), *Bowl with Figures*, 68, *69*

*Ondine* (Ashton), 111–12

*Oriental Fantasy*, Bakst costume for Pavlova, 135, 285n29

Other/the other: African Americans as, 84–85, 258, 258–59; Eastern exoticism and, 288n63

Oustinoff, Elizabeth, 281n23

outdoor settings, and men, 39, 231

paganism: overview and definition of, 95, 107, 132, 279n1; Ballets Russes and, 135, 137, 140; Dionysian Bacchanal and, 96, *97*, 99, *99*, 104, *105*, 115; eroticism of dance and, 100–101, *101*, 102, *102*, 104, *104*; faun image and, 138, *139*, 140, *141*, 141–42, 151–52, 284n4; high society intersection with visual arts and, 101, *102*; literature and, 99–100, 279n10; modernism in dance and, 44–45, *45*, 107, 108, 159,

Turkey Trot, 11, 189, 190. *See also* African
American dance and music
Twain, Mark (Samuel Clemens), 123, 223
typography images, 204–7, *205*

United States. *See* America; *specific cities,
regions, and states*
urban settings: everyday life images, 76–78,
*78*; women sophisticates' virtue and,
40–41, *41*. *See also specific cities*

Valentino, Rudolph, 192
Van Alen, William, 201
VanDerZee, James: *Dancing School*, 73, *74*;
photographs of African American dancers, 71, 73, *74*
Van Gogh, Vincent: *Bal à Arles [Dancehall
at Arles]*, 76, *76*, 277n19; *Potato
Eaters*, 76
Van Vechten, Carl: on African American
social dances, 11, 68, 70; on Ballets
Russes, 135; on Futurism in ballet, 203;
on *Marseillaise* (Duncan), 242; photograph of Abraham Walkowitz standing
outside the Isadora Duncan Memorial,
239, *239*
vaudeville: abstraction of figures and, 124–
25, *126*; African American dance and,
62–63, 74, *75*; Cakewalk and, 62–63;
high and popular culture boundaries
and, 190; immigrant experience images
and, 26; modernism in dance and, 160,
161; national identity and, 228; visual
arts as influenced by, 212; women's
careers and, 288n62. *See also specific
vaudeville performers*
Velázquez, Diego, 112, 115, 117, 119, 164
Virginia, and racial social constructs and
country dance, 34, 34–35
Virgin Mary, and modernism in dance,
44–45, *45*, 46
visual arts and artists: overview of, 3;
abstraction of figures and, 210, 269;
absurdity of life and, 269; African
American dance and music influences
on, 85, 87, *88*, 89; African American
studies and, 278n39; archaic circle
dance and, 105, 129–30, 269, 280n18,
282n34, 282n37; Cakewalk's relationship with, 5, 62–64, *63*, *64*, 144;

children's art and, 298n44; collaborations between dance and, 270,
302nn12–13; country dance images as
antidote to weight and fixity of composition in, 31–34, *32*, *33*, 36; cultural
heritage of America as influence on,
48, 49, *50*, 50–52, *51*; cultural meaning and, 3; dance as, 7, 167; dance as
influence on, 48, 49, *50*, 50–52, *51*;
dance's relationship with, 3–5, 102,
148, *148*, 171, 265, 285n28, 289n79;
documentation of immigrant experience in dance scenes by, 22–27, *25*, *26*,
*28*, 29, 29–30, 63, 144; as embodiment of social practice, 4, 132; energy
of dance in, 150–51; European influences on, 76–77; gauzy costumes and,
224; gender social constructs and,
11–12; "high" art, 3, 131, 283nn40–
41; high society intersection with, 101,
*102*; Japanese dance-drama influences
on, 144, 168; light effects and, 177–
78; liminal effect and, 266; modernism in dance images and, 150, 180,
182–83, 238–39, 241, 299n61; modernism in dance influences on, 48, 49,
*50*, 50–52, *51*, 144, 161, 180, 182–
83, 218; movement in dance and, 178,
*178*, 267–68, *268*, 269, 290n4, 302n7;
music and dance synthesis with, 135,
151–52, 184–85, 302n12; narrative
function liberation and, 267–68, *268*,
302n7, 302n9; natural movement in
dance and, 95, 279n3; passing moment
and, 174, 187, *188*; preservation of
dance and, 6, 145, 148, 168, 172, 205,
285n29; racial social constructs and,
11–12; Romantic ballet as influence on,
109–10, 138, *139*, *141*, 141–42, *142*,
150–51, 280n4, 280n6; space and, 5–6;
Spanish dance influences on, 109, 112,
119, 280n3, 282n26; spontaneity and,
119, *120*, 268–69; support of dancers by, 165, *165*, 288n68; vaudeville as
influence on, 212; vitality of life in, 27,
29, 29–30. *See also* African American
dance and music; cultural heritage of
America; *specific visual arts*
vitality of life: burlesque as metaphor for,
*259*, 259–60; dance marathons and,